Veterans: Benefits, Issues, Policies and Programs

New York

Veterans: Benefits, Issues, Policies and Programs

Health Care for Veterans: Background, Education, System Reform and Improvements
Juliette Binet (Editor)
ISBN: ISBN: 978-1-53617-530-1
eBook ISBN: 978-1-53617-531-8

Veterans Affairs Information Technology: Progress, Modernization and Challenges
Bryan Barton (Editor)
ISBN: 978-1-53616-452-7
eBook ISBN: 978-1-53616-453-4

More information about this series can be found at
https://novapublishers.com/product-category/series/veterans-benefits-issues-policies-and-programs/

Gina P. Sharpe
Editor

Supporting Our Veterans

Comprehensive Care for Mental Health and Substance Use Disorders

snova
New York

NOTICE TO THE READER

Library of Congress Cataloging-in-Publication Data

ISBN: 979-8-89530-504-1 (Hardcover)
ISBN: 979-8-89530-522-5 (eBook)

Published by Nova Science Publishers, Inc. † New York

Contents

Preface

Many veterans carry the invisible wounds of war. For some, these wounds manifest as mental health challenges; for others, they lead to substance use as a way to cope with the burdens of service. Often, these struggles are intertwined, with one exacerbating the other. According to recent data, approximately 1.1 million veterans are affected by both substance use disorder and mental illness. This book explores how we can improve access to effective, quality care for veterans dealing with substance use disorders and mental health conditions. It aims to highlight the interconnectedness of these issues and examine comprehensive strategies to better support veterans on their path to recovery.

Chapter 1

Combatting a Crisis: Providing Veterans Access to Life-Saving Substance Abuse Disorder Treatment*

Committee on Veterans' Affairs

Tuesday, April 18, 2023
U. S. House of Representatives,
Subcommittee on Health, Committee on Veterans' Affairs,
Washington, D.C.

The subcommittee met, pursuant to notice, at 10:20 a.m., in room 390, Cannon House Office Building, Hon. Mariannette Miller- Meeks [chairwoman of the subcommittee] presiding.

Present: Representatives Miller-Meeks, Van Orden, Luttrell, Kiggans, Brownley, Budzinski, and Landsman.

Opening Statement of Mariannette Miller-Meeks, Chairwoman

Ms. MILLER-MEEKS. Good morning again. This oversight hearing for the Subcommittee on Health will now come to order. Our country has been experiencing a substance abuse and overdose epidemic, and we are seeing historic highs in overdose deaths and our Nation's veterans are not immune. One death from substance use disorder is one too many. It is a somber reality that many lives are taken by this treatable mental disorder. One hundred sixty-five million people in the United States alone struggle with drug and alcohol abuse, and over 100,600 Americans died from drug overdose in 2021.

As a 24-year veteran, I have seen the unique challenges that many of my fellow service members and veterans face. Among the veteran population, we have sadly seen a 53 percent increase in drug overdose mortality rates from 2010 to 2019. Four in 10 veterans struggle with illicit drug use, seven in 10 struggle with alcohol use, and one out of eight struggles with both.

This is an enormous obstacle that we need to address. Had the VA sent us testimony in a more timely manner, let me emphasize that, had the VA sent us testimony in a more timely manner, I would have liked to have addressed the initiatives they are talking about today. In

* This is an edited, reformatted and augmented version of Hearing Before the Subcommittee on Health of the Committee on Veterans' Affairs, U.S. House of Representatives Serial No. 118–9, dated April 18, 2023.

In: Supporting Our Veterans
Editor: Gina P. Sharpe
ISBN: 979-8-89530-504-1

spite of that, I would like to acknowledge the VA Mental Health Residential Rehabilitation Treatment Program, also called MHRRTP, that provides rehabilitative and clinical care to veterans that need intensive specialty treatment for mental health and substance use disorders. The MHRRTP continuum includes more than 70 programs for the treatment of substance use disorder and more than 40 programs for the treatment of posttraumatic stress disorder, with the expectation that all programs provide integrated, concurrent treatment for co-occurring substance use disorder and mental health treatment needs.

That being said, veterans through the Mission Act should be eligible to receive in and outpatient substance abuse treatment in the community when it is appropriate course of action.

I am very concerned about how the VA has interpreted and differentiated between institutional and uninstitutional extended care. It is becoming increasingly clear that once again bureaucracy has overcome intent. VA continually repeats that there is no wrong door for veterans seeking substance abuse care. However, we will hear from our witnesses on the second panel that that is inaccurate and bureaucratic hyperbole with that statement.

I would like to point out three instances where the VA has not embodied their no wrong door declaration. First, we have heard from a specific veteran who struggles with Post Traumatic Stress Disorder (PTSD) and alcohol abuse. After many attempts and 3 months of trying to receive care, this veteran was not able to get the help they needed. This was essentially a locked door. This veteran spoke with multiple congressional offices and with the VA central office. They were eventually referred to community care. However, it was rescinded as the VA ensured that this veteran could receive the care they need. This veteran still struggles with their sobriety today.

Next is an example of the VA presenting no door to a veteran. As we will hear during our second panel, there was another instance where a veteran sought care in the community. However, VA noted that they could not refer this veteran to the community if a VA bed was available within 30 days. Veterans can and should not have to wait 30 days to receive care that they desperately need. The program attempting to assist this veteran was told that veterans must first go to a domiciliary, then grant per diem programs such as VA homeless shelter, and then to the Salvation Army. Then after all of these options have been exhausted, they could be referred into the community.

That is a disgrace. As a state senator, I specifically introduced legislation to get rid of preauthorization for medicated assisted treatment. So, within immediate. To find that this is existing with our VA system is unacceptable.

Finally, we have heard from a veteran who has struggled with PTSD, substance use disorder, and a history of traumatic brain injury. This specific veteran was searching for a residential program for substance use disorder at the VA. However, this veteran was denied because they did not have a history of seeking help through the VA. Because this veteran had not been to the VA since 2017, their record was closed and they were never contacted about receiving care. This appears to be a case where a veteran experienced a missing door. Luckily, a Veterans Service Organization (VSO) paid for a treatment program for this veteran.

There is no excuse for any of the neglectful and harmful care that these veterans are experiencing and we need to hold the VA to a much higher standard. I am saddened and I am frustrated that this is how VA has been managing care for those who have selflessly served our country. Thank you all for being here and I look forward to our discussion on both panels to best identify ways to improve access. With that, I yield to Ranking Member Brownley for her opening statement.

Opening Statement of Julia Brownley, Ranking Member

Ms. BROWNLEY. Thank you, Madam Chair, for holding this morning's important hearing. As of Fiscal Year 2022, more than 550,000 veterans receiving VA healthcare, or about 8.5 percent of all veterans using VA healthcare services, had substance use disorder diagnoses. Often, veterans have turned to alcohol or drugs to try to relieve stress or symptoms of PTSD and other co-occurring mental health disorders. As a result, substance use disorder is a significant challenge among the veteran population. This challenge was only compounded by the COVID–19 pandemic, which increased feelings of social isolation, anxiety, and depression, and caused many adults to start or increase their use of alcohol or drugs.

At the same time, access to intensive residential treatment at VA and in the community declined as providers limited admissions and placed residents in single occupancy rooms in an effort to minimize the spread of COVID–19. I am perplexed by the two very different stories that were told in the written testimony of VA and the other witnesses we will hear from today. If we are to take VA at its word, veterans receive timely access to residential treatment, admission within 72 hours for veterans requiring priority admissions, and within 30 days for routine admission. The VA Office of the Inspector General, however, has found that VA "faces significant challenges in meeting the needs of individuals with substance use disorders."

This finding is echoed in the testimony of our second panel of witnesses. I hope today's hearing will help us better understand the true state of veterans' access to residential treatment for substance use disorder. I do not doubt that there are instances where veterans would benefit from referral to residential treatment from community providers, particularly when there are excessive wait times for beds in VA programs, or when veterans can access timely care in the community closer to home. However, we must ensure that veterans receive high quality evidence-based care when they are sent to the community.

I hope today's hearing will also shed some light on the extent to which VA ensures that the community providers to which it refers veterans meet clinical practice guidelines and accreditation standards for delivering such care. While we will focus much of our attention today on access to residential treatment, I hope we will also take some time to consider the full continuum of care, including the extent to which veterans are successfully transitioning from residential care to outpatient treatment and independent living.

As the VA Office of Inspector General points out in its testimony, care coordination between VA and community providers is critically important for high-risk patients like those receiving treatment for substance use disorder. When patients receive care in the community, they are not always as easily able to access other VA benefits, such as housing and employment support as they would if receiving care at a VA facility.

In 2019, I visited a truly impressive program operated by the VA Boston Healthcare system called the Women's Veterans Trust House, which provides excellent care, coordination, and continuity of care for women veterans who had completed residential treatment for substance use and posttraumatic stress. The typical stay is about 12 months, during which time women veterans participate in individual and group psychotherapy, compensated work therapy, and recreational community outings. Through this program, they are learning how to develop healthier coping mechanisms and constructive interpersonal relationships. Unfortunately, at the time I visited, the Trust House could accommodate just seven women at a time, and they were traveling from all over the country, first to participate in VA's residential treatment program and then this transitional program. Undoubtedly, more women veterans, indeed all veterans, would benefit from greater access to transitional programs like this.

I hope that we can learn more today about the extent to which VA is trying to expand its capacity in this area as well. I have legislation that aims to do just that, and I hope today's hearing will help inform my planned reintroduction of the bill. Thank you again, Dr. Miller-Meeks, for organizing this important hearing and I yield back.

Ms. MILLER-MEEKS. Thank you, Ranking Member Brownley. I would now like to introduce the witnesses. Joining us today from the Department of Veterans Affairs is Dr. Tamara Campbell, who is the executive director of the Office of Mental Health and Suicide Prevention (OMHSP). Accompanying Dr. Campbell today is Dr. Sachin Yende. I apologize for any mispronunciation. The chief medical officer in the Office of Integrated Care. We also have Dr. Julie Kroviak, the Principal Deputy Assistant Inspector General of Healthcare Inspections in the office of the Inspector General. Dr. Campbell, you are now recognized for 5 minutes to deliver your opening statement.

Statement of Tamara Campbell

Ms. CAMPBELL. Good morning, Chairman Miller-Meeks, Ranking Member Brownley, and distinguished members of the subcommittee. Thank you for the opportunity to discuss VA's mental health, substance use disorder, residential rehabilitation treatment programs, and community care referrals. Accompanying me today, as mentioned, is Dr. Sachin Yende, Chief Medical Officer, Office of Integrated Veteran Care.

Over the past decade, potent and dangerous drugs became more widely available and misused in the United States. In response to the rise in substance use morbidity and mortality, prevention and treatment efforts have been established. VA is making a positive difference in veterans' quality of life by enhancing motivation and building confidence in their treatment and recovery process. Veterans receiving treatment for their substance use disorder in VA are experiencing benefits in terms of their mental and physical health across many other aspects of their lives that impact social determinants of health. VA's mental health Residential Rehabilitation Treatments (RRTPs) are a critical component of VA's broader efforts to address the needs of veterans with substance use concerns.

Mental health residential programs are institutional extended care and are not subject to designated access standards. They do, however, have access requirements that inform when consideration for referral to the community should occur. These access requirements are defined by Veterans Health Administration (VHA) Directive 1162.02 and more recently by implementation of the Comprehensive Prevention, Access to Care, and Treatment (COMPACT) Act for Crisis Residential Care.

The ability to pay for community care mental health residential treatment has resulted in an increase in the number of programs available to veterans. From Fiscal Year 2021 to Fiscal Year 2022, referrals to the community increased from 7,000 to 11,000 uniques, with expenditures exceeding 1.2 billion since 2021. Concurrent with these increases, VHA has observed instances of community programs marketing directly to veterans and providers, resulting in confusion by veterans when informed of the availability of VHA to meet their needs. We believe the solution to this lies with increasing familiarity with the process and with VA's mental health residential resources, while also addressing concerning marketing practices when they are identified.

Timely access to residential treatment has been a priority area of focus for VHA. This has been critical as the residential programs experienced significant reductions in capacity early in the pandemic. I am pleased to share that today MHRRTP capacity is rebounding, with wait times decreasing and census increasing.

Recognizing a need to ensure access to this critical level of care, OMHSP worked collaboratively with the Office of Integrated Veteran Care to verify authority, to provide residential treatment in the community, and to provide a mechanism by which VHA could pay for such care. VHA policy requires that when a veteran is assessed as requiring residential treatment and the program is unable to meet the veterans' needs, an alternate treatment program must be offered. Alternate treatment may include treatment within VA or within the community. VA is thankful for the independent investigation of the Office of Inspector General in the review of the Domiciliary Substance Use Disorder (SUD) Treatment Program and residential community care referrals.

The ability to refer to mental health residential treatment in the community is a relatively new process with the first Standard Episode of Care for the Mental Health Residential Treatment, released in October 2020, and updated in August 2021. OMHSP worked collaboratively with Veterans Integrated Services Networks (VISNs) during this time to clarify requirements and expectations for when referrals for mental health residential care in the community may occur. These efforts have continued with targeted efforts to ensure awareness of requirements and processes for ensuring access to residential treatment in the community when indicated.

In conclusion, we appreciate the committee's continued support and partnership in this shared mission. Nothing is more important to VA than supporting the health and well-being of our veterans and their families. This critical work is lifesaving, and my colleagues and I are now prepared to respond to any questions you may have. Thank you.

[The prepared Statement of Tamara Campbell appears in the Appendix]

Mr. LUTTRELL. [Presiding] Thank you, Dr. Campbell. Dr. Kroviak, you are now recognized for 5 minutes to deliver your opening remarks.

Statement of Julie Kroviak

Ms. KROVIAK. Thank you. Ranking Member Brownley and subcommittee members, thank you for the opportunity to discuss the Office of Inspector General's (OIG's) oversight of VHA's substance use disorder treatment program. The OIG's Office of Healthcare Inspections reviews the quality and safety of healthcare provided across VHA and communicates the findings through public reports. We are unique in the IG community because of our ability to conduct this oversight. With over 250 clinical staff, the majority having significant experience providing direct care to veterans, our reports can provide in-depth clinical analyses and identify issues that impact healthcare delivery.

Take our mental health team, staff with board-certified psychiatrists, psychologists, and licensed clinical social workers. They are proactive and vigilant in conducting oversight work that supports veterans in need of mental health treatment. We are in the last stages of developing a new cyclical review that will initially focus on VHA's inpatient mental health units. These units treat acutely ill psychiatric patients. And our teams have developed tools to evaluate the safety and efficacy of these settings to ensure veterans are receiving the high-quality care they need and deserve.

Substance use disorders have devastating effects on veterans, their families, and caregivers, and often require intensive, multidisciplinary interventions to support a meaningful recovery. In addition, veterans with substance use disorders often have additional mental health diagnoses that can place them at higher risk for suicide. Given that VHA's top clinical priority is to reduce veteran suicide, evidence-based, substance use disorder treatment programs are critical to addressing these clinical needs.

To meet the increasing demand for these services, VHA depends on community care. When VHA and community care providers are comanaging these patients, the coordination must be seamless and collaborative. The OIG has identified persistent administrative errors and communication failures among VHA, its third-party administrators, and community care providers, as well as between the care providers and their patients. These deficiencies challenge the efforts of VHA personnel to ensure that seamless experience for veterans.

Many OIG reports have described the challenges and, most importantly, the risks when patients are referred to the community. These risks are amplified for patients with high-risk mental health issues or complex disease. For example, my written statement details our January 2023 hotline inspection that substantiated the allegation that in 2020 and 2021, VA North Texas staff did not follow VHA policy requiring that patients be offered alternative options for care within VHA or the community when the wait time for a needed service exceeds 30 days. This practice potentially delayed treatment for these veterans and has the long-term potential to fracture trust between patients and the healthcare system upon which they rely. We also determined that the VISN's chief mental health officer lacked authority to ensure staff adherence to these policies.

We made five recommendations, with one specifically ensuring that staff comply with community care referral requirements and another recommending a review of the facility's management of community residential care referrals. All of these recommendations are open, and we will begin the follow-up process with VHA at the end of this month.

While this report highlights issues with offering community care to veterans, it does not provide a complete picture of the concerns we have found when veterans are receiving community care. Our office has published reports related to community care detailing delays in diagnosis and treatment, lack of information sharing or miscommunication between providers, and significant quality of care concerns. While we recognize the importance of VHA staff consistently informing and offering veterans all options available to meet their care needs, ignoring that the current community care framework does not adequately address critical gaps in coordination will further increase risk to patients. We are piloting a new community care review that will provide data to support VHA's leaders' efforts to reduce these risks.

The OIG will continue to provide meaningful oversight to support and improve the quality of healthcare provided to our Nation's veterans. We also recognize the need to enhance and adapt our work to best support this dynamic healthcare system. We remain grateful for the participation and cooperation of VHA staff across the country, and we commend their commitment to caring for those who have served. Members of the subcommittee, this concludes my statement. I would be happy to answer any questions you may have.

[The prepared statement of Julie Kroviak appears in the appendix]

Mr. LUTTRELL. Thank you, Dr. Kroviak. We will now proceed to questioning. I now recognize the ranking member, Ranking Member Brownley, for any questions she may have.

Ms. BROWNLEY. Thank you, Mr. Chairman. The first question I have is to Dr. Campbell. I understand VA currently has two dedicated residential substance use disorder treatment programs for women veterans. Is that correct? Two?

Ms. CAMPBELL. I did not hear, I am sorry, the first part of the question.

Ms. BROWNLEY. I understand that VA currently has two dedicated residential substance use disorder treatment programs for women veterans. Is that true?

Ms. CAMPBELL. We have 13 programs across nine locations specializing in treatment for women at the residential level.

Ms. BROWNLEY. I had difficulty finding those. Where do I go to find those?

Ms. CAMPBELL. You can locate them on our website. They are in VISN 110, and I believe 17.

Ms. BROWNLEY. I understand that all of these are not substance use disorder treatment programs.

Ms. CAMPBELL. There is a mixture, and thank you for that question, of substance use disorder as well as PTSD. We understand that those diagnoses typically coexist, and so we ensure that our programs are treating both the PTSD and substance use at the same time.

Ms. BROWNLEY. Just to get back to my original question, there are currently two dedicated residential substance use disorder treatment programs for women veterans. True or false?

Ms. CAMPBELL. I would have to go back to get that exact number. What I have is 13 programs across nine locations, five programs that specifically focus, and two additional that are in for implementation for Fiscal Year 2024.

Ms. BROWNLEY. Okay. I also understand the Fiscal Year 2024 budget request indicates the Department has two additional women-only residential programs in development. Is that correct?

Ms. CAMPBELL. Yes, ma'am, that is correct.

Ms. BROWNLEY. In what locations will they be?

Ms. CAMPBELL. I will have to get back about those locations.

Ms. BROWNLEY. How did you decide where the locations should go?

Ms. CAMPBELL. We are in the process now of making that determination.

Ms. BROWNLEY. Okay. In my opening comments, I talked about transitional programs and the continuity of care for our patients. Does the VA, you know, I know today we are focusing much more on intensive residential treatment, but wanted to know how many transitional programs across the VA do exist. I mentioned one in Boston.

Ms. CAMPBELL. Thank you for that question. I would have to get back with you about the specific numbers. In terms of transitional programs, we have compensated work therapy and community re-entry programs within all of our domiciliary programming. Is that what you are referring to?

Ms. BROWNLEY. Yes, I mean, for those kinds of services. In a transitional, you know, in a transitional space environment, you know, where women would be co-located going through with these particular kinds of services offered to them. The one I referenced in Boston lasted for almost a year of transition. That is what I am looking for. Apparently we do not have the answers to that. I will have to wait until you can get back to me on several of these questions about numbers of residential treatments for women and the two additional women clinics, where they are and how they were decided upon in terms of location.

My last question to Dr. Kroviak. In terms of veterans being referred to in the community, what are some of the hallmarks of quality residential substance use disorder treatment programs? How does coordinating this kind of care in the community differ from coordinating a medical procedure such as surgery?

Ms. KROVIAK. There are some accrediting bodies that are important to the residential programs, like are for Joint Commission. VA is required to ensure that when they are referring a patient to this type of treatment, that those facilities are certified by one of the two institutions as well as the state in which they are operating. In terms of referrals, the referral process is quite similar. You know, a patient can self-refer. Any provider can refer a patient when they are appropriate and engaged in that level of care.

Ms. BROWNLEY. Just this accreditation process or, you know, approval from these outside agencies and as far as you are concerned, the VA is adhering to those requirements?

Ms. KROVIAK. We have no concerns that VHA is not, meaning that we have not heard allegations on that front. Those are appropriate accrediting standards to ensure.

Ms. BROWNLEY. Thank you. I yield back, Mr. Chairman.

Mr. LUTTRELL. Thank you, ranking member. The chair recognizes Congresswoman Kiggans.

Ms. KIGGANS. Thank you, Mr. Chair. Thank you committee members just for being here, our board members. Just a question about reimbursement for community care providers. We got to hear from them and just some of their struggles with why are they not accepting some of our patients that we are referring to. They had concerns about their reimbursement rates and about the time it was taking for them to be reimbursed. Can you tell how competitive we are when looking at community care compared to the VA system? Is the compensation competitive or do we look at that even when we are thinking about compensation?

Mr. YENDE. Thank you for that question, Congresswoman. In terms of processing claims in general, VA has been pretty good about processing clean claims. I believe over 95 percent of these clean claims are processed within 30 days. I do not have the exact numbers for RRTP programs, but we can get back to you if needed. In terms of a reimbursement, we follow Medicare rates in general, but there are lots of nuances about reimbursement. I believe we are competitive. If there are specific questions about a particular Current Procedural Terminology (CPT) code or those kind of details, we are happy to work offline and try to clarify those questions.

Ms. KIGGANS. It was just a comment that I have heard more than once about why they can not take VA or they do not want to contract with the VA because our reimbursement rates were not competitive for them. There is such a shortage of mental health providers in the community and throughout the country that, you know, I just want to make sure we are prioritizing staying competitive so that they are incentivized to be able to see our patients.

I represent Hampton Roads and recently got to talk to and visit the Hampton VA, which is doing a great job. Their two complaints were that they wanted more space and they needed more people, which I think is kind of are universal complaints. Their mental health department, I think they are doing good work. Overall, I just want to say thank you, you know, to them. I know it is a hard job. I know that as a nurse practitioner, I know nurses especially have been asked to do a lot during the pandemic, especially in the mental health field and all providers. I want to thank them because they are doing good work out there.

One of the things I hear about and that I am concerned about as well is when we have these great inpatient programs that we send our veterans to for substance abuse for any mental health as depression, anxiety, suicidal ideations, we stabilize them and have them there for however long it takes, and then we release them back to the community, back to their homes. That continuity of care piece, you guys talked about it a little bit, but, you know, we see it. I saw it, you know, in my practice. It is like we lose them to the community, right? How are we ensuring that when these patients are discharged, I am sure there is a discharge planner that makes sure they have a follow-up appointment, that make sure they go home with their meds. On the State House level, I know we were pushing for things like home health to actually visit the home because leaving the motivation just with this patient and they are already probably struggling, and their family, and a lot of questions, new side effects of medication, transportation issues, all those things.

My desire was to have someone actually visit the home. There is so much benefit. We can get to see what that home environment looks like. That continuity of care piece, whatever that looks like, is it home health? What is the VA doing to just ensure that? Is it utilization of nurse managers, you know, to make sure that we are really thinking of all the issues that veterans struggle with once we get them stabilized so that we do not lose them to the community?

Ms. CAMPBELL. Thank you for that question. We do have full comprehensive continuum of care that includes, as we mentioned, inpatient, which is the most restrictive all the way to outpatient services, as well as leveraging our peer specialists and that provide a lot of coaching. The uniqueness about VA peer specialists is that they have a veteran lived experience and so they are able to rapidly build rapport with our veterans.

We certainly are able to leverage telehealth services so that when the veteran reintegrates in the community and is competitively employed, we can utilize that service so they do not have to spend time away from a job that they have been newly employed to. Then we have multiple award-winning apps that can be downloaded for the veterans use. Thank you.

Ms. KIGGANS. They are utilizing those things. Someone is going behind them and making sure they are utilizing one of those great services.

Ms. CAMPBELL. Yes, we are.

Ms. KIGGANS. Thank you. Thank you, I yield back.

Mr. LUTTRELL. Thank you. Congresswoman Budzinski, you are recognized for 5 minutes.

Ms. BUDZINSKI. Thank you, Mr. Chairman and thank you, ranking member. Thank you to the panel for being here today. I represent a predominantly rural district in Central and Southern Ill nois. I just got back from a 2-week recess working at home in-district and heard from many of the veterans while I was in-district that are struggling still in accessing VA services, specifically in our rural areas. This is very concerning to me as the rate of veterans with substance use disorders continues to climb, especially post pandemic. Rural vets simply do not have the access to as many SUD treatment programs and facilities as they do in urban areas. My first question is really two-part and it is for Dr. Campbell. What are the steps the VA is taking to ensure rural veterans with substance use disorders are able to access high quality VA treatment programs? What is being done to address the infrastructure and access shortages for our rural vets?

Ms. CAMPBELL. Thank you for that question. We do realize that that is a challenge for our rural veterans. Whenever we can, we leverage our telehealth services. Sometimes we know that there could be bandwidth problems with that. Veterans are still able, certainly, to see individuals face to face as needed. The Office of Mental Health and Suicide Prevention has partnered with rural health and our clinical pharmacy service to help us leverage additional prescribers for medication assistant treatment for our veterans.

Ms. BUDZINSKI. Thank you. I wanted to add on to what Ranking Member Brownley had just asked about some of our women veterans in particular. As you know, the number of women in the military is increasing and women are the fastest growing demographic within the VHA. It is why within my district I am going to be specifically assembling a women's veterans council so I can hear specifically from the women veterans in the district because female veterans are experiencing many of the same problems as males.

There is emerging evidence showing that women veterans may be more likely to experience substance use disorders than their male counterparts. This is due to additional factors for women veterans tending to experience such as higher chances of experiencing sexual assault, and harassment, rape, and intimate partner violence. Again, my question is for Dr. Campbell. The VA has acknowledged it needs to improve VA services for women veterans, but what are some specific steps that the VA is taking to improve and expand specialized care for women veterans experiencing substance use disorders?

Ms. CAMPBELL. Thank you again for that question. Wherever we can in terms of our full continuum of treatment, we are making sure that those individuals who are specialized to address women health needs are right in those clinics, such as the primary care mental health integration clinics, certainly on our residential treatment programming clinics. Then we are also ensuring that our women's advocacy is shored up that they have the time to devote to make sure that there is seamless flow of treatment for women within VA.

Ms. BUDZINSKI. Okay, thank you. Since I have a little bit more time, I am actually going to shift to residential rehabilitation treatments. To just note, you know, I understand some of the concerns my colleagues have voiced regarding access standards for residential SUD treatment, as this can lead to longer wait times and longer travel times for our vets, which I know we have been talking about. The ability to have all levels of SUD treatment available, including outpatient, residential, and hospital inpatient services is still strained for all veterans. However, more so again concerning for women veterans and for rural veterans.

I also understand that we need to ensure our veterans have protections from fraudulent community providers who have taken advantage of vulnerable patients seeking treatment and who have prioritized profits over the safety of their patients. Veterans deserve, as I believe, high quality evidence-based care if they are sent to community providers for SUD treatment.

Dr. Campbell, I know not all veterans have a substance use—require a substance use disorder residential treatment. For those who do, how can the VA help to ensure those veterans are able to access the intensive SUD care they need while also making sure they are protected from fraudulent providers or entities? Thank you.

Ms. CAMPBELL. Thank you again for that question. We are in the process of continuing to educate within our own organization, and certainly with the community, the standards that we expect in terms of particularly SUD treatment. We have completed regional conferences to make sure that our staff is aware of the policies as it pertains to community care, as well as holding quarterly meeting with our VSO stakeholders to make sure that they understand where our programs are and to listen and learn regarding the concerns they have.

I wanted to mention another certainly concern of our women veterans is that they need to feel safe when they come to our facilities. Within our residential units, we have secured wings just for female veterans with closed circuit TV monitoring at exit entrances so that we can keep monitoring as closely as we can. Dr. Yende can——

Mr. YENDE. Just to add to Dr. Campbell's point, from a community care side, in addition to the accreditation requirements that Dr. Kroviak mentioned, we also have standardized processes where our Transition Patient Advocates (TPAs) are expected to review LEIE list. If a provider has engaged in fraudulent activities and that has been confirmed, they will be part of the List of Excluded Individuals and Entities (LEIE) list and they are expected to be excluded from that.

Ms. BUDZINSKI. Thank you. I think we are overtime. Thank you for your generosity, Madam Chair.

Ms. MILLER-MEEKS. Thank you. The chair now recognizes Representative Luttrell for 5 minutes.

Mr. LUTTRELL. Thank you, Madam Chairman. Dr. Campbell, I understand—I am going to go off what the ranking member asked. The VA currently has two dedicated residential substance use disorder treatment programs for women veterans. Then the question was asked, there are two additional residential programs in development. Where are they and are they admitting patients? How did the VA decide on these location programs because the budget itself is already out?

I do respect and appreciate the weight that you have to carry, but we have to go back to our district. When these questions come from our constituents. The fact that you were not able to answer those questions in front of us today is disheartening, because now we have to go back and tell them that the VA does not know. You want to respond to that?

Ms. CAMPBELL. I would. Thank you again for that question. I certainly understand the responsibility that we all have to our veterans for these answers. I will certainly get that answer to you as quickly as I can regarding where the two additional programs will be located. The other programs that I mentioned specific to women are in VISN 110 and 17. I will check that, though, to make sure that that is accurate.

Mr. LUTTRELL. Thank you, Doctor. I appreciate it. Dr. Kroviak, are you familiar with VHA Policy 1162.02 regarding mental health residential rehabilitation treatment programs?

Ms. KROVIAK. I am somewhat familiar. I certainly did not draft it, but I would be happy to take your question.

Mr. LUTTRELL. What do you know about it? Give me the wave top.

Ms. KROVIAK. I am sorry?

Mr. LUTTRELL. Can you give me what the wave top description is? The way you think that is?

Ms. KROVIAK. The referral time you mean?

Mr. LUTTRELL. Well, I will just go this way. It states, the directive states that any veteran with a scheduled wait time of greater than 30 calendar days must be offered alternative residential treatments on another level of care to meet the veterans needs and preferences at the time of screening. Where did 30 days come from?

Ms. KROVIAK. That was legislated to my understanding.

Mr. LUTTRELL. Do you think that that is a good——

Ms. KROVIAK. Oh, I am sorry. I might be confusing with the Mission Act. I think the 30 days was just a measurable metric developed to assess progress toward providing the care that was not available at the time of the referral.

Mr. LUTTRELL. Given the issues that we see in suicide and substance abuse, the psychiatrists, and psychologists, and doctors in the VA still think 30 days is a reasonable timeframe?

Ms. KROVIAK. I would have to defer that question to VHA in terms of the 30-day standard of what their providers assume is appropriate.

Mr. LUTTRELL. As the Inspector General, I would assume that you were digging into this problem.

Ms. KROVIAK. In terms of the 30-day standard, that was not established by the IG.

Mr. LUTTRELL. No, I know.

Ms. KROVIAK. We just do oversight to hold——

Mr. LUTTRELL. I guess my question——

Ms. KROVIAK [continuing]. VHA accountable.

Mr. LUTTRELL [continuing]. is, do you think that that timeframe is too long?

Ms. KROVIAK. I think it depends on the diagnosis that you are describing. I think it is a clinical decision. I think 30 days is somewhat arbitrary for a lot of these issues that veterans are referred for specialty care.

Mr. LUTTRELL. Some do not like the Community Care Network. However, the intent of the new COMPACT Act is to provide immediate access to those services anytime, anywhere, largely expanding access to community care. What is the view of the VA on implementing the COMPACT Act? Is there any rulemaking to write directives and policy to implement the act itself?

Ms. CAMPBELL. Thank you for that question. COMPACT has been implemented, as you mentioned, that it allows the veteran to be treated for an acute suicide episode at any community facility or within VA. I will defer to Dr. Yende for more information on COMPACT.

Mr. YENDE. Congressman, implementation started in January of this year. Implementation of the COMPACT Act started in January of this year. To date, we have provided care for over 11,000 veterans since the program started.

Mr. LUTTRELL. Eleven thousand?

Mr. YENDE. Yes. This is both on the direct care side as well as on the community care side.

Mr. LUTTRELL. Okay, final question. I am just going to throw this out to the three of you. Are any of you aware of a new VA community care policy or process and/or guidance within the last 10 months surrounding a mental health residential rehabilitation treatment program that restricts, inhibits, or deters community care referrals? I say that because I actually have verbal and written statements by VA employees that State that they are under this new policy.

Mr. YENDE. To our knowledge, Congressman, we have no policies that would restrict. If they meet criteria for referring the patient to alternative treatment facilities for RRTP programs, which includes community care, they should be referred in a timely manner.

Mr. LUTTRELL. My time is up, ma'am. I would like to preserve the opportunity to submit additional questions.

Ms. MILLER-MEEKS. So recognized. The chair now recognizes Representative Landsman for 5 minutes.

Mr. LANDSMAN. Thank you, Madam Chair, and thank you all for being here. My district, which includes the city of Cincinnati, Southwest Ohio, is home to a great VA. We offer, you know, some of the best veterans care in the country for PTSD, suicide prevention, and other mental health issues.

When I have spent time with folks at the VA in Cincinnati, they talk a lot about the evidence-based programming, and it is really compelling. When it comes to specialty treatment for substance use disorder, veterans across the country are not getting the care they deserve. This may have already come up. I have seen statistics that suggest more than 550,000 veterans diagnosed with substance use disorder last year, of those, 62 percent received outpatient treatment. Those numbers drop off drastically as the level of services increase. Less than 25 percent received specialty care and even fewer received intensive care at 4 percent. You see, there is a drop off in terms of if a veteran needs additional treatment outside of the outpatient treatment.

I have two questions. One has to do with, you know, do you have a sense as to the drop off? What you know, have you seen, is it staffing, is it other issues? Then the second has to do with a general question as it relates to all of the VA services. This is true for a lot of public services, nonprofit services, and that is that we really do struggle to get to folks who are not getting to us. You know, this is particularly true for veterans, particularly veterans who are just not coming in, you know, and have real issues.

I have been pushing in these hearings for the kind of programming outreach that gets the VA to where folks are. I am curious what you think has worked, could work in terms of meeting veterans where they are, and connecting those who are currently disconnected. Two questions, one has to do with the drop off and the second outreach. Thank you.

Ms. CAMPBELL. Thank you, sir, for those questions. I will take the first question in terms of the dropout. The dropout may not necessarily mean that that veteran is not in some type of other care. I think what you were referring to is a drop off when it concerns more intense care, such as residential treatment. The veteran may still be involved in an outpatient treatment, may be involved with teleservices, and sometimes, for various reasons, the veteran has elected a later date to come into treatment. That decision regarding the level of care is always between that individual veteran patient and the provider that is helping with the medical disposition and clinical decisionmaking. We do realize, especially where community care is concerned, because SUD is such a specialized treatment, that it may not be available in every location where that veteran is.

In terms of your second question regarding being able to touch veterans who are not already in our care, we are certainly hoping that the legislation that has been passed with COMPACT, allowing veterans to be treated wherever the need is without any cost to them will help with that. We have fantastic media campaigns, Don't Wait Reach Out, where we are utilizing veterans to help veterans understand what it is like to come into VA for care. Then certainly leveraging everywhere we can our peer support specialists who have that lived experience that can help us bring in care.

Mr. LANDSMAN. Thank you very much. I have additional que tions if I can submit them. Thank you.

Mr. VAN ORDEN. Dr. Campbell, good afternoon. How long has your office been in existence? I know you have been there since 2022, but how long has the Office of Mental Health and Suicide Prevention been in existence?

Ms. CAMPBELL. I am sorry, sir, I did not hear the entire.

Mr. VAN ORDEN. How long has the Office of Mental Health and Suicide Prevention been in existence?

Ms. CAMPBELL. Been getting?

Mr. VAN ORDEN. Been in existence?

Ms. CAMPBELL. Oh, been in existence. At least 34 years.

Mr. VAN ORDEN. Thirty-four years. Very well, thank you. How many people work for you?

Ms. CAMPBELL. I have about 140 people within my office.

Mr. VAN ORDEN. Got it, thank you. Do your reporting numbers reflect, for veteran suicide, do they reflect overdoses?

Ms. CAMPBELL. That is a separate report in terms of overdoses that we hope to be able to publish the end of June.

Mr. VAN ORDEN. In your opinion, Doctor, if someone kills themselves by overdose or gunshot wound, are they still dead?

Ms. CAMPBELL. They are still dead, sir.

Mr. VAN ORDEN. Okay. Do your metrics for veteran suicide include overdose?

Ms. CAMPBELL. The metrics that we reported recently on our annual report does not include overdose.

Mr. VAN ORDEN. Okay. That is a problem. What are your established metrics of success for your Office of Mental Health and Suicide Prevention?

Ms. CAMPBELL. We have various metrics depending on the service that we are looking at in terms of outcomes. We have hundreds of metrics that we use. It depends on specifically what you are asking about in terms of outcome.

Mr. VAN ORDEN. Do you think, and please take this as it is intended, Morgan and I have had multiple friends commit suicide. Over 21 now, for me personally. Veterans have committed suicide. Do your metrics include veterans that do not commit suicide? I know it is kind of hard to prove a negative. What I am wondering is, after 34 years of existence with over 140 employees, if your office ceased to exist, would more veterans be alive tomorrow? I mean, is your office preventing veterans from committing suicide or not? Or are we just spending money and hiring people so that they can get together, come to these committee meetings, talk a bunch, submit reports, metrics that can not be defined? Are you moving the needle?

Ms. CAMPBELL. Sir, we do. Thank you for that question. I certainly can understand the frustration. This is a very complicated area. We are certainly ourselves saddened by any—

Mr. VAN ORDEN. Doctor, please——

Ms. CAMPBELL [continuing]. suicide.

Mr. VAN ORDEN. — I have a limited amount of time.

Ms. CAMPBELL. I do believe we are moving the needle on this. We have a full public health approach where suicide prevention is concerned. The field of mental health and psychology, psychiatry has evolved over the past 30 to 40 years. As we continue to evolve, we are learning new things, new methods, new evidence-based approaches that we can use.

Mr. VAN ORDEN. Thank you. That leads to my next question. How many non-evidence-based treatment modalities do you guys support, specifically religious and faith-based programs similar to the incredibly successful Mighty Oaks Foundation? How many faith-based nonevidence programs are currently being administered by the Veterans Administration?

Ms. CAMPBELL. Thank you again for that question. Within VA, we certainly value scientifically based evidence-based programs. That does not mean, however, that we do not collaborate with our chaplain services that certainly help us with specifically the moral injury side of PTSD and other mental health disorders.

Mr. VAN ORDEN. Doctor, what I am hearing from you is that the Veterans Administration is not helping these wildly successful programs that can quantify, like, actually quantify the amount of veterans lives that they are saving because they are faith-based, which, according to you guys, are non-evidence-based. Living veterans, that is evidence of a program's functioning.

I just want to be real clear. You are telling me the Veterans Administration is not allowing non-evidence-based, specifically faith-based programs like the incredibly successful Mighty Oaks Warrior Foundation to function within your organization, even though they have proven to save thousands of veterans lives? Is that accurate?

Ms. CAMPBELL. Sir, we are certainly willing to sit down and have a conversation with this organization to see how we can partner with them.

Mr. VAN ORDEN. Thank you very much for your time, ma'am.

With that, I yield back.

Ms. MILLER-MEEKS. Thank you. The chair now recognizes herself for 5 minutes of questioning. The Independence Fund will testify that in the past 23 months, their case workers intervened for 110 veterans who ran into issues accessing complex mental health care and 59 of those required substance use care. In fact, in the last Congress, we passed a bill, the Brandon Act, because a veteran in my district went to the VA Center, was denied care, and 5 hours later committed suicide. Would you agree that these veterans, frustrated by access to critical care, would be at elevated risk for suicide? Dr. Campbell, yes or no, please?

Ms. CAMPBELL. Yes, I would agree that they are at high risk, and veterans at high risk certainly would be at high risk for suicide.

Ms. MILLER-MEEKS. Dr. Yende.

Mr. YENDE. Yes, chair, Congresswoman.

Ms. MILLER-MEEKS. Dr. Campbell, the committee has been made aware of a policy that was supposedly rolled out internally, as was mentioned, that required that if a VISN's Veterans Administration Medical Center (VAMC) could not meet the 30-day appointment availability window, it must confer with other VISN VAMCs for VA residential substance use disorder bed availability before leveraging community care in order to keep care in house. I certainly have experienced these complaints in my own district in Iowa. It was also reported that five VAMCs must be contacted to fulfill the directive. Can you either confirm or deny this policy?

Ms. CAMPBELL. There is no policy, Madam Chairwoman, denying veterans access to community care. The Standard Episode of Cares (SEOCs) regarding residential treatment were newly established. SEOCs is a standard episode of care for community care in October 2020. The process is somewhat new for us. We understand there are challenges in making sure that people are educated about the appropriate referrals to community care. We do not have a policy denying people community care access.

Ms. MILLER-MEEKS. Would you call these veterans liars?

Ms. CAMPBELL. No, I would not call the veterans liars. What I would say is that we need to do a better job of educating our veterans, our staff, and the community about the appropriate procedures for referrals to community care.

Ms. MILLER-MEEKS. Well, I can certainly say as both a physician who has taken care of veterans through the community care system, the Mission Act, and as a veteran myself, that it is unacceptable. When people report and come to the decision to obtain substance use disorder treatment, they should be addressed and acknowledged and get care immediately. This also goes for complex mental health. I can tell you the family of our veteran who committed suicide 5 hours after being at a VA hospital, would also agree with that.

Dr. Campbell, we have heard of multiple instances where veterans have been approved for a community care referral, as I said, only to have that referral overruled by administrative or other senior staff. Can you explain why a decision for a specific course of medical care as determined between the veteran and their provider would be reversed by an official outside of their clinical chain? What recourse does the referring physician have when their clinical judgment is overruled? How are you going to address this deficit?

Ms. CAMPBELL. Thank you for that question. Each case, as we mentioned, is an individual case that is a decision between that provider and the patient or veteran. I am not aware of policies where decisions are being overturned. I will turn to Dr. Yende to see if he has more information regarding community care.

Mr. YENDE. Congresswoman, if the provider determines that the veteran should go to the community, then that decision should be followed through. Our policies do not require that that care should be provided in the VA in that instance. If there are instances, we are happy to look into it.

Ms. MILLER-MEEKS. Let me just speak for the entire committee. We expect better of the VA medical care system. Our veterans deserve better. Through this oversight, you know, some of the comments that have been revealed are really astonishing. We hold oversight because what is occurring at the VA Medical Center and what is occurring in referrals for community care when veterans are in need, especially complex mental health and substance use disorder, needs to be addressed and addressed rapidly. We will continue to ask for both collaboration and verification, as we have said. What you have learned today should in fact put you on notice and on record.

On behalf of the subcommittee, seeing that there are no other Representatives who wish to ask questions, I want to thank you for your testimony and for joining us today. You are now excused. We will wait for a moment as the second panel comes to the witness table.

Welcome, everyone, and thank you for your participation today. On the second panel, we have Dr. Daniel Elkins, the chief of staff with the Independence Fund, Mrs. Jen Silva, chief program officer with the Wounded Warrior Project, Mr. Thomas Sauer, chief executive Officer and owner of Miramar Health. Accompanying Mr. Sauer is Mr. Brendan Dowling. Mr. Elkins, you are now recognized for 5 minutes to deliver your opening statement.

Statement of Daniel Elkins

Mr. ELKINS. Good morning Chairwoman Meeks, Ranking Member Brownley, and members of the subcommittee. On behalf of Sarah Verardo, Chief Executive Officer (CEO) of the Independence Fund, we would like to thank you for your kind invitation to provide testimony at today's hearing. As a currently serving Green Beret in the National Guard and the chief of staff of the Independence Fund, I have seen firsthand my brothers and sisters in desperate need be denied access to care, fall through the cracks of bureaucracy, and suffer alone with the wounds from war. It is this denial of access and subsequent isolation that often culminates in death by suicide, a death that could be prevented.

This hearing could not be more timely as our casework staff have been receiving a significant number of inquiries nationwide who are experiencing frustration and hardship when seeking the most critical services for acute mental health conditions. The geographic dispersion and similarity of factors presented in many of the cases indicate that these cases are not merely anecdotal but may be indicators of a more widespread problem for mental health within the hospital network. We would like to thank VA's VSO liaisons for their support and assistance and help with these cases. However, there is work that needs to be done.

In our written testimony, the Independence Fund has provided extensive case study examples of the inconsistencies currently present within VHA care. Each of these cases involves a veteran who was in acute need and required priority treatment for substance abuse disorder in PTSD. These veterans were denied access to care, even community care referrals, in direct conflict with the spirit. In some cases, incidents of the letter of the law of Mission Act. We have found that the Veterans Health Administration was unable to provide these veterans with proper continuity of care, failing to meet the most basic of industry standards.

Indeed, it was not until October 2021 that the Independence Fund discovered that VHA does not consider the access standard authorities of Mission Act when veterans are seeking help for substance use disorders. Yes, you heard that correctly. Veterans do not have Mission Act's regulatory protections for wait times, travel distance when seeking treatment for substance use disorders as these treatments fall within VHA's residential rehabilitation treatment program.

According to the VA, this program is instead under the authority of VHA Directive 1162, which requires that VA admit a veteran seeking inpatient residential care within 72 hours for priority patients, and no more than 30 days after a VA assessment for any patient needing residential care. Based on our experience, however, that is not unusual. It is not unusual for veterans to wait beyond this time limit. Furthermore, it has been our observation that even after those time limits are exceeded, VHA exercises latitude to further delay access to treatment when looking for an available bed in another VA facility, even if that facility is several states away. More troubling, the Independence Fund has found that some VHA administrators or senior clinical staff overrule referrals of care for the community, in spite of VA-appointed providers for the veteran. There have also been some cases where our casework team were told by an administrator that community care was not offered. At times, the administrative staff did not understand community care was even a lawful option. In certain circumstances, VA staff do not discuss community care options with the veteran without prompting or until a case worker inquires a VA administrator or patient advocate.

It is important for us all to keep in mind that many veterans do not know their full care options and have already taken a monumental step in seeking help. More work needs to be done. In our written testimony, we offer six recommendations to the subcommittee on how to resolve these issues that create barriers to care for veterans seeking treatment for substance use disorder and PTSD and other conditions that are highly indicative of death by suicide. I will highlight what we believe should be the foremost priority for this subcommittee.

We must ensure that all criteria for community care wait times, travel distance, and access standards under Mission Act govern VHA Directive 1162 or eliminate VHA Directive 1162 entirely and defer to Mission Act's original authorities and intent to support all levels of specialty care, including rehabilitation services. Once this goal is achieved, it will substantially improve the quality, timeliness, and effectiveness of care for veterans in acute need of treatment for substance use disorder, whether that be in a VHA provider or community care provider.

Thank you for this opportunity to share with you all the struggles of our Nation's heroes, and I look forward to answering any questions you may have.

[The prepared statement of Daniel Elkins appears in the Appendix]

Ms. MILLER-MEEKS. Thank you, Mr. Elkins. Ms. Silva, you are now recognized for 5 minutes to deliver your statement.

Statement of Jen Silva

Ms. SILVA. Thank you, Chairwoman Miller-Meeks, Ranking Member Brownley, and the distinguished members of the Health Subcommittee for this opportunity to speak before you. Since our founding 20 years ago, Wounded Warrior Project has been helping post-911 wounded, ill, and injured veterans address their biggest challenges and reach their highest potential through impactful no cost programming and advocacy. Today, those two paths intersect to highlight how veterans who need inpatient care for mental health or substance use are not receiving access to the prompt and in some cases, lifesaving care that they need and deserve.

The VA Mission Act was signed into law with broad support in the potential to provide veterans and their advocates with clear, useful, and timely information that could inform their health care decisions. In January 2019, VA published access standards that included limits on wait times and travel for mental health care. However, as time has passed, it has become clear that these access standards have a critical gap for veterans seeking care in inpatient programs, most specifically VA's mental health residential rehabilitation treatment programs, or their community-based equivalents. As discussed in our written statement, VA's Mission Act derived access standards do not extend to these crucial inpatient mental health programs. Instead, veterans and their advocates are left to interpret a VHA directive that we have discussed. In our experience, this directive provides little predictability about the course of their treatment and their options for care along the way. Unless Congress or VA act to address this policy gap, many of these veterans will continue to face obstacles in connecting to the care they need, placing them at heightened risk for negative outcomes the longer they wait.

My remarks today are largely informed by Wounded Warrior Project's Complex Case Coordination Team, or C3. This team offers a high touch service to warriors with complex challenges that are often multifaceted and require urgent action. The team connects warriors to our internal support programs and to VA and community care treatment options, all with the goal of providing immediate assistance and case coordination.

In just the last four years, our team has helped nearly 1,200 warriors with complex cases navigate VA and community treatment options. However, our support simply cannot reach the scale required to assist all veterans who need this heightened level of care and intervention. The team's single biggest challenge since inception has been helping veterans access VA inpatient mental health care. The lack of a consistently applied access standard has essentially resulted in no true access standard for residential treatment. Local policy variations have resulted in unpredictable referral decisions. Wait times are not uniformly calculated and can be impacted by inconsistent policies about a veteran first having to complete significantly less intensive treatment options. Staffing challenges can also limit communication and bed availability.

Alternative treatment options that would result in a community or even intra-VA referrals and faster access are not uniformly accepted by VA administrators.

In totality, many veterans are not accessing the care they need when they are ready to receive it. Delays in finding appropriate care in a timely manner not only fails to capitalize on the veteran's desire to change their life circumstance, but in some cases causes further damage to their mental and physical health, declines in family and social relationships, and even involvement with the justice system. As illustrated in VA's most recent National Veterans Suicide Prevention Annual Report, substance use disorder continues to be a significant factor in veteran suicide. While the report showed overall reduction in the veteran suicide rate, subpopulations struggling with opioid, cocaine, cannabis, and stimulant disorders showed increased suicide rates.

To mitigate the risks associated with inpatient care access and ensure consistent VA help throughout the enterprise, we believe that Mission Act access standards must apply to the delivery of inpatient mental and substance use disorder care. We want and we need the VA to be successful in this. Simply put, for us, VA is our most critical partner in connecting veterans to the inpatient care they need. In closing, I want to thank the subcommittee for this invitation to testify, and I welcome your questions.

[The prepared statement of Jen Silva appears in the Appendix]

Ms. MILLER-MEEKS. Thank you, Ms. Silva. Mr. Sauer, you are now recognized for 5 minutes to deliver your opening statement.

Statement of Thomas Sauer

Mr. SAUER. A broken record here, all right. Thank you very much. Chairman Miller-Meeks, Ranking Member Brownley, and members of the subcommittee, my name is Tom Sauer, and I am honored to testify before you today. I am a Navy and Marine Corps veteran, and for the better part of my life, I have been wearing the cloth of the Nation. I am a former listed Marine infantryman, a 2006 Naval Academy graduate, and a former Navy explosive ordinance disposal officer. Today, however, I am the owner and CEO of Miramar Health, a veteran-owned and operated community care provider for intensive substance use disorder and mental health treatment exclusively for America's veterans.

Mental health and addiction treatment are deep passions of mine because depression and addiction killed my dad. Five days before I graduated from high school and 3 weeks before I shipped out for the Marines in 1999, a methamphetamine overdose took his life after decades of struggle, just like so many millions of Americans suffering from our country's disastrous mental health and addiction crisis. I would also like to point out that 4 days ago, my father-in-law died of addiction. He was an Air Force veteran.

Thanks to recent legislation, thousands of veterans have enhanced access to lifesaving mental health care and addiction treatment within the VA's Community Care Network. We provided intensive, custom tailored, world class mental health and addiction treatment for nearly 250 veterans from a dozen VA medical centers across the western United States, typically for 30, 60, sometimes 90-plus day stays. This treatment is for our veterans who are truly suffering, in crisis, and often near death from suicide or overdose resulting from this disastrous mental health and addiction crisis. In 3–1/2 years, we have grown from one small clinic with six employees to eight residential facilities and one large outpatient facility. These facilities are staffed by nearly 100 phenomenal physicians, nurses, psychologists, therapists, medical technicians, case managers, and support staff, many of whom are veterans themselves. One is sitting right to my left as well. I could not be any prouder of them.

I did not come all the way out here just to tell you all this, just so I could pat myself on the back, but rather to simply convey the sincerity of our intentions and to lay out how important this challenge is. Miramar believes in our partnership with the VA by bridging both capability and capacity gaps within certain VA medical centers and in being an advocate to veterans in need, all while providing them with the highest quality of care. In other words, we do not consider ourselves to be just another government contractor. We are partners and we are teammates with the VA, and we are here asking for your help to ensure our Nation's veterans receive the lifesaving care they need and deserve by helping us to strengthen that partnership.

The overwhelming majority of frontline, boots on the ground VA personnel we directly interact with are fantastic, dedicated, life-saving public servants. Some of these guys deserve medals and parades. There are many who deserve medals and parades. I am here to add today to advocate for veterans in need to be able to access care anywhere immediately and we can figure out that paperwork later.

The current VA policy of 30 days to wait to find a bed in a given region does not meet the urgent level of this crisis. I think you have been hearing this before, a recurring theme. Specifically, we have encountered several occasions where, despite community care being available for a veteran in crisis, they are either put on a waiting list for up to 30 days before receiving care when they do not have 30 minutes without becoming a very real risk to suicide or overdose. Chairwoman Miller-Meeks, I think you have highlighted such a case. We have cases that can highlight that as well too.

I have firsthand knowledge of these suicide and overdose deaths since I have owned Miramar, so I can understand the devastation this policy can cause. We believe this issue could rather be easily corrected through either through a legislative carve out for community care eligibility, as with urgent care, or when it comes to urgent care for community care, when it comes to mental health and addiction treatment. This could be done by clarifying ensuring the COMPACT Act is being implemented as intended and that veterans are aware of this option for receiving care.

We urge you to seek to ensure that our veterans have access to care they need when they need it through the Community Care Network. We appreciate your consideration of this matter, and we are willing to work with you to address these issues to ensure that our guys and gals get the care they need so desperately. Thank you, Chair, and members of the subcommittee, each of you, your staffers, and the committee staff are champions for America's veterans. I am exceptionally grateful to you and to your commitment to serving them and that you are holding this important hearing today. In conclusion, thank you so much for addressing these issues, and I am more than happy to answer your questions.

[The prepared statement of Thomas Sauer Appears in the Appendix]

Ms. MILLER-MEEKS. On behalf of all the committee, Mr. Sauer, our condolences on the loss of your father, and I thank you for your testimony. I will go last in the lineup of questions. I now recognize Ranking Member Brownley for any questions she may have.

Ms. BROWNLEY. Thank you, Madam Chair. Ms. Silva, I just wanted to stay on a theme of women veterans for a minute, and I know we are talking about access, so I was wondering if you could speak at all to your experiences in trying to get women veterans the gender specific care that they need programs, inpatient programs, and if you could speak to that within the VA and within the community.

Ms. SILVA. Well, thank you for the question. I believe the women specific care adds an element that complicates this already kind of urgent action approach to this. We have a very short window for care. If a veteran comes to us and needs that—we are talking, specifically mental health and substance use disorder—the co-occurring with either military sexual trauma makes them at a heightened risk, as we talked about in the previous panel for this.

I have a vignette that I think is a pretty interesting one, where a female veteran was trying to get care for Military Sexual Trauma (MST) and substance use disorder, so co-occurring, and the opportunities were not available. They were available in that Community Care Network area. Unfortunately, in this situation, the VA said it seemed too resort-like and were not able to get her into that care. They did not allow for that.

What she did, but they did have an intra-VA option and she moved her entire family across a couple of states in order to get into that care. She was into VA care. I think in my experience, once they are in the care, so all those barriers of maybe females not being comfortable, once they are in there, it has been very productive and the outcomes are fantastic. We have got to work on— it does not have to be that difficult where you have got to move across states. Maybe it had to work in this situation. I think we can do better though.

Ms. BROWNLEY. Well, I think it is true for men as well as women, but I think for particularly women, I think you just highlighted one of the, I think, big obstacles to access, and that is a woman to get the proper resources and treatment that she needs, many times has to travel outside of her state in order to receive that within the VA. You know, what does a woman do with her family? All of that. It becomes a tremendous burden for them to, you know, to leave family, to leave responsibilities in order to get the appropriate treatment. I feel like we need to address some of those issues as well.

As a consequence, we need more, I believe, more gender specific programs for women. I wonder if you could just comment a little bit. I know we are talking more about access, but just in terms of your experiences with getting referrals inpatient within the VA and within the community, can you speak to—it is my sense that when I have spoken to people, once they get into the VA and inpatient care, it is pretty good and the success is there. Can you talk a little bit about quality of care compared to, you know, inpatient VA versus community care? Can you give any kind of conclusions?

Ms. SILVA. Ma'am, I actually agree with what you said. Once they are into care, whether it is in the VA and in the community, it has been very positive overall. It is the connective tissue in order to get them into that care is lacking. They are willing oftentimes they have to go to a less intensive program before they are—even if the clinical decision is that they need this inpatient approach, it needs to be quick. That window of opportunity, especially when we are talking about these complex cases, most of them co-occurring or the substance use disorder it is a really short window. You have got to act as everyone would agree.

You have to have that availability. There is a shortage, et cetera. If the community can provide that, then that is the best way to go, in my opinion, because ultimately the veteran has a positive experience. It is still a VA referral. I think from a customer perspective, it actually keeps your customer, if I can use that term, happy with the overall care, even if it is not within the VA Medical Center.

I know within—back to the military sexual trauma or women specific care, we have found within our Warrior Care network, it is extremely important to many of the women that are served through our intensive outpatient program that they receive it outside of the VA or outside of maybe if they are still active duty. That is a gigantic barrier to care. If that is the best option for that female veteran, then let us do it. We have VA liaisons there that can get them back into VA care. It is really not outside. It is just the connective tissue is a really positive experience for that veteran.

Ms. BROWNLEY. Thank you. I yield back.

Ms. MILLER-MEEKS. Thank you, Ranking Member Brownley. I now recognize Representative Luttrell for any questions he may have.

Mr. LUTTRELL. Thank you all for your service to this country and your continued service to our veteran community. I really appreciate that. Sir, I am very sorry for your loss.

Given the previous testimony on the previous panel's testimony, Mr. Sauer, can you just explain to us as a veteran why it is you do what you do today?

Mr. SAUER. Well, thanks for the question, Mr. Luttrell. I found really no higher calling than helping fellow service members. That is what it comes down to. When it came down to all this. I realized that there is a bigger crisis, you know, especially you two gentlemen up there on the dais, that we probably lost more friends and colleagues to suicide and addiction than we did on the battlefields overseas. I saw this as an incredibly growing problem.

The opportunity for a TriWest contract was presented. I did not know this was something that was even available. I like looked at this phenomenal opportunity that serves this growing dramatic public need. When one of my partners, who is my Naval Academy classmate, and I work with folks like Mr. Dowling here from the special operations community, like what a phenomenal group of people. Just to absolutely save lives.

I can tell you right now that, you know, as a former Navy Explosive Ordnance Disposal (EOD) officer, I spent a long time in uniform, that the work that we are doing herein today is far more valuable and to the Nation, and to the country, and frankly, for the world at large than anything I ever did wearing the uniform.

Mr. LUTTRELL. Congressman Van Orden brought up a very valid point. He said that the Suicide and Prevention Office in the VA has been in place for 34 years. My question that I did not get to ask then was has the suicide rate gone up in those 34 years? It has, absolutely. I think that lends itself to the efforts that this panel is making to protect our brothers and sisters in the veteran space.

If there were one change that you could make that would increase veteran access to lifesaving substance abuse and mental health inpatient care, what would that be?

Mr. SAUER. I think it is a pretty simple one right now is that to change that wait time from 30 days. When they do not have 30 minutes, ordinarily I would suggest 24 hours. You know what, to kind of be—to be a little understanding of the VA, 72 hours, that is one business day. When a veteran shows up to their VA provider in a mental health or addiction crisis that the VA is, you know, their standard must be that they put that veteran into a bed, get them off the X, so to speak, because lots of—we do not know exactly that the severity of the need of care. Get them off the X and they have the opportunity to be in a residential treatment program, whether or not that is in an in-house VA facility. If those facilities are full, not available right away, then you get them into a community care facility within 72 hours, one business day, preferably 24, frankly.

If we can do that right there, because obviously, one, we need to be able to ramp down the level of care as far as like if somebody has to wait 30 days, but then they can do telehealth, like that is ramping up the level of care. You need to get them off the X right away, get them into a highly intensive level of care, and then you can assess and start ramping down those levels of care. However, I would say that is what you got to do right there, just immediately get them off the X in that care, 72 hours. Yes, I think that is it right there. I mean, in a simple word, is not 30 days. You have got 72 hours, whether it is in the VA or outside with community care. Mr. LUTTRELL. For us on the panel and having dealt with the VA at multiple levels, is it in your professional opinion that the referral process is failing at a lower level or at the higher leadership level, at the higher level?

Mr. SAUER. Absolutely. It is not the social workers we deal with. I have encountered many who have told me, you know, over the phone, told people like Brendan over the phone as well, or even over email saying, this program looks fantastic. I would love to write you referral. You know, instead they would say, however, the residential rehabilitation care has a different Mission Act eligibility criteria than other specialty services and then they cite 1162.02. In that particular case, I took that particular veteran on scholarship. He was a retired Marine, spent a long—former infantryman—and we took him on scholarship. We also have a former Navy Seal who is in our facility today on scholarship as well, because he was denied care and denied access. We saw we had to do the right thing. We know when I speak to these social workers nearly every single time, they are the ones who say we would love to be able to refer them, but we can not. They will not let us.

Mr. LUTTRELL. If you do not mind, I would like to circle the wagons and get those names and the positions they hold so I can address them directly. I yield back.

Ms. MILLER-MEEKS. Thank you, Representative Luttrell. I now recognize Representative Van Orden for 5 minutes.

Mr. VAN ORDEN. Dr. Campbell, I see you in the back there. I want to thank you for staying here. Just so you are aware, I think Brendan, you are an enlisted guy, right? Yes, you did not go bad like, you did not go bad like Sauer?

Mr. DOWLING. Yes, I was.

Mr. VAN ORDEN. Yes, yes, noted. Ma'am, so as enlisted people, we need to make the rubber meet the road. Although those questions appear to be harsh, they are for a very specific reason so that we can quantify a problem and then move forward. Our purpose here, my sole legislative agenda as the chair of a Subcommittee for Veterans Economic Opportunity is to prevent veteran suicide. I thank you for staying here. I appreciate that greatly.

What I have noticed, gentlemen and gentlewoman, is that the issue is not with the Veterans Administration in many cases. It is with the Department of Defense (DOD). What I would like to ask you specifically is what is your access to the Transition Assistance Program? We will just start with Mr. Elkins, the Green Beret.

Mr. ELKINS. Well, as an enlisted guy, it is always a pleasure to be in the company of other enlisted, as well.

Mr. VAN ORDEN. Okay. I did not realize that. I thought you went bad too. Go ahead.

Mr. ELKINS. Working with the Transition Assistance Program at many levels, having gone through it multiple times, we will have to go through it again in the next several months, as I am about to transition out of my role to deploy for the third time in the last several years. There is definitely gaps that need to be addressed.

Mr. VAN ORDEN. Let me ask you something specifically, does your organization have access to the Transition Assistance Program so that you can speak to active duty service member as an upstream solution to prevent them from committing suicide and having drug and alcohol addiction issues after they retire?

Mr. ELKINS. Yes.

Mr. VAN ORDEN. You do?

Mr. ELKINS. Yes.

Mr. ELKINS. Okay. Ma'am, Ms. Silva. Ms. SILVA. No, we do not.

Mr. VAN ORDEN. You do not. Okay. Mr. Sauer.

Mr. SAUER. No, sir, we are not. We are dealing usually directly with VAs, and by the time a veteran comes to us or we are made aware of a veteran that in need, that they have already gone down. They are already in a bad spot.

Mr. VAN ORDEN. Then, Brendan, what class were you in?

Mr. DOWLING. I was in Buds Class 242.

Mr. VAN ORDEN. New guy. Oh, with you? OK. When you went through the Transition Assistance Program, were you made aware of any of these external organizations that may help you bridge the gap from being active-duty service member to becoming a productive veteran?

Mr. DOWLING. No, I was not. My Transition Assistance Program experience was unremarkable. I did not really pull anything from it——

Mr. VAN ORDEN. Okay.

Mr. DOWLING [continuing]. of use.

Mr. VAN ORDEN. Then just for everybody across the board, do you feel like you have access to the Department of Defense and ready access to the Veterans Administration on a coequal basis because we have to get upstream solutions. Do you guys have points of contact that you can call? Do you feel like the DoD is responsive to your guys' inquiries? If you needed to, can we help? If you do not, can we facilitate that for you so that we can start up here and then work our way to the veteran status?

Mr. ELKINS. We do have access. In some cases, it is very timely, and other times, we will use you and your office for assistance.

Mr. VAN ORDEN. Okay. That is absolutely open at any time.

Ma'am?

Ms. SILVA. I would say we have developed, on the DoD side, we have developed relationships with different commands. We have heavy involvement in Alaska due to the increased suicide rates there, and we have been able to be part of that solution, working with the community there. And then different—it is very commandrelated. That is the difference, in my opinion, between DoD and VA. Most of the warriors that we serve are already on the veteran side of the equation, and so our bigger contacts are with the VA. We certainly would love more collaboration with the transition piece of DoD.

Mr. VAN ORDEN. Okay, excellent. Mr. Sauer.

Mr. SAUER. Miramar is contracted with TriWest Healthcare Alliance, which, you know, currently has the sole contract with the Department of Veterans Affairs. We have no formal relationship with DoD. However, as you may be aware, TriWest Healthcare Alliance won the contract for Tricare West, so we will, beginning next year, it is my understanding we will be able to treat active duty and their families, which we look forward to. We are close to Camp Pendleton. There is a large population of active duty there, and we welcome the opportunity to strengthen those relationships for that transition.

Mr. VAN ORDEN. Okay. Hey, my time is expiring. I just want to tell you that my office is yours. I know that there is no one on this panel, Democrat or Republican, who is unwilling to step out to make sure that we can facilitate your organizations to work in conjunction with Dr. Campbell back there to help prevent veteran suicide. With that, God bless you, and thank you for your work very much. Ma'am, I yield back.

Ms. MILLER-MEEKS. Thank you, Representative Van Orden. I thought about removing your time because I take offense as a former enlisted who became an officer.

Mr. SAUER. Same here.

Ms. MILLER-MEEKS. Ms. Silva, who is a West Point grad, that I did not go to the dark side when I got pinned my lieutenant bars. I now yield myself 5 minutes for questions.

You know, this is a very sobering hearing in many ways. Let me just say that as a veteran and as an ophthalmologist and I did both care, active duty military. I did Veterans Administration care. I was an assistant professor in academic medicine and as well as private practice, and I was an ophthalmologist. Let me just say that when I would get calls from a patient for a red eye, I would see that patient that same day. That is a red eye. Nowhere near the gravity of what we are talking about now. That was my personal standard. It was not a standard imposed upon me by an insurance company, by the institution for which I worked, nor by Members of Congress.

Mr. Elkins and Mr. Sauer, in both of your testimonies, you mentioned being made aware of a VA policy stating that the VA has 30 days to place a veteran with substance use into an inpatient mental health residential rehabilitation program when working cases for veterans in crisis. Can you explain further your experiences with the VA when policy is not adequately or inaccurately conveyed?

Mr. ELKINS. Thank you for that question. Thirty days is too long to ask a veteran to wait on the availability of an RRTP facility or care in the community. In a 30-day period, the risk of suicide or destabilization can drastically increase. We recommend a clinically sound, lesser number of days because PTSD in conjunction with SUD require swift intervention and services. Additionally, in some cases, veterans lack trust with the VA based on past experiences and the mere fact that you have to go through an RRTP facility first and fail and then afterwards go to the community care, needs to be addressed.

Ms. MILLER-MEEKS. Thank you. Mr. Sauer, I will just kind of dovetail on that and then go to you. Both of you in your work with veterans, have you heard anything about a recent direction from the VAMC that if they can not meet the 30-day appointment availability, they have to confer with other VISNs. They have to try to get them into care at another location. Or that five VAMCs must be contacted to fulfill the directive. Have you all heard that?

Mr. SAUER. Yes, we have. A matter of fact, Mr. Dowling, to my left is the one who directly dealt with that when after speaking with a VAMC therapist who was one who also managed many community care referrals or made the consults that would later become referrals. Brendan can definitely speak about it in more detail if you have questions. It was that if a VISN's VAMC—it went to effect on I think October 1 is what they were told. We were told this in verbally. This was not in a writing or policy, that if a VISN's VAMC cannot meet the 30-day appointment availability window, it must confer with the other VISNs for bed availability before leveraging community care in order to keep the care "in house." He further reported that five VAMCs must be contacted in order to fulfill the directive. He advised this new policy would highly impact referrals throughout the community. Is there something else you wanted to add, if I may? Is it is all right, to Mr. Dowling? It is Okay if not. Understood.

Ms. MILLER-MEEKS. Have you experienced the same thing?

Mr. ELKINS. Yes, we have experienced the same thing in multiple cases over the last several months. As of January, we have seen a significant increase in the amount of cases we are seeing where there are unnecessary delays.

Ms. MILLER-MEEKS. Thank you. It is surprising then that our bureaucracy has not heard the similar thing.

Mr. Sauer, we often hear that the VA care is the best care because those who work at the VA understand the veteran. I am going to refer to a community organization I have in one of my largest cities in my district in Davenport, where an entirely volunteer veteran organization assisted a veteran who had not seen their family or come for any kind of care for 20 years, had not seen their family. The veteran showed up there to this total voluntary organization, no one taking a salary, and contacted his family for the first time in 20 years. How does your experience and the experience of your staff, such as those with Mr. Dowling's background, equip you to serve our Nation's veterans?

Mr. SAUER. It is a big question, ma'am. I would say that we are incredibly honored for this opportunity to do this. I will say that there is nothing that is more rewarding. I know that when Brendan joined the team last year, he saw the mission we were doing. I mean, he can speak for himself on that one. Most certainly we go pretty far out of our way for a number of cases. We have taken, for what it is worth, as well, when we have cases where a veteran has for any number of reasons, but usually due to the reasons that we are here for which we are here today, they are unable to get care, we take them on scholarship.

Now, I still have 100 employees — nearly 100 employees. I have to make payroll to keep the lights on. I can not do that continually, but I am happy to do that, you know, in certain situations. We have done that about seven or eight times that I can think of in the past year or two. We just do it because it is the right thing to do, that is it.

Ms. MILLER-MEEKS. Thank you. I yield. Ranking Member Brownley, would you like to make any closing remarks since I see no other members here?

Ms. BROWNLEY. Yes. Thank you, Madam Chair. Really, thank you very much for having this hearing. It is very much an important hearing of which I still feel like we need to do even a deeper dive on it to really get down to the bottom of things. I really thank this panel for your testimony. This is one of these hearings where I wish we had panel two first and the VA second, because there is so much that you have raised that now I would like to ask the VA. I think there is clearly a disconnect between the VA's testimony and your testimony, and we need to get to the bottom of that. I have a feeling that some of the problem has to do with how VA really addresses access and how they account for access and missing some data points, perhaps.

I do want to acknowledge that what I am hearing from panel two as well is that the quality of care within the VA once the veteran gets into the VA is very good. I want to, you know, applaud the VA for the quality care. The access piece and when we are talking about suicide and other kinds of things, that getting, you know, when someone is in crisis and they come to the VA or come to any of you, if there is not a bed, they still need to be in a room. They do not get to leave the hospital at that particular point. They are in the care of the VA. Never should a veteran walk out of that VA in crisis. I think clearly something has to be done here around these access points.

Mr. Sauer, too, I want to congratulate you, too, on, you know, the quality of community care that you are providing in your area. We thank you for that. Again, my condolences to you with regards to your father. With that, I will yield back.

Ms. MILLER-MEEKS. Thank you, Ranking Member Brownley. I would like to thank everyone for their participation in today's hearing and for their productive conversation. I would like to especially thank our most recent panel for submitting their witness testimony in a timely fashion so Members of Congress could read it.

As a veteran, as a doctor, as a former director of the Department of Public Health, and someone who is very active in mental health and substance use disorder, it is one of my top priorities. I know the same goes for my colleagues on both sides of the aisle to take care of all veterans and to ensure that they have timely care, especially for those who are struggling with complex mental health issues and substance use disorder. No one here on this panel—witness up on the dais today has impugned the quality of care delivered at the VA. The most important metric, not hundreds of metrics, the most important metric of success is whether the suicide rate has gone down, and unfortunately, it has gone up. No veteran should be turned away when a decision is made to seek help. I look forward to working on these issues. I look forward to working with my colleagues on the other side of the aisle and many more with the department, stakeholders, and my colleagues on this subcommittee.

The complete written statements of today's witnesses will be entered into the hearing record. Questions will be submitted, and we will ask that they be responded to in a timely fashion. I ask unanimous consent that all members have 5 legislative days to revise and extend their remarks and include extraneous material. Hearing no objection, so ordered. This meeting is now adjourned.

[Whereupon, at 12:03 p.m., the subcommittee was adjourned.]

Appendix: Prepared Statement of Witnesses

Prepared Statement of Tamara Campbell

Good morning, Chairman Miller-Meeks, Ranking Member Brownley and distinguished Members of the Subcommittee. Thank you for the opportunity today to discuss VA's substance use disorder treatment programs through Mental Health Residential Rehabilitation Treatment Programs (MH RRTP) and through community care referrals. Accompanying me today is Dr. Sachin Yende, Chief Medical Officer, Office of Integrated Veteran Care (IVC).

Veterans are increasingly struggling with substance use disorders (SUD). From fiscal year (FY) 2018 to FY 2022, the number of Veterans diagnosed with a SUD and receiving treatment in the Veterans Health Administration (VHA) increased from 522,544 to 550,412. This increase also reflects an increase in Veterans with a diagnosis of alcohol use disorder receiving care in VHA which increased from 393,531 to 411,615 over the same time period. Of the over 550,000 Veterans receiving care from VHA in FY 2022, or 8.5 percent of all patients who received care from VHA, received treatment for a substance use disorder. While the annual number of Veterans receiving treatment from VHA for opioid use disorder has stabilized at about 67,000 patients per year, a rising number of VA patients are receiving treatment for cannabis use disorder and amphetamine stimulant use disorder, which includes methamphetamine use disorder. The number of patients treated in VHA for amphetamine stimulant use disorder has climbed by almost 8 percent over the previous 5 years to more than 40,000 patients annually, while the number of patients treated in VHA for cannabis use disorder has increased by more than 12 percent to more than 139,000 patients annually. The number of Veterans who have been diagnosed with an alcohol use disorder over the same time period has increased by nearly 5 percent. Together with each of you, VA is totally committed to providing a wide range of interventions that are supported by evidence to cater to the requirements of every Veteran.

Care for Veterans who have co-occurring SUD and mental health issues is a crucial component of general health care. Because it has an integrated health care system, VA is in a unique position to meet the requirements of Veterans with SUD by offering assistance for co-occurring medical, mental health, and psychosocial issues, including by providing supports for employment and housing. Due to the complexity of SUD, neither a single remedy nor solely clinical or VA interventions will suffice to solve address the issue. To reduce the burden of SUD in the veteran population, it is important to use broad-based national preventative and treatment strategies. To achieve its goals, VA uses both whole-of-Government and whole-of-Nation approaches. These are exemplified by VA's interagency collaborations. As an illustration, the Department of Defense (DoD) and VA collaborated to produce clinical practice guidelines for the management of substance use disorders. To meet the needs of Veterans with or at risk of substance use disorder, VA also collaborates closely with several other Departments and agencies, including the Departments of Health and Human Services, Energy, Justice, and Housing and Urban Development. Also, VA is incorporating Oak Ridge National Laboratory data into predictive models for targeted prevention programs so we can better identify Veterans with the greatest challenges to recovery and get them the additional support they need. Through collaborations with the Lawrence Berkeley, Los Alamos, and Sandia National Labs, VA is making better use of medical record information to identify high- risk VA patient populations. Through work with JJR Solutions in Dayton, Ohio, a service-disabled Veteran-owned small business, VA has found that provider education sessions on opioid safety practices lead to more effective treatment for Veterans in primary care and reduction in overdoses.

Overview of SUD Treatment at VA

There has been an upsurge in morbidity and mortality from substance use disorders during the past 10 years or more as powerful and hazardous illicit drugs have become more widespread in the United States. Federal, State and community prevention and treatment efforts have been developed in response, particularly aimed at reducing overdose deaths and addressing the opioid epidemic.

Within VA, patients with at-risk alcohol use or the SUDs of mild severity may be treated with evidence-based brief interventions and/or medical management in primary care or general mental health. For those with more severe disorders impairment, specialty SUD treatment programs provide intensive services including withdrawal management, evidence-based psychosocial treatments, SUD medication, case management and relapse prevention provided in outpatient, intensive outpatient and residential settings of care. VA has developed services specifically focused on engagement in care for vulnerable Veteran populations. VA efforts include universal screening for at-risk alcohol use, urine drug screening for at-risk Veterans, the provision of peer support services, integration of SUD treatment within homeless programs, and collaboration with Veterans' courts and the work of our re-entry specialists to engage Veterans with SUD involved with the legal system.

These efforts also have required close collaboration with other Federal partners in support of priorities defined by the Office of National Drug Control Policy (ONDCP). In alignment with ONDCP's National Drug Control Strategy, VA is working to expand access to evidence-based treatment for SUDs and enhancing evidence- based harm reduction efforts aimed at reducing overdose fatalities. VA offers a comprehensive continuum of specialty SUD services for Veterans. Our VA/DoD Clinical Practice Guidelines,[1] updated in fiscal year (FY) 2021, provide the foundation for evidence-based treatment within VA and have positioned VA to respond to emerging drug use trends. Current policy requires facilities provide access to a comprehensive continuum of SUD treatment services ranging from early intervention and harm reduction services through intensive outpatient and, when needed, residential or inpatient treatment for SUD. In addition, current policy requires facilities provide same day outpatient access for Veterans with emergent substance use treatment needs. This care may be provided in several settings including general mental health, primary care mental health integration clinics, and SUD specialty clinics. Core characteristics of SUD services include timely same day triage, a no wrong door approach, concurrent treatment for co-occurring needs and Veteran-centered and individualized treatment based on the needs and preferences of the Veteran.

With national initiatives like Stepped Care for Opioid Use Disorder, Train the Trainer, and the Psychotropic Drug Safety Initiative, VA emphasizes access to evidence-based treatments for SUDs. These initiatives also aim to increase access to both evidence-based pharmacotherapies and evidence-based psychotherapies for substance use disorders. According to the National Survey on Drug Use and Health conducted by the Substance Abuse and Mental Health Services Administration, only 22 percent of the general population with opioid use disorder received medication for opioid use disorder in 2021. In calendar year 2022, VA more than doubles that rate, with over 47 percent of patients with opioid use disorder receiving medications for opioid use disorder from VA within the last 12 months. Appropriate use of FDA- approved medications for opioid use disorder can lower the risk of illicit opioid use, overdose, suicide, and other mortalities.

In 2022, VA provided psychosocial or behavioral therapy for SUD to almost 172,000 Veterans. VA is using national training initiatives to ensure that these treatments are as effective as possible, expanding access to highly evidence-based cognitive behavioral therapies and contingency management programs. Notably, contingency management is the most effective, evidence-based treatment for stimulant use disorder and has shown success in treating cannabis use disorder, two substance use disorders that are increasingly common in the VHA patient population. More than 6,200 Veterans have received contingency management treatment since 2011. Over 90 percent of the nearly 80,000 urine samples that those Veterans submitted tested negative for the target drugs, which are frequently stimulants and occasionally cannabis (THC). For Veterans with alcohol use disorder, VA offers both evidence-based medications as well as evidence-based psychotherapies separately or in combination depending on the shared decision-making between each Veteran and his/her treatment provider.

VA recognizes that not all Veterans with SUD will embrace abstinence among their recovery goals. Furthermore, SUD, like hypertension or diabetes, is a chronic, relapsing condition; even Veterans who are striving to abstain from substances may not always be consistently successful. Because any exposure to substances can be fatal for individuals with SUD, VA provides Veterans with evidence-based interventions to protect them from harms,

[1] https://www.healthquality.va.gov/guidelines/MH/sud/.

like overdose or infectious diseases like HIV and hepatitis, that could otherwise lead to their death. In just the past year, VHA equipped over 70,000 Veterans with naloxone to reverse potentially fatal opioid overdoses. Furthermore, nearly 1 million naloxone prescriptions have been provided to Veterans since 2014, when we launched our Overdose Education and Naloxone Distribution (OEND) initiative. This initiative has led to more than 3,700 overdose reversals. As part of this effort, VA uses data-driven modeling to identify Veterans at high risk of overdose and conducts clinical case reviews to inform their customized treatment plans. Support from Congress has been critical for the success of VA's overdose prevention efforts with passage of the Jason Simcakoski Memorial and Promise Act allowing VA to provide naloxone at no cost to Veterans at risk for overdose.

In support of its comprehensive approach to the treatment of SUD, VA has developed a wide array of substance use education programs in its efforts to expand SUD education and outreach. The programs are being implemented across the Department and can be classified as follows:

- Initiatives to educate primary care practitioners on the diagnosis and treatment of alcohol use disorders.
- Harm reduction approaches to reduce negative consequences of substance use including planned/developed mobile and internet-based treatment to expand VA's efforts related to SUD treatment, education, and outreach.
- Programs developed for Veterans and Veterans' families.
- Clinician training and consultation programs to improve their knowledge, skills, and abilities to treat Veterans with SUD.
- SUD training programs for trainees participating in clinical training with VA.

In addition, VA is supporting SUD training for our future workforce and is imple- menting novel harm reduction approaches including the development of mobile and internet-based applications. Beginning with the President's Budget for fiscal year 2022, VA has requested support to directly respond to national priorities defined by ONDCP. The plan directly addressed the unique needs of Veterans with substance use concerns within the context of broader national priorities.

VA honors Veterans' autonomy in determining their recovery goals, and our providers support them with evidence-based treatments and subject matter expertise. Consequently, VA is making a positive difference in Veterans' quality of life by building confidence in their treatment and helping motivate them in their recovery. Indeed, Veterans receiving treatment for their SUD in VA are experiencing benefits in terms of their mental and physical health and across many other aspects of their lives such as housing stability, employment, and improved interpersonal relationships (See DeMarce et al. for an example of such impact).[2] These are the goals VA is pursuing. We want to help Veterans do more than just survive – we want to help them learn how to thrive.

---

[2] Josephine M. DeMarce, Maryann Gnys, Susan D. Raffa, Mandy Kumpula & Bradley E. Karlin (2021) Dissemination of cognitive behavioral therapy for substance use disorders in the Department of Veterans Affairs Health Care System: Description and evaluation of Veteran outcomes, Substance Abuse, 42:2, 168–174, DOI: 10.1080/08897077.2019.1674238.

FY 2024 President's Budget Expands Access to Treatment for Substance Use Disorders (SUD)

President Biden's FY 2024 Budget proposes continued support for initiatives started during FY 2022, with over 1,100 additional staff awarded enterprise-wide to help meet VA's SUD treatment priorities to include the following:

- Stepped Care to expand access to evidence-based treatment for SUD in settings outside specialty SUD Care;
- SUD Residential Treatment to reduce wait times and improve the quality of SUD care with expansion of staff and programs;
- SUD Telehealth to expand access to evidence-based SUD treatment via tele-health;
- Homeless Program SUD Treatment Coordinators to engage Veterans with SUD into VA SUD outpatient and residential services;
- Supported Employment Specialists to expand access to employment opportunities for Veterans in recovery; and
- SUD Peer Specialists to increase engagement and retention in evidence-based SUD treatment.

As of March 7, 2023, over 55 percent of the more than 1,100 positions have been filled or are in the final steps of the hiring process. VA continues to respond to emerging illicit drug threats to ensure the needs of Veterans experiencing substance use concerns are met. VA will establish program management leads for harm reduction and will work collaboratively to develop policy and national tools to support implementation of targeted harm reduction strategies throughout VHA addressing critical issues such as stigma and the need for technical assistance for the field to support implementation.

Mental Health Residential Rehabilitation Treatment Programs (MH RRTP)

VA's MH RRTPs are a critical component of VA's broader efforts to address the needs of Veterans with substance use concerns. With origins that date back to the National Homes for Disabled Volunteer Soldiers, the Domiciliary Care programs have evolved over time to meet the changing needs of Veterans. Today, residential treatment for mental health and substance use concerns in VA is provided through Mental Health Residential Rehabilitation Treatment Programs (MH RRTP) located throughout the country. The MH RRTP continuum includes Domiciliary Care (SUD, Posttraumatic Stress Disorder (PTSD), General and Domiciliary Care for Homeless Veterans – DCHV) as well as Compensated Work Therapy-Transitional Residence programs, which provide transitional housing for Veterans actively engaged in vocational rehabilitation and participating in either transitional work or supported employment. There are currently more than 250 MH RRTPs across 121 locations of care with more than 6,700 operational beds. This includes more than 70 programs for the treatment of SUD and more than 40 programs for the treatment of PTSD with the expectation that all programs provide integrated, concurrent treatment for co-occurring SUD and mental health treatment needs (dual diagnosis services) as more than 90 percent of all Veterans served by the MH RRTPs have a SUD diagnosis.

All Domiciliary Care programs within VHA provide 24/7 professional and peer support with comprehensive services addressing mental health, medical and psycho-social needs provided by an interdisciplinary team; these programs are accredited by The Joint Commission and the Commission on Accreditation of Rehabilitation Facilities. VHA Directive 1162.02 defines expectations for clinical services within the programs with the Domiciliary SUD (DOM SUD) programs expected to adhere to the VA/DoD Clinical Practice Guidelines for the Management of SUD. Given the nature of the care provided in the residential programs, VA's MH RRTPs often are at the forefront in implementation of critical services for Veterans. For example, efforts to support implementation of OEND within VA have their origins with work that was started by the MH RRTPs in 2012, as part of the first Culture of Safety Stand Down, which was established in response to concerns about opioid overdose. At that time, only 11 percent of Veterans served by the MH RRTP received medications for opioid use disorder. During FY 2022, more than 40 percent of Veterans received medications to treat opioid use disorder during their stay. Further, during FY 2023 to date, more than 70 percent of Veterans with an opioid use disorder have received a prescription for naloxone[3] during their MH RRTP stay. Several studies have demonstrated the impact of VA residential treatment.[4] Studies completed within the SUD residential programs have shown sustained reductions in substance use and changes in other factors related to recovery (e.g., Blonigan & Macia, 2021;[5] Boden & Moss, 2009;[6] Lash et al., 2007,[7] 2013[8]).

---

[3] We note that U.S. Food and Drug Administration (FDA) recently approved the first non-prescription naloxone product. See FDA Approves First Over-the-Counter Naloxone Nasal Spray, U.S. FOOD &DRUG ADMIN. (Mar. 29, 2023), https://www.fda.gov/news-events/press-announcements/fda-approves-first-over-counter-naloxone-nasal-spray#:?:text=Today percent2C percent20thepercent20U.S.percent20Foodpercent20and,for percent20use percent20withoutpercent20a percent20prescription.

[4] Smith, N. B., Sippel, L. M., Rozek, D. C., Spangler, P. T., Traber, D., Straud, C. L., Hoff, R., & Harpaz-Rotem, I. (2020). Courses of suicidal ideation among military veterans in residen- tial treatment for posttraumatic stress disorder. Depression and anxiety, 37(3), 273–284. https:// doi.org/10.1002/da.22993 Holliday, R., Smith, N. B., Holder, N., Gross, G. M., Monteith, L. L., Maguen, S., Hoff, R. A., & Harpaz-Rotem, I. (2020). Comparing the effectiveness of VA residential PTSD treatment for veterans who do and do not report a history of MST: A national investigation. Journal of psychiatric research, 122, 42–47. https://doi.org/10.1016/j.jpsychires.2019.12.012 Cook, J. M., Schnurr, P. P., Simiola, V., Thompson, R., Hoff, R., & Harpaz-Rotem, I. (2019). Adoption by VA Residential Programs of Two Evidence-Based Psychotherapies for PTSD: Effect on Patient Outcomes. Psychiatric services (Washington, DC.), 70(7), 553–560. https://doi.org/10.1176/appi.ps.201800338.

[5] Blonigen, D. M., & Macia, K. S. (2021). Personality change during substance use disorder treatment is associated with improvements in abstinence self-efficacy post-treatment among U.S. military veterans. Journal of Substance Abuse Treatment, 120, 108187. https://doi.org/ 10.1016/j.jsat.2020.108187.

[6] Boden, M. T., & Moos, R. (2009). Dually diagnosed patients' responses to substance use disorder treatment. Journal of Substance Abuse Treatment, 37(4), 335–345. https://doi.org/10.1016/j.jsat.2009.03.012.

[7] Lash, S. J., Stephens, R. S., Burden, J. L., Grambow, S. C., DeMarce, J. M., Jones, M. E., Lozano, B. E., Jeffreys, A. S., Fearer, S. A., & Horner, R. D. (2007). Contracting, prompting, and reinforcing substance use disorder continuing care: A randomized clinical trial. Psychology of Addictive Behaviors, 21(3), 387 397. https://doi.org/10.1037/0893–164X.21.3.387.

[8] Lash, S. J., Burden, J. L., Parker, J. D., Stephens, R. S., Budney, A. J., Horner, R. D., Datta, S., Jeffreys, A. S., & Grambow, S. C. (2013). Contracting, prompting and reinforcing substance use disorder continuing care. Journal of Substance Abuse Treatment, 44(4), 449–456. https:// doi.org/10.1016/j.jsat.2012.09.008.

Access to Mental Health Residential Treatment within VHA

VHA affirms the critical importance of timely access to residential treatment for mental health and substance use concerns and has taken steps to remove barriers to care. Veterans may self-refer or may be referred by their provider (internal or external to VHA) to mental health residential treatment. In accordance with nationally defined admission criteria, Veterans must be screened for appropriateness for admission with a decision provided within 7 business days. VHA's goal is to admit Veterans as quickly as possible, and the admission date should take into consideration the Veteran's preference. Timely access to residential treatment has been a priority area of focus for VHA with several efforts underway to ensure Veterans have access to residential treatment when clinically indicated. One such effort included development of a process to facilitate access to residential care in the community. Prior to the time of enactment of the VA MISSION Act of 2018 (June 6, 2018), residential treatment in the community was not readily accessible, with a limited number of care providers and no direct pathway to authorize and pay for such treatment. When care did occur, it was provided either through inpatient programs for the treatment of substance use disorder or through contracts with community care providers. Recognizing a need to ensure access to this critical level of care, VA worked to verify authority to provide residential treatment in the community and to provide a mechanism to pay for such care. The Mental Health Residential standardized episode of care (SEOC) and the technical mechanism to place a consult for this care were released to VA medical centers in October 2020.

VHA's formal guidance to facilities defined how and when referrals for residential care in the community should occur. This guidance was informed by VHA Directive 1162.02, which defines requirements for ensuring timely access to residential treatment. While the MH RRTPs are considered institutional extended care and not subject to the designated access standards established by VA at 38 CFR § 17.4040, which can establish eligibility to elect to receive care in the community, access standards for MH RRTPs still do exist. VHA policy requires that when a Veteran is assessed as requiring residential treatment and the program is unable to meet the Veteran's needs (72 hours for Veterans requiring priority admission and 30 days for Veterans assessed as appropriate for routine admission) an alternate treatment program must be offered. Alternate treatment may include another MH RRTP in the Veterans Integrated Service Network (VISN), a comparable program appropriate to meet the Veteran's needs (e.g., a homeless grant and per diem program) or referral for care in the community. The policy in question does not reflect a new policy requirement but rather was the first step to provide a clear expectation for provision of residential treatment within the community and a mechanism to facilitate access. Through the second quarter (Q2) of FY 2022, the average time between screening and admission for all Veterans admitted for residential treatment was 23 days, with half of Veterans admitted within 12 days of being screened for admission. For the DOM SUD programs the average time was 24 days, but with half of Veterans admitted within 9 days of being screened for admission. It is important to note that a small subset of Veterans request or require a later admission date (18 percent for DOM SUD programs during FY 2022). VHA is committed to ensuring timely access to care with a focus on moving toward same day/next day admission consistent with priorities defined by the National Drug Control Strategy. Through Q2 of FY 2023, 40 percent of Veterans were admitted either directly from an inpatient mental health stay or within 1 day of screening.

Further, since the publication of the MH Residential SEOC, the number of Veterans receiving residential care in the community has increased rapidly. During FY 2021, there were more than 7,000 referrals for mental health residential care in the community using the new SEOC, with that number increasing to roughly 11,000 unique referrals during FY 2022 and exceeding 6,800 to date during FY 2023. Expenditures for residential care in the community since 2021 have exceeded $1.2 billion. By comparison, during FY 2022, VA's Domiciliary Care programs overall served more than 20,000 unique Veterans with the DOM SUD program serving more than 9,800 Veterans.

Community care residential treatment programs are critical resources when a facility is unable to furnish residential treatment for a Veteran within the VISN. Facilities are actively working with community providers to ensure that when a Veteran is referred to a residential treatment program, the program meets quality standards and that there are clear processes for referral and for engagement in post-discharge continuing care with VHA. Collaboration with community providers also has allowed VISNs to communicate about specific treatment needs where residential treatment options may be limited in VHA.

Beyond ensuring that mechanisms exist to ensure Veterans have access to community residential treatment when applicable, VA is committed to addressing internal access challenges. The MH RRTPs were significantly impacted by the pandemic with many programs reducing capacity to ensure both Veteran and staff safety. VA began communicating on the importance of ensuring access to MH RRTP services as early as July 2020, with a focused effort to resume MH RRTP services and increase capacity initiated in February 2021. Since that time, VA's Office of Mental Health and Suicide Prevention (OMHSP) has been working collaboratively with the VISNs to increase capacity and reduce wait times with the average number of days between screening and admission approaching pre-pandemic levels. However, VHA recognizes the need to establish accelerated targets informed by Veteran feedback. Beginning in August 2022 and concluding in December 2022, VHA conducted regional meetings specifically focused on access to residential care emphasizing a goal of providing same day or next day admission when clinically indicated. Since the start of those conversations in August 2022, the average daily census has grown from around 3,300 Veterans to just over 3,800 Veterans in March 2023.

In addition to efforts to return MH RRTP capacity to pre-pandemic levels of operation, several new DOM SUD programs have recently been established or are under development and expected to open within the next few years. During FY 2022 and FY 2023 year to date, 55 DOM SUD beds have been established at 3 new locations of care with 14 additional beds at 2 additional programs projected to open during FY 2023.

Compliance with Community Care Referrals for Substance Abuse Residential Treatment

VA is grateful for the independent investigation of the Office of Inspector General (OIG) in the review of the DOM SUD treatment program and residential community care referrals.[9] As

[9] Department of Veterans Affairs Office of Inspector General. "Noncompliance with Commu- nity Care Referrals for Substance Abuse Residential Treatment at the VA North Texas Health Care System". Report No. 21–03864–34. January 31, 2023.

noted in VHA's response in the OIG report, the ability to refer for mental health residential treatment in the community is a relatively new process with the first SEOC for mental health residential treatment released in October 2020 and updated in August 2021. OMHSP worked collaboratively with VISNs during this time to clarify requirements and expectations for when referrals for mental health residential care in the community may occur. These efforts have continued with targeted efforts to ensure familiarity with access requirements and processes for ensuring access to residential treatment in the community when indicated.

Specifically, in response to recommendations in the report, VA has taken several steps to ensure a clear understanding by all programs of access requirements and when referrals for mental health residential treatment in the community should be completed. Further, in response to the OIG report, VA has ensured clarification on the existing guidance regarding the role of the mental health treatment coordinator and expectations for engagement with the coordinator as part of the referral and admission process for Veterans requiring mental health residential treatment. Further, VA has several efforts currently underway to address access for MH RRTP services, with a workgroup convening to determine potential changes in national policy responsive to access challenges that have been communicated by stakeholders with the expectation that a formal plan and path forward would be finalized within 45 days of the workgroup convening. In addition, OMHSP is working to put in place a process that leverages existing monitoring efforts to inform procedures for notifying VISN leadership when there are concerns with conformance to national policy.

Implementation of Veterans COMPACT Act, Section 201

The Veterans COMPACT Act created a new authority in 38 U.S.C. § 1720J for VA to provide emergent suicide care to eligible individuals in acute suicidal crisis at no cost both in VA and in the community. This authority increases access to care, including residential care, and is in full alignment with VA's National Strategy for Preventing Veteran Suicide.[10] Building upon VA's comprehensive public health approach, this new emergency suicide care and treatment health care benefit enhances our ability to provide critical treatment for eligible individuals experiencing a suicidal crisis. Eligible individuals in suicidal crisis can go to any VA or community health care facility for emergent suicide care. VA is responsible for providing, paying for, or reimbursing for this care, depending on the setting it is provided in, and therefore, this care is provided to eligible individuals at no cost. Eligible individuals receiving emergent suicide care will also have the costs of ambulance transportation and related prescriptions covered. Emergent suicide care can be provided in multiple settings, including inpatient or crisis residential care for up to 30 days and crisis-related outpatient care for up to 90 days. The access standards for mental health residential treatment outside of an acute suicide crisis (72 hours for priority admission and 30 days for routine admission) would not apply. This health care benefit has the potential to increase access to acute suicide care to an additional 9 million unenrolled Veterans and reduce the number of Veteran suicides by offering immediate care when Veterans are most vulnerable.

---

[10] U.S. Department of Veterans Affairs. (2018). National Strategy for Preventing Veteran Suicide. http://www.mentalhealth.va.gov/suicideprevention/docs/Office-of-Mental-Health-and-Sui-cide-Prevention-National-Strategy-for-Preventing-Veterans-Suicide.pdf.

On January 17, 2023, VA published an interim final rule outlining eligibility for emergent suicide care and immediately began providing this new benefit to eligible individuals. As part of implementation, VA developed a robust communications plan targeted toward eligible individuals, Veterans, and community providers. VA continues to aggressively address critical cross-platform information technology enhancements to ensure that multiple administrative and clinical systems work seamlessly together to ensure timely and efficient care at no cost. The Veterans Crisis Line serves a critical role in the coordination of life-saving resources, such as emergency dispatch for Veteran crisis care. VHA provided external resources for Veterans and providers, as well as internal resources and training for VA staff on section 201 of the COMPACT Act. We are committed to ongoing education and training efforts within VA and in the community as we deploy this new, life-affirming benefit in our ongoing suicide prevention efforts.

Conclusion

We appreciate the Committee's continued support in this shared mission. Nothing is more important to VA than supporting the health and well-being of the Nation's Veterans and their families. VA has employed broad, evidence-based strategies to address the opioid epidemic, including patient and provider education, pain management and access to non-pharmacological modalities, risk mitigation strategies, and addiction treatment for Veterans with SUD. This critical work saves lives.

My colleagues and I are prepared to respond to any questions you may have.

Prepared Statement of Julie Kroviak

Chairwoman Miller-Meeks, Ranking Member Brownley, and Subcommittee Members, thank you for the opportunity to discuss the Office of Inspector General's (OIG) oversight of the Veterans Health Administration's (VHA) domiciliary substance use disorder treatment program. The OIG's Office of Healthcare Inspections reviews the quality and safety of health care provided across VHA and communicates the findings through a variety of public reports. These include results from hotline inspections, national reviews, comprehensive healthcare inspections, vet center inspections, and Veterans Integrated Service Network (VISN) reviews. For each of these reports, OIG clinical review teams provide recommendations for improving processes or further reducing risks to the veterans who entrust their health care to VHA.

VHA faces significant challenges in meeting the needs of individuals with substance use disorders. The devastating effects on veterans, their families and caregivers, and communities cannot be overstated. Veterans with substance use disorders often have co-occurring mental health issues that can place them at higher risk for suicide. Given that VHA's top clinical priority is to reduce veteran suicide, evidence-based substance use disorder treatment programs are imperative to addressing the clinical needs of these high-risk patients. When both VHA and community care providers are engaged in managing these patients, the coordination must be seamless and collaborative.

This testimony focuses on OIG reports that have identified challenges with community care access and coordination for high-risk patients. The OIG believes the findings and recommendations should be considered by all VHA providers and leaders managing patients with complex mental health needs including substance use disorders.

Noncompliance with Community Care Referrals for Substance Abuse Residential Treatment at the VA North Texas Health Care System

In August 2021, the OIG hotline received allegations that staff for the domiciliary substance use disorder treatment program (DOM SUD) at the VA North Texas Health Care System (VA North Texas) placed patients on waitlists for two to three months and failed to offer non-VA community residential care referrals for substance use disorder treatment.[11] The complainant also alleged that VA North Texas staff denied patients' requests for community residential care referrals, whereas patients from another VISN 17 facility, the Central Texas Veterans Health Care System (Central Texas VA), received community residential care treatment. During the course of the OIG staff's review of the allegations (including examining 15 VA North Texas DOM SUD consults (referrals) and electronic health records for 10 patients), the team identified additional concerns related to compliance with required scheduling procedures and the assignment of mental health treatment coordinators to patients awaiting admission. To understand the context for the resulting report's findings, it is important to consider VHA's program goals and requirements.

Background

Mental health residential rehabilitation treatment programs (MH RRTPs) provide 24-hour treatment and rehabilitative services to patients with a range of treatment needs and include domiciliary substance use disorder programs. MH RRTP is an umbrella term for the range of residential programs that provide treatment to patients experiencing homelessness, substance use disorders, posttraumatic stress disorder, as well as other medical and mental health conditions. To be eligible for an MH RRTP referral, veterans must need a higher level of care than an outpatient program but not be at imminent risk to themselves and others, and not meet criteria for a medical or acute mental health admission. VHA requires that each facility provide access to care at MH RRTPs through service agreements with other VA facilities or through referral to non-VA community residential care facilities.

VA North Texas, part of VISN 17, includes a 40-bed DOM SUD at the Dallas VA Medical Center and a 69-bed DOM SUD at the Sam Rayburn Memorial Veterans Center in Bonham, Texas. The Central Texas VA is in Temple, Texas, and has a 169-bed general domiciliary that offers substance use disorder treatment as a "track."

According to VHA's requirements, patients referred to MH RRTPs must be screened within seven business days by a team that includes a licensed mental health professional and a medical provider to determine whether admission is appropriate. If accepted, the patient must

[11] VA OIG, Noncompliance with Community Care Referrals for Substance Abuse Residential Treatment at the VA North Texas Health Care System, January 31, 2023.

receive a tentative admission date and a point of contact at the MH RRTP.[12] So VHA can track admission wait times, the patient must be added to the pending bed placement list.[13] Since 2018, VHA has required staff to include information in the patient's electronic health record to improve tracking of program wait times and capacity.[14]

Community Care Program Eligibility Criteria

The John S. McCain III, Daniel K. Akaka, and Samuel R. Johnson VA Maintaining Internal Systems and Strengthening Integrated Outside Networks Act of 2018 (MISSION Act) mandated changes to VHA's community care program.[15] Those changes led to VHA's Office of Community Care issuing implementation guidance stating that "wait time and drive time access standards are only applicable to primary care, specialty care, and non-institutional extended care services." The guidance further said MH RRTPs "are considered institutional extended care services" and do not follow the same wait-time standards.[16] When MH RRTP care is not available within VA facilities for an eligible patient who "elects to receive care in the community," VHA will authorize community residential care. Further, for MH RRTP admission wait times greater than 30 calendar days, facility staff must offer the patient alternative care that addresses the patient's needs and preferences including a referral to community residential care or another VHA program. Additionally, facility staff should discuss outpatient care options with the patient while the patient awaits MH RRTP admission. It is important to note that the COVID–19 pandemic put additional stresses on VHA and that the Texas facilities were not alone in facing long wait times. In February 2021, VHA estimated that 3,500 patients nationally were pending admission with an average wait time of more than 150 days. At that time, VHA required MH RRTP staff to provide alternatives, including community residential care, if unable to admit patients within 30 days.[17]

VA North Texas DOM SUD Wait Times Exceeded Requirements and Staff Failed to Refer Patients to Community Residential Care as Required

The OIG team reviewed 15 VA North Texas DOM SUD consults to determine admission wait times and evaluate whether staff offered community residential care. The team substantiated

---

[12] VHA Directive 1162.02, Mental Health Residential Rehabilitation Treatment Program, July 15, 2019. Tentative admission date refers to the MH RRTP staff's expected date of bed availability.

[13] VHA Directive 1002, Bed Management Solution for Tracking Beds and Patient Movement Within and Across VHA Facilities, November 28, 2017.

[14] VHA Deputy Under Secretary for Health for Operations and Management (10N) memo, ''Mental Health Residential Rehabilitation Treatment Programs (MH RRTP) CPRS Note Tem- plates Implementation,'' July 30, 2018.

[15] MISSION Act, Pub. L. No. 115–182, 132 Stat. 1393 (2018).

[16] VHA Office of Community Care, ''Field Guidebook: Specialty Programs,'' updated November 3, 2021. The Office of Community Care determines a patient eligible for community mental health care when the wait time is greater than 20 days or the drive time is greater than 30 minutes for a VHA outpatient mental health appointment.

[17] VHA Assistant Under Secretary for Health for Clinical Services memorandum, ''Ensuring Access to Residential Treatment for Veterans with Mental Health and Substance Use Disorders during the Pandemic,'' February 11, 2021.

the allegation that VA North Texas staff placed patients on waitlists for two to three months and failed to offer community residential care referrals during most of fiscal years 2020 and 2021, inconsistent with VHA requirements. It is important to note that the OIG did not identify any adverse clinical outcomes due to the patients' delayed access to residential care.

In March 2020, due to the pandemic, facility leaders restricted access to the Dallas DOM SUD to local veterans, in accordance with VHA guidance. The Dallas DOM SUD subsequently reopened to a broader group of patients but still with reduced capacity in September 2020. The Bonham DOM SUD remained open during the pandemic at reduced capacity until January 2022, when admissions were halted until June 2022 due to COVID–19 concerns. VHA data indicated that the Dallas and Bonham DOM SUDs' average wait time was 30 days or greater from the third quarter of fiscal year 2020 through the second quarter of fiscal year 2021, likely due to pandemic-related restrictions.

Of the 10 North Texas patients' records the OIG reviewed, five had one DOM SUD consult placed and the other five had two consults placed during the review period, resulting in a total of 15 consults examined. Of the 15 consults, 13 were referrals to the Bonham DOM SUD and two were referrals to the Dallas DOM SUD. Seven consults were closed when the patient was admitted within 30 days, declined screening, or was not approved for admission. Among the eight remaining consults, two were closed when the patients declined admission and six resulted in patients waiting an average of 79 days before VA North Texas staff offered DOM SUD admission or removed the patient from the pending bed placement list. For seven of the eight consults, staff documented that the "anticipated admission date exceeds 30 days; however, there is no available alternative to consider at this time."

The OIG determined that the VA North Texas chief for Patient Administration Services, who oversees community care, misinterpreted community care guidance and provided inaccurate information to VA North Texas leaders and staff. Specifically, the Office of Community Care's guidance states that community care wait time standards were not applicable to MH RRTP. Facility staff should have instead followed VHA policy requiring a patient with a schedule wait time of greater than 30 days be offered alternative residential treatment or another level of care. Alternative residential treatment could include a referral to a community program, another program in the VISN, or another program in another VISN.[18]

However, the Patient Administration Services chief told the OIG team during the review that MH RRTPs are "excluded from the MISSION Act" and not eligible for community care based on access standards—reflecting an inaccurate understanding of the Act. In contrast, the national director of the MH RRTP reported that although drive time and wait time standards do not apply to DOM SUDs, community care referrals are expected when a patient is determined to require a residential level of care and VHA is unable to provide treatment within the required timeframe.

In September 2020, the MH RRTP national program office released guidance that included instructions for community care referrals. In February 2021, VHA provided guidance that VISN chief mental health officers and facility leaders must ensure that patients who require a residential level of care are offered a VA MH RRTP bed or community residential care. VHA further required that each facility provide the operational status of MH RRTP beds and "information on the availability of community based residential treatment options."[19] VISN

---

[18] VHA Directive 1162.02.

[19] VHA Assistant Under Secretary for Health for Clinical Services memorandum.

17's response to the February 2021 guidance indicated that the Dallas and Bonham DOM SUDs were not making community residential care referrals.

In December 2021, the OIG informed VISN 17 and VA North Texas leaders of staff's failure to comply with community residential care referral expectations and requested corrective action be taken to address staff education and potential patient treatment needs. VA North Texas leaders communicated referral requirements to Office of Community Care and Mental Health Services staff and reviewed all community residential care consults placed from October 1, 2019, through November 30, 2021. Additionally, in response to the OIG's request, VA North Texas staff completed a clinical review to ensure appropriate follow-up for patients referred from October 1, 2019, through December 31, 2021, to the Dallas and Bonham DOM SUDs whose wait times were greater than 30 days.

The OIG made a total of five recommendations in this report.[20] The first recommendation is for the VA North Texas director to ensure that staff provide alternative treatment options, including community care when MH RRTP admission wait times exceed 30 days. The second recommendation calls on the director to conduct a comprehensive review of the management of community residential care referrals. They concurred in principle with this recommendation. The remaining three recommendations are described below.

VA Central Texas Compliance

In contrast to the VA North Texas's failures, the OIG's review of two patients referred to the Temple DOM SUD by VA North Texas staff indicated the VA Central Texas staff placed consults and scheduled patients in accordance with VHA policy. Further, VA Central Texas developed procedures for community residential care referrals when MH RRTP wait times were greater than 30 days.

Inadequate VISN Oversight

The OIG determined that VISN 17 leaders did not ensure VA North Texas leaders' adherence to the national MH RRTP policy. According to the MH RRTP directive, each VISN mental health lead is responsible for ensuring that all VISN MH RRTPs collect data sufficient for oversight related to VHA policy implementation.[21] Additionally, the national director of the MH RRTP confirmed the VISN has oversight responsibility to ensure eligible patients have access to a residential level of care, although there are not defined expectations related to community care utiliztion monitoring. The VISN 17 chief mental health officer provided guidance to VA North Texas leaders on three occasions in 2021 regarding the use of community residential care. However, she reported that the VISN role did not have the authority to ensure policy adherence or "direct oversight" because "oversight is at the local facility management

[20] The OIG considers all five recommendations currently open pending the submission of suffi- cient documentation that would support that adequate progress has been made on implementa- tion to close them. The OIG requests updates on the status of all open recommendations every 90 days, which are then reflected on the recommendations dashboard found on the OIG website. For this report, the OIG will request the first update on or about May 1, 2023.

[21] VHA Directive 1162.02, Mental Health Residential Rehabilitation Treatment Program, July 15, 2019.

level." The third report recommendation is for the under secretary for health to make certain that VISN leaders provide adequate oversight to ensure that access to care for MH RRTPs is provided consistent with VHA policy.

Bonham MH RRTP Nonadherence with VHA Scheduling Requirements

During the inspection, the OIG team also identified that the Bonham MH RRTP standard operating procedure was inconsistent with VHA's minimum scheduling effort requirements, as it instructed schedulers to close a consult after three failed scheduling contact attempts rather than the four required. Since 2016, VHA has required providers to document a request for other services in the referred patient's electronic health record. The second attempt must use a different method of contact and can be completed the same day as the first attempt, while the third and fourth attempts must be on different days. To allow the patient time to respond, staff must wait a minimum of 14 calendar days from the second contact attempt before determining the action on the consult request, such as closing the consult. Additionally, the Bonham MH RRTP staff were attempting to contact patients by phone and not using other modes of contact. Failure to adhere to VHA minimum scheduling requirements may hinder efficient patient scheduling and contribute to the barriers patients experience in accessing DOM SUD services. The fourth recommendation is for the VA North Texas director to ensure that Bonham MH RRTP scheduling procedures are consistent with VHA minimum scheduling effort requirements.

Mental Health Treatment Coordinator Assignment

Finally, the OIG found that VA North Texas policy did not include information about the requirement for MH RRTP staff to assign a mental health treatment coordinator for patients awaiting admission to a residential program. Since 2012, VHA has required facility staff to assign a mental health treatment coordinator to patients who are receiving treatment in an outpatient mental health setting, have been admitted to an inpatient mental health setting, or are "waiting to engage in a different level of care" including an MH RRTP bed. However, in an interview, the national director for the MH RRTP acknowledged not having an assignment process for patients pending MH RRTP admission. This failure to develop a national-level process likely contributed to the VA North Texas MH RRTP leaders' lack of knowledge that the VA North Texas policy should address the identification and assignment of a mental health treatment coordinator for accepted patients awaiting admission. This lack of policy awareness may not only contribute to a coordinator not being assigned but can also diminish the likelihood of patients' engagement in out- patient care while awaiting admission. The fifth report recommendation relates to strengthening coordinator assignment procedures for patients waiting for an MH RRTP bed.

Other OIG Reports Citing Concerns with Community Care Coordination of Veterans with Complex Mental Health Needs

Coordinating medical care between the VHA care system and community providers remains a challenge, particularly for managing patients with complex mental health needs. The OIG has identified persistent administrative and communication errors or failures among VHA, its third-party administrators, and community care providers, as well as between the care providers and their patients. These deficiencies challenge the considerable efforts of VHA personnel to ensure a seamless experience for veterans. Many OIG reports have described the frustrations and, most importantly, the risks associated with patients referred to the community. The following reports exemplify the consequences that poor care coordination contributes to for high-risk patients.

In a report on the deficiencies found in the care and administrative processes for a patient who died by suicide, the review team found that administrative errors and confusion in the Phoenix VA health care facility's community referral process delayed specialized psychological testing for a veteran. The veteran died by suicide never having received the appropriate testing and resulting targeted treatment.[22] Another oversight report focused on a patient who ultimately died by suicide after not receiving several authorized community care counseling sessions. This was due to deficiencies in the coordination of the patient's care between the Memphis VA facility's community care staff, providers in the community, and the third-party administrator.[23] In addition, the patient suffered from hyperthyroidism, a condition that can aggravate anxiety. The patient declined a referral to endocrinology at the facility, due to the distance from home, but was never offered a referral to the community.

Conclusion

High-quality care demands that patients receive the necessary care provided by qualified clinicians in a timely manner. This is even more critical for individuals deemed to be at high risk due to their mental health and substance use conditions.

The pandemic disrupted healthcare delivery in all settings, including addiction treatment, yet at the same time increased the demand for such interventions. VHA will continue to rely on community providers to deliver care when a veteran's needs cannot be met within VA's own facilities. The reports highlighted in this testimony call attention to the risks introduced when that care is not offered and even more concerning, when the care is not coordinated.

Chairwoman Miller-Meeks, Ranking Member Brownley, and members of the Subcommittee, this concludes my statement. I would be happy to answer any questions you may have.

---

[22] VA OIG, Deficiencies in Care and Administrative Processes for a Patient Who Died by Sui- cide, Phoenix VA Health Care System, Arizona, March 31, 2021.

[23] VA OIG, Deficiencies in Care, Care Coordination, and Facility Response to a Patient Who Died by Suicide, Memphis VA Medical Center in Tennessee, September 3, 2020.

Testimony of Daniel Elkins, Chief of Staff
The Independence Fund

House Committee on Veterans Affairs Subcommittee on Health Hearing
"Combatting a Crisis: Providing Veterans Access to Life-saving Substance Abuse Disorder Treatment"
April 18, 2023

Mr. Elkins is the Chief of Staff at The Independence Fund (TIF), the leading Veteran Service Organization in helping America's most severely wounded Veterans. TIF serves the Warfighter Community by providing innovative programs and services to support the physical, mental, emotional, and spiritual independence and dignity of our Service Members, Veterans, Caregivers, Families, and Service Allies. Mr. Elkins works directly with TIF CEO, Sarah Verardo, to ensure the Fund's mission success, tracking completion of objectives, as well as coaching and motivating staff in order to Mr. Elkins is a subject matter expert on Special Operations, national security, covert and clandestine capabilities, military transition, preservation of the force and family, the National Guard, suicide prevention, military and veteran healthcare, student veterans, the Post-9/11 G.I. Bill, Federal Tuition Assistance, and for-profit and nonprofit education policy. Mr. Elkins maintains strong relationships with the White House, multiple Veteran Service Organizations, Congress, and the Departments of Defense, Education, and Veterans Affairs. These key relationships often place him at the forefront of policy decisions that impact members of the Special Operations community.

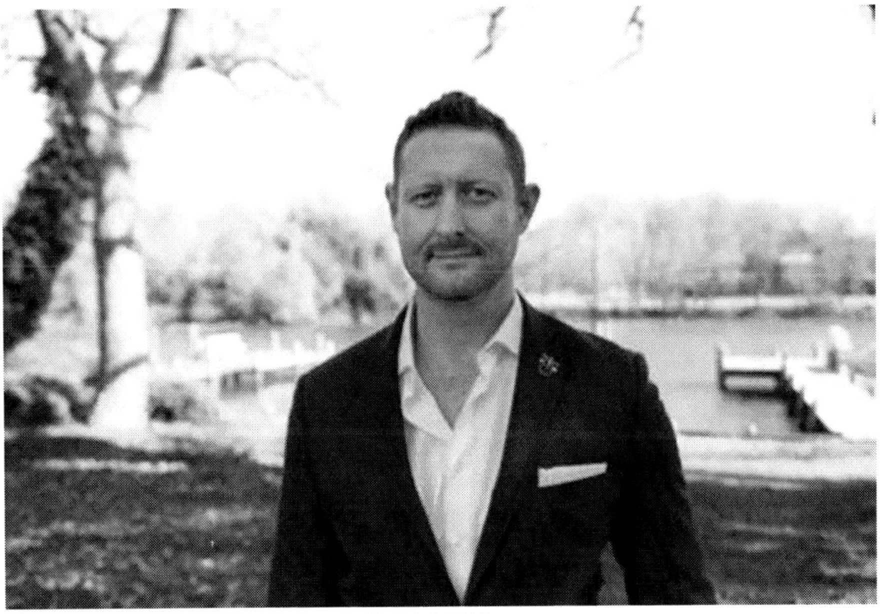

Daniel Elkins

Mr. Elkins is also a currently serving Green Beret in the National Guard and proud recipient of multiple military awards and decorations, including the Combat Infantryman Badge,

Parachutist Badge, Special Forces Tab, Military Free Fall Parachute Badge, and the Afghanistan Campaign Medal with Campaign Star.

Prior to serving with TIF, Mr. Elkins founded the Special Operations Association of America (SOAA), the only Veterans Service Organization in Washington D.C that engages in policy and legislation advocacy on behalf of all of the men and women in the Special Operations community and their families. In his role at SOAA, Mr. Elkins frequently engaged Congress, the White House, the Department of Defense, the Department of Veterans Affairs, and other key stakeholders in the Administration on behalf of the Special Operations Forces (SOF) community.

Before SOAA, Mr. Elkins had served as the Executive Director for the Veterans Education Project (VEP) where he directed nationwide grassroots outreach to ensure the protection of military benefits. He was also responsible for monitoring all legislative activities on Capitol Hill, with a focus on oversight and implementation of policy. His day-to-day responsibilities included developing new relationships with key stakeholders on Capitol Hill, maintaining relationships with the Administration, and serving as an expert witness to both congressional and federal offices.

Mr. Elkins serves as a board member for Equinox Innovative Systems, a company specializing in the integration of drone technology into Special Operation Forces for low intensity conflict. Furthermore, he retains positions on the boards of both SOAA and VEP where he serves as the president of the board. Prior to working as an advocate for Veterans and serving in the military, Mr. Elkins spent five years working overseas with nonprofit organizations to solve complex issues related to human trafficking across South America, Sub-Saharan Africa, Europe, and the Middle East.

Mr. Elkins is a proud life member of the Special Forces Association, the Enlisted Association of the National Guard of the United States, and Veterans of Foreign Wars. Mr. Elkins is originally from Western Maryland, and primarily splits his time between Charlotte, NC, and Washington, DC.

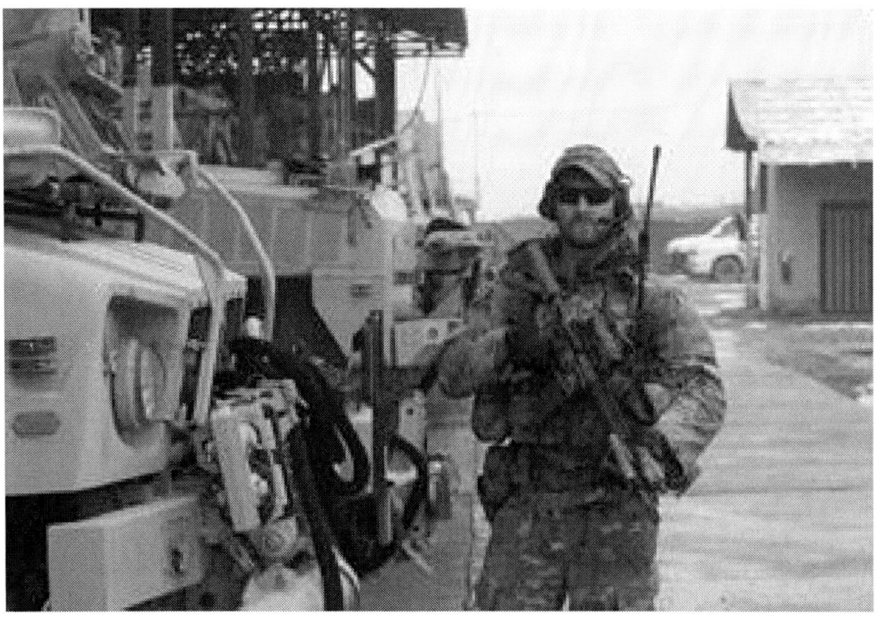

THE INDEPENDENCE FUND

Dear Chairwoman Meeks, Ranking Member Brownley, and Members of the Subcommittee:

On behalf of Sarah Verardo, CEO of The Independence Fund, we would like to thank the Subcommittee for your kind invitation to provide testimony at today's hearing, "Combatting a Crisis: Providing Veterans Access to Life-saving Substance Abuse Disorder Treatment." My name is Daniel Elkins and I joined TIF, the leading Veteran Service Organization (VSO) in helping America's most severely wounded Veterans as the Chief of Staff in 2022. I also currently serve as a Green Beret in the National Guard. For over a decade I have fought on behalf of the Warfighter Community to support the physical, mental, emotional, and spiritual independence and dignity of our Service Members, Veterans, Caregivers, Families, and Service Allies through Advocacy. I am also a Veteran of Operation Freedom's Sentinel. As a result of my many years of Advocacy within the Military and Veteran Community, I maintain strong relationships with the key leaders from the White House, multiple Veteran Service Organizations (VSOs), Congress, and the Departments of Defense, Education, and Veterans Affairs and am a Subject Matter Expert on a wide array of issues including military and veteran healthcare and suicide prevention. Prior to my tenure with TIF, I founded the Special Operations Association of America (SOAA) and Veterans Education Project (VEP) helping the Special Operations community and their families and Veterans with their higher education goals. As a combat Veteran, I have experienced firsthand the transformative and vital role the VA plays in healing the seen and unseen wounds of war. It is through this testimony that I would like to share our perspective, experiences and recommendations to ensure the often touted "worldclass healthcare" of the Department of Veterans Affairs (VA) is caring for our most vulnerable and at-risk Veterans.

TIF has been, and is, intimately involved advocating for and advising Veterans across the Nation when they encounter difficulties accessing appropriate care for mental health (MH) treatment and substance abuse disorder (SUD) and seek our counsel and intervention with the VA. This hearing could not be timelier because our Casework staff have received a significant number of inquiries from Veterans in the past two years that involve obstacles to timely and clinically appropriate care for their MH conditions. The geographic dispersion and similar factors present in many of these cases lead us to surmise these cases are not merely anecdotal rather they may be indicators of a more widespread access to care and care coordination problem for MH within the Veterans Health Administration's (VHA) hospital network.

TIF was founded in the halls of Walter Reed National Military Medical Center to provide greater mobility and independence for severely wounded and injured military personnel returning from Iraq and Afghanistan. We began by providing motorized all-terrain wheelchairs, fitted with treads, to Veterans for easier movement across everyday wheelchair barriers, like a playground or the backyard, and to also give disabled Veterans a chance to get back to the unpaved outdoors, whether it be the beach, the woods, or mountain trails. We just ordered our 2,640th chair this month, representing more than 42 million dollars alone for track chairs to

America's severely disabled Veterans. We have also been centrally involved in the evolution of the Caregiver program because our CEO, Sarah Verardo, is the wife and caregiver to Sergeant Michael Verardo, U.S. Army (Retired). Michael was catastrophically wounded in Afghanistan by an IED blast, his left leg and left arm were severely injured, and he suffered burns, complex polytrauma, traumatic brain injuries, and a host of other wounds. Michael is alive today because of the great care he received from the Army and the care he continues to receive from VA.

As a result of Michael Verardo's experiences and those of his fellow soldiers from the 82nd Airborne Division, many of whom returned from multiple deployments with invisible wounds like Traumatic Brain Injury and Post Traumatic Stress, TIF has been sharply focused on MH and suicide prevention. The need for peer-to-peer engagement and compassionate care led to the establishment "Operation Resiliency," a multi-day event where combat units are reunited under the formation they deployed under for fellowship and candid discussions concerning their MH. We conduct these reunions with the support of VA MH professionals.

Our Casework team, based in Charlotte, North Carolina, is led by a Licensed Clinical Social Worker who is an Air Force Veteran with prior service in Afghanistan. Her team focuses on the individual Veteran at the center of each unique case, conducts due diligence on the case, and acts as a liaison to VA and Community providers. This quick-response care model assists Veterans, Caregivers, and their families in finding solutions to issues that are beyond their ability, knowledge, or experience to solve on their own at the local level. TIF provides assistance in the areas of service-connected benefits, VA medical eligibility, Caregiver assistance, upgrading discharge status, Community resources, medical referrals to Community providers, Vocational Rehabilitation, unresolved medical issues, access to medical care, and legal resources. Our team of professionals frequently provides case management services to support and aid individuals in navigating the complexities of VA policy and regulations while routinely interacting with VA leaders and employees in medical facilities and program offices to develop and cultivate strong community relationships and ensure the right resources are available for a Veteran's care in a timely manner. The team fields calls daily from Veterans across the Nation seeking advice and aid with problems or impediments they are experiencing with access to VA care relative to a MH diagnosis or an emergent MH concern, substance use, traumatic brain injury, and suicidal ideation.

Casework Observations on Residential MH Care Access Related to SUD

In the past 2 years, our Casework team records indicates we received 1,304 cases for action with 110 of those, or 11.8%, stemming from a problem a Veteran was experiencing seeking timely access to complex MH care from VA through Intensive Outpatient care or Residential Inpatient care and requesting help from our Casework team to obtain a resolution that involved either VA- based care and/or a referral from VA to Community-based care. Fifty-nine of those 110, or 53%, were Veterans with SUD. Twenty-one of those 59 have been recorded since January of this year. It is important to note that MH cases and SUD cases specifically consume the vast majority of our Casework team's time and energy due to the sometimes-fragile condition of these Veterans, and difficulties they have comprehending the intricacies of VA regulations and processes. These 59 cases spanned 26 states and involved 29 VA medical facilities.

The casework narratives for these cases frequently depict, to varying degrees, multiple laudatory and concerning aspects with local VA facility responsiveness to Veterans' needs and conditions. In many cases the Veteran has taken what is for them a major step by voluntarily asking for care in a structured setting or program. When they are met with a sense of urgency and responsiveness that can make a significant difference in how they respond to treatment, but when they experience a lack of empathy and an inability to listen from VA employees, or a lack of clarity and consistency regarding the care process, a Veteran's trust in VA can decline rapidly. That is often when our Casework team is contacted by a Veteran, while they are seeking admittance to a VA facility or a program or soon after they are admitted, and they begin to feel unheard or receive contradictory direction and expectations from VA clinical staff. Our Caseworkers understand there are often many sides to how human interactions are perceived, so they tread carefully and try to understand all sides.

Until October 2022 our Caseworkers operated under the assumption VA's MH care in a residential/domiciliary setting - which includes SUD treatment - in what VA calls MH RRTP or the MH Residential Rehabilitation Treatment Program, was covered by the access standard authorities in the 2018 MISSION Act for travel distance and wait times. It was only by accident that our caseworkers discovered this law does not apply to MH RRTP access standards and practices. A copy of the MH RRTP policy was sent to us by a senior clinician at a facility that could not provide care to a Veteran and that facility had denied a referral to an approved and willing Community Care provider.

This VHA Directive #1162 requires that VA admit a Veteran seeking inpatient, residential care within 72 hours for priority patients and no more than 30 days after a VA assessment of any patient needing residential care. Based on our experience, it is not unusual for Veterans to wait beyond 72 hours or 30 days for care and it has been our observation that even after those limits are exceeded, a facility has the latitude to continue to seek an available bed in another MH RRTP facility sometimes several states distant, rather than approve a referral to a community provider with those services in the Community Care Network (CCN).

In some interactions with VA administrators at local facilities, our Casework team has found that the primary care provider for the Veteran, a VA physician, has approved a referral to a CCN provider, but that referral is overruled by administrative or senior clinical staff. There have also been some cases where our caseworkers were told by an administrator that Community Care is not offered for residential MH treatment and other interactions where the VA administrative staff do not understand Community Care is a lawful option and are unfamiliar with how a referral is generated. In certain circumstances VA staff have not discussed CCN care options with a Veteran without prompting or until a caseworker inquires of a VA administrator or patient advocate.

It is important to emphasize that the VA healthcare system is often complex and confusing to many Veterans who do not understand their care options or their rights. Our caseworkers work diligently to educate them in real-time and advocate for appropriate and timely care, regardless of whether that care is to be provided by VA or a CCN provider. Given the staffing and capacity limitations in MH RRTP, it is not unusual for our caseworkers to attempt to identify an available and qualified CCN provider that can render necessary care in order to avoid the Veteran waiting beyond the limits of the MH RRTP policy or to request a referral before those limits are reached, if the Veteran is in crisis and the VA facility concedes it hasn't found an available bed for the Veteran.

Another key concern with the MH RRTP policy of 73 hours and 30 days is the difficulties our caseworkers have encountered determining when the "clock starts" for those prescribed time limits and who in each facility is designated to monitor the elapse of time relative to the policy and ensure the process is being adhered to by VA clinical and administrative staff. This opacity has often lead to frustration and distrust. In one instance of delayed and poorly coordinated care, it was discovered that the VA staffer responsible for entering patient communications with RRTP staff into the electronic record had not done so, leaving significant gaps. Consequently, when our casework staffer attempted to reference those communications there was no way to reference them to help reach an informed and timely resolution of the case.

Casework Narratives

The following casework narratives are provided for a more detailed understanding of what our caseworkers encountered with a range of SUD, MH RRTP cases and how the cases were managed. Some were resolved within days, others in weeks or months, and some remain unresolved:

Case #1: OIF Combat Veteran, PTSD/SUD, Maine; October 2021 (Resolved)

History: Veteran needed dual treatment, detox, and experienced suicidal ideations. Veteran had to leave a facility in Florida due to reports of abuse (to date, Caseworker received three reports of abuse from different Veterans). Veteran is from Maine, used heroin, history of six overdoses, suicidal ideations, and chronic pain. Veteran contacted Caseworker and asked for support leaving the facility on Thursday evening.

Case Coordination: Caseworker reached out to VHA staff and left a message. Veteran became dangerous to himself during detox. Veteran wanted treatment and Maine VA stated they could not provide referral in the VHA network within 60 days.

Resolution: Caseworker discussed the case with Provider and Community Care authorization was issued to support the Veteran's continued treatment.

Duration of Case: six days to resolution.

Case # 2: OEF Combat Veteran, SUD, Houston, TX; January 2022 (RESOLVED)

History: Veteran sought MH therapy at the Debakey Clinic for post-traumatic stress disorder (PTSD) related to combat experiences in January 2022. Veteran was told he could only receive an appointment for April 2022.

Case Coordination: Caseworker reached out to provider team and was told that Veteran was indeed eligible for Community Care for local services. Scheduler subsequently reached out to the Veteran and said he could stay in the VA system if he wanted services. Caseworker reached out to the Patient Advocate, and the Patient Advocate stated that this was a huge oversight and that the Community Care team dropped the ball and could not believe he was getting issued referrals, only to have them stopped twice by Community Care staff. Caseworker called the Community Care department and discussed Veteran's need to see a provider. Community Care scheduler called Veteran and finally scheduled appointment only after MH Provider had to place another referral in the system.

1. Miscommunication on Veteran's need for therapy; had a referral to Community Care canceled twice while Veteran had over three-month wait to receive inside VHA services.
2. Lack of accountability with Houston/ Debakey staff meant that Veteran's case continuously was being dropped, referral was canceled, and no communication was made on behalf of VHA to explain to Veteran.

Duration of Case: took four weeks to receive Community Care after schedulers initially refused to offer Community Care.

Case #3: OEF Combat Veteran, PTSD/SUD, February 2022 (Resolved) History

Veteran needed dual treatment, detox, and was unable to work or support family financially or physically as he was continuously intoxicated and making poor choices. MHcondition escalated to the point of considering ending his life. The Veteran was previously involved in Operation Resiliency. Reached out to Casework to ask for support getting access to treatment quickly after driving to children's school and falling asleep intoxicated.

Case Coordination: Caseworker reached out to VA Patient Advocate and discussed the previous attempts of the Veteran to stabilize with therapy and medication. VHA staff agreed that a dual diagnosis facility would be the best option and considered Veteran's preference in the request.

Resolution: VHA issued Community Care referral and Veteran was admitted in less than a week.

Duration of Case: seven days to resolution.

Case #4: Post 9-11 Veteran, SUD, Mountain Home, TN; March 2022 (Unresolved)

History: March 2022 Veteran requested Community Care for inpatient MH treatment as he frequently drank to the point of blacking out and went through the evaluation process to assess SUD at VA. Veteran was told to wait 45 days until May 2022 for appointment.

Case Coordination: Caseworker called and spoke to SUD MH team and scheduled and advocated for Community Care.

Duration of Case: No resolution. Veteran dropped Casework services due to relapse and inability to get into MH services.

Case #5: Post 9-11 Veteran, SUD, Mountain Home, TN; May 2022 (Unresolved, Incarcerated)

History: May 2022 Veteran was denied inpatient SUD support after VHA stated he should receive VA care. Admission date was two months away and Veteran presented in a dangerous cycle of blacking out, PTSD, and using methamphetamines.

Case Coordination: Casework attempted to advocate with local recovery coordinators (LRC). LRCs denied ability to admit sooner and denied the possibility of Community Care services.

Resolution: No resolution. Veteran ended up in jail for possession after two weeks of asking for inpatient Community Care referral.

Duration of Case: No resolution.

Case #6: OEF/OIF Combat Veteran, PTSD/SUD, Texas and New York; July 2022 (Resolved)

History: Veteran needed dual treatment, detox and experienced suicidal ideations. Family and friends took him to a VA community partner, concerned that without immediate intervention the Veteran would succeed in ending his life.

Case Coordination: Veteran was from NY, stayed with family in TX as he struggled to overcome his suicidal ideations associated with PTSD triggers and depression with SUD withdrawal. The family contacted Caseworker and asked for insight; stated over the weekend Veteran became dangerous to himself. Family consulted a Community Care partner and asked if they would havea bed available; they did. Veteran was admitted. The family stated that insurance would still charge $6,000 co-pay. Asked Caseworker for support with any VHA coverage.

Resolution: Caseworker reached out to the provider at NY VAMC. VHA Primary Care Physician (PCP) reported that she would do everything to assist Veteran and was very supportive of dual diagnosis program based on Veteran's history. PCP initiated referral and authorization, and Veteran was supported financially throughout his treatment.

Duration of Case: three days to resolution.

Case #4: OEF/OIF Combat Veteran, PTSD/SUD, Salisbury, NC; July 2022 History

Veteran needed dual treatment, detox, and was incarcerated due to drug use and destructive behavior.

Case Coordination: Veteran was from NC, struggled with SUD. Veteran contacted Caseworker wanted assistance with seeking support related to his PTSD and SUD. Stated he experienced anger issues and couldn't control it without help.

Resolution: Caseworker reached out to Salisbury VAMC MH team who promptly issued a Community Care referral observing his needs for dual diagnosis.

Duration of Case: five days to resolution.

Case #5: OEF Combat Veteran, PTSD/ SUD/MST; July 2022

History: Veteran needed support for combat PTSD and SUD use of heavy narcotics and fentanyl. Veteran reported blacking out, overdosed numerous times, and knew he was "going to die" if he kept using.

Case Coordination: TIF partner contacted the team and put Caseworker in touch with Veteran. Veteran badly wanted help but reported that he could only stay sober in the mornings. Veteran reported that military sexual trauma (MST) had never been discussed with his VHA MH team, but he had been gang raped by male Veterans on his squad. Caseworker reached out to Social Worker at VHA. Discussed the MST and concern for Veteran reporting feeling unsafe around male Veterans.

Resolution: Social Worker worked quickly to obtain Community Care referral. Veteran was able to receive treatment in a safe environment and is now a leader in peer support.

Duration of Case: ten days to resolution.

Case #6: Post 9-11 Veteran, PTSD/SUD, Togus, ME, July 2022 (Resolved by 3rd Party)

History: Single-amputee combat, Army Veteran who received his amputation after service due to an infection incurred by service and, in his own words, "ignored" by Military doctors.

Case Coordination: Casework originally began working with him in June 2021 with other familial support. Recently reached out on July 2022, asking for help to obtain residential treatment for alcohol substance use and combat PTSD. Veteran has been under the care of a VA Psychiatrist and MH counselor at the Togus, ME VAMC but had only recently admitted that his challenges were significant enough to seek treatment in a residential setting. Presented to caseworker identifying that his psychiatrist was supportive and recognized his need for a higher level of care. The psychiatrist placed the referral for inpatient help through the national nonprofit Warriors Heart; however, it was denied by Community Care leadership. This triggered a complex and evolving call to advocacy on his behalf.

1. *An Extended Delay:* Since Veteran contacted us in July, Veteran and TIF Casework have worked to advocate for support for SUD and PTSD residential support. At almost 90-days since the request, Veteran was told he could not receive Care through a Community partner, but had to seek VA care first. When he elected to seek care in a VA facility, he was told he could not get approved for a facility in Sarasota, FL, close to his family.
2. *Stress on the Veteran:* Veteran attempted suicide in September due to inaccessibility to treatment and support. He prepared a noose and ingested large volumes of alcohol preparing to hang himself, his wife walked in on him during the attempt.
3. *Failure to Care:* Veteran was discharged from VA after a 72 hour hold without a follow- up treatment plan.
4. *Policy Conflicts:* Contact has been sporadic with Togus VAMC staff, and the goal posts continued to move. Even with the combined Advocacy of TIF, Rep. Jared Golden's (D- ME) office, and the VA Central Office, there was no resolution. Togus VAMC's leadership challenged the MISSION Act, stating that Community Care is not warranted unless the Veteran completes VA first and fails out of it. They further asserted that residential treatment did not fall within the MISSION Act rather fell under different criteria specified in the VHA Office of Integrated Veteran Care (IVC) Community Care Field Guidebook Specialty Programs.
5. *Care Implementation Timeline:* VA leadership at Togus VAMC asserted that Veteran should seek VA Care first- but when pressed, has no known timeline of when a VA bed could be available.
6. *Communication / Documentation Errors:* VA leadership stated that when Veteran requested Care through Sarasota, it was never documented in the system and was never mentioned internally as a discussion for options for Veteran's treatment.

Resolution: Veteran received financial support from a nonprofit partner paying for his admission at Warriors Heart in October 2022.

Duration of Case: three months to resolution.

Cases # 7 & # 8: Veteran One, OEF/OIF Combat Veteran PTSD/SUD (Alcohol), St. Cloud, MN; August 2022 (RESOLVED) Veteran Two, OEF Combat Veteran PTSD/ SUD (Heroin); St. Cloud, MN; August 2022 (Unresolved)

History: Both cases presented as referred to TIF on August 2022, before Labor Day weekend, by a Community Care partner. Veterans one and two were staying in a non-VA, community sober living facility where a friend and fellow Veteran recently died by suicide. They reported finding him after the deceased Veteran asked for help multiple times, having disclosed to them that he was in an intimate relationship with the facility director and it had become abusive. Veterans one and two reported feeling unsafe remaining at the community facility under the present circumstances, but had no place to live otherwise. Both Veterans stated their safety and well-being concerns to St. Cloud VAMC Staff. They were advised by VA staff that they would have to wait through the Labor Day weekend to receive a VA assessment for care and were advised to go to an Urgent Care outlet for any immediate health concerns. Veteran two subsequently left the community facility on a weekend pass and used heroin. Veteran one was assessed by VA on 8/31/2022 and Veteran two was assessed by VA on 9/1/2022. Veteran two reported that he felt the urge to use heroin again and was having memories of the corpses he had retrieved in Iraq. Veteran one was experiencing reported panic attacks.

Case Coordination: TIF Caseworker contacted VAMC Director prior to the Labor Day weekend and requested an expedited referral to Community Care via #1162, under a criterion of unsafe living conditions (which allows 72 hours to treat veterans per the Directive) and given that a VA Community Care partner with qualified and parallel programming was willing to admit both Veterans immediately. Facility director stated to Caseworker there was no provision for Community Care in those circumstances within St. Cloud VA System.

Resolution: Veteran one was admitted to St. Cloud VAMC on 9/6/2022; delay for VA care did not exceed the post-screening, 72-hour limit as stipulated in #1162. Veteran two relapsed and lost contact with VA and local casework partners. Veteran one and Veteran two reported to TIF they felt they were being "forced" to accept VA care and were told by VA staff that Community Care options were not something their local VA considers when referring for MH and addiction treatment.

Additional Information: Dr. Nichole Welle, Director of CBOC issued the following authority on St. Cloud's willingness/ ability to provide MH community services: "Veteran and I discussed the limitations for VHA Care in the Community (CITC) covering the cost of MH residential programs in the community. Minneapolis VAHCS CITC leadership clarified that VHA does not fund MH residential programming outside the VHA system when VHA provides the service."

Case # 9: OIF Combat Veteran, PTSD/SUD, East Orange, NJ: September 2022 (Resolved)

History: Veteran needed support for combat PTSD and SUD use of heavy narcotics and fentanyl. Veteran was engaging in high-risk behavior as a cry for help.

Case Coordination: Casework partner contacted the TIF team to discuss Veteran's case. Veteran was hospitalized for OD and nearly died. Upon discharge home, Veteran's parents told him to "go f*cking die" and set the Veteran off again. Veteran went missing for 24 hours. TIF Casework staff notified VHA staff and discussed the case. Veteran called into Casework two days later and asked for help. VHA staff worked quickly to support a Community Care referral to dual facility in TX. The veteran was admitted two days later after discussion with Caseworker and VHA staff.

Duration of Case: five days to resolution.

Case # 10: OEF Veteran, SUD, Portland, OR; September, 2022 (Resolved)

History: Veteran was, at the time of contact with TIF, homeless, in need of inpatient treatment and receiving care through the Portland VAMC. The Veteran was sent to detox by Portland VAMC, but was told he did not have priority to receive authorization for residential substance abuse treatment, which is typically provided immediately following detox to eliminate possibility for a relapse. Veteran disclosed to TIF he was discharged on 9/12/2022 from detox and had already used drugs since then while calling the Portland VAMC multiple times to request treatment; Veteran's SUD was service-connected.

Case Coordination: On 9/16/2022 TIF Caseworker and Veteran had a conference call with an employee at the Portland VAMC-Substance Abuse Department. VA employee shared that Veteran's appointments were on 11/3/2022 and 11/23/2022 for the initial Substance Abuse Evaluation. Veteran expressed his need for earlier appointments. Caseworker asked the VA employee if there were cancellations to allow an earlier date or dates. VA employee shared that there are rarely cancellations and that most individuals didn't show up with any notice. Veteran and TIF Caseworker inquired about the Community Care program as an option. The VA employee stated that "substance abuse does not qualify for the care in the Care in Community program and recommended the Veteran call VA MHMH RRTP - Vancouver, WA. Veteran said he had done so and MH RRTP did not have an opening until January 2023. The VA employee said there was nothing else she could do to assist the Veteran prior to his appointments in November 2022.

Resolution: Portland VAMC initially provided a wait time of four months for this Veteran to be admitted into a residential program and Portland VAMC staff stated Community Care was not an option at their location. This Veteran was homeless and at higher risk which should have initiated a priority request for care within 72 hours, per the VHA regulation. After TIF contacted the VA MH RRTP Program director, the Veteran was admitted within seven days, but still outside of the 72-hour limit stipulated in #1162.

Additional Information: While conducting Casework, Advocacy and Research to assist one of the Veterans cited above, The Independence Fund was provided a VA policy excerpt by a VAMC employee that explains the referral process to a Community Care provider for inpatient MH treatment.

The policy states, in part:

> "By national policy, MH RRTPs are Veterans Integrated Service Network (VISN) resources. VISNs should ensure adequate access to MH RRTP care across the VISN. When the care cannot be provided by a MH RRTP, and the Veteran meets the eligibility standards for MH RRTP care and elects to receive COMMUNITY CARE, VA will authorize that care to be provided by a community provider with whom VA has contract for the provision of the necessary services."

Further specifics in the policy are as follows:

"When can a Veteran be referred to COMMUNITY CARE:

- A Veteran who meets criteria for a priority admission (within 72 hours) that cannot be accommodated by a MH RRTP. Referrals to an alternate MH RRTP should be exhausted before a community referral.
- A Veteran who must wait greater than 30 days for admission to a MH RRTP. Referrals to an alternate MH RRTP should be exhausted before a community referral.

General requirements for MH RRTP/Community Residential Care referrals:

- Veteran is assessed as not meeting criteria for acute psychiatric or medical condition(s).
- Veteran has attempted a less restrictive treatment alternative, or one was unavailable.
- Veteran is assessed as requiring the structure and support of a residential treatment environment.
- Veteran is assessed as not being a significant risk of harm to self or others.

Wait time and drive time access standards are only applicable to primary care, specialty care, and non-institutional extended care services. MH RRTP services are considered institutional extended care services and therefore these standards are not factors that require consideration for a community referral."

Case # 11: Post 9-11 Veteran, SUD, Columbia, SC; September 2022 (Unresolved)
History: September 2022 Veteran has attended VA directed MH RTTP four times and Intensive Outpatient Program (IOP) seven times. VA Chief of Substance Abuse clinic refused to offer community services citing that there were VA options with beds available to Veteran. The Veteran was not considered in previous attempts to attend VA care. Veteran is still unserved after six months. The Veteran completed MH RRTP and believed it did not help through the VA and wanted to explore other options.

Case Coordination: Caseworker reached out to clarify the Veteran's interest in Community Care options and the VA Chief stated that there were four VA systems the Veteran could use. Veteran reported that those programs did not help him as evidenced by his inability to stay sober. Veteran refused to attend VHA care again and Chief of MH at Columbia VAMC, Dr. Brian Apple refused to offer Community Care referral. Dr. Apple was adamant he would not consider it as indicated below:

- "He has received outpatient care with the VA in the past. We can offer this service again, including Suboxone. We can refer him to a Methadone Clinic if he desires that service on an outpatient basis.
- The VA has an inpatient program we can send him to. He can pay for other services outside the VA if he wants, but we need to try the Residential programs within the VA first.
- He was approved for admission to the Salisbury VA, but they could not contact him in March of this year (he was incarcerated). We can place a consult there again.
- We can also place consults to Asheville, Atlanta, Dublin, and Augusta. Previous inpatient treatment in the VA was found in his records. There is no indication he was not successful.

- He was in the Buffalo VA RRTP in 2020; he was in the Asheville VA RRTP in 2019; he was in the Salisbury VA RRTP in 2013 and 2014.

Resolution: No resolution.

Case # 12: OIF Combat Veteran, PTSD/SUD, Columbia, MO; October 2022

History: Veteran needed support for combat PTSD and IOP program. Veteran attempted to get IOP through VA, but the nearest in person program was 2.5 hours away in another state. Veteran completed MH RRTP and needed to follow up with IOP services to remain successful.

Case Coordination: The Veteran called Caseworker and requested support to navigate and get IOP. Caseworker called Social Worker at VHA and Social Worker agreed based on PTSD related presentation, Veteran would be better in an in-person IOP.

Resolution: Referral was issued shortly after discussion with Social Worker.

Duration of Case: three days to resolution.

Case # 13: OIF Combat Veteran, PTSD/ SUD, East Orange, NJ; October 2022 (Resolved)

History: Veteran needed support for combat PTSD and SUD use of methamphetamines. Veteran was in trouble after passing out with meth on person within a vicinity of school zone. Veteran needed assistance getting into treatment facility but was told he would have to wait over thirty- days locally or travel out of state.

Case Coordination: Veteran reached out to Caseworker for legal support and was also connected with Veterans Justice Initiative (VJI), a TIF Program that works with law enforcement to avoid the unnecessary criminalization of mental illness, substance abuse, and incarceration of veterans. An advocate from VJI was able to discuss Veteran receiving treatment in lieu of incarceration as there was no intention to distribute.

Resolution: Casework team reached out to VHA staff and discussed treatment options to ensure probation was facilitated. The Veteran was connected with a referral for Community Care in the local community which allowed him to adhere to restrictions issued in court by the magistrate.

Duration of Case: nine days to resolution.

Case # 14: Post 9-11 Veteran, SUD, St. Louis, MO; October 2022 (Resolved)

History: Veteran requested MH services and was denied access to care within 30 days. Casework staff subsequently reached out and assisted Veteran in obtaining Community Care services within the month.

Case Coordination: VHA staff stated it could take over 30 days to receive MH RRTP services. Nationally recognized CCN provider offered specific dual diagnosis resources within thirty minutes of Veteran's home, other VHA options would take Veteran hours away. Lack of urgency to provide a referral to Veteran even though screened as needing MH RRTP support.

Resolution: Veteran was able to obtain referral after discussing the urgency and severity of struggle with symptoms and after conference with VHA MH staff and Caseworker.

Case # 15: Gulf War Era Veteran, SUD, Dallas, TX; October 2022 (Unresolved)

History: Veteran was sexually assaulted by male counterparts in service. He was using heroin, fentanyl, and drinking to escape the memories of his trauma. Wife threatened to leave him if he didn't stop using. The Veteran reported if he didn't get help soon he was going to likely "die" and "destroy" his life. Numerous attempts to contact the MH staff and ask for support, but the VHA wanted him to travel a minimum of four hours to Dallas to receive services. Veteran had been to treatment twice within VHA before and requested a Community Care referral.

Case Coordination: Caseworker and Veteran reached out to VHA staff regarding Veteran's need for support. Both Veteran and his Peer support person reported the Chief of MH, screamed at him, and stated Community Care was not an option she would consider. Chief of MH never responded to Caseworker's emails or telephone messages asking for support.

Veteran reported that the Chief of MH called him again and told him if he denied VHA care, he was declining care. Veteran responded he could not travel and did not want to be around other Veterans due to the culmination of his experiences (Veteran has complex sexual trauma). Veteran reported he was not being considered at all in his own treatment.

Resolution: No resolution.

Need for New or Revised Regulations and Policy for SUD and Mental Health Access to Care and COMPACT Act

Based on past and ongoing casework interventions TIF has undertaken on behalf of Veterans with SUD and other MH needs and our Casework team's interaction with VHA administrators and clinicians, there appears to be a lack of uniformity, consistency, and adherence to VHA Directive #1162 across several VHA facilities in different VISN regions. The administrative barriers and impediments to receiving timely care within an MH RRTP or a timely referral to a CCN provider with the same services are incongruent with trauma-informed care and unaligned with the intent of the MISSION Act's "best medical interest" proviso. The following recommendations are provided in an effort to revise and align #1162 with the MISSION Act and ensure the processes and procedures for access to care are focused first and foremost on the Veteran who is seeking that care within the original spirit and intent of the MISSION Act:

1) Include all criteria for Community Care wait time, travel distance, and access standards under MISSION Act in #1162 to govern residential rehabilitation programs or eliminate #1162 entirely and defer to MISSION Act's original authorities and intent to support all levels of VHA provided specialty care, including residential rehabilitation services.
    a) Mandate patient assessments be conducted within a uniform window of time after care is first requested by the Veteran or his/her primary care provider. Require no more than 72 hours to conduct that assessment.
    b) Reduce the maximum wait time for access to a facility. Thirty days is too long to ask a Veteran to wait on the availability of MH RRTP or residential Community Care. In a thirty-day period, risk can rise and a Veteran's condition destabilize. Recommend a clinically sound, lesser number of days because PTSD and SUD require swift interventions and services.
2) Rescind any formal or informal VHA guidance or directives that require a Veteran to complete a program in an MH RRTP and "fail" before they can be referred to a CCN

provider. In some cases, Veterans lack trust in VA based on past experiences. If a Veteran has a fear or concern about an inpatient MH program or has attended a program in the past and indicates they do not want to return, there is potentially diminishing value for the Veteran to be required to enter MH RRTP again. That is not trauma-informed care.

3) Expand COMPACT Act to cover non-suicidal crises like SUD and allow civilian providers inside and outside the CCN to authorize care for SUD residential services.
4) Conduct outreach and education on COMPACT Act authorities and the request for the approval process to the following:
   a) All Executive Directors for the Veterans Service Organizations in The Military Coalition based in Washington DC.
   b) All local Veterans Service Organization leaders for the localities where a VAMC is located and the catchment area for those VAMCs.
   c) All CCN and non-CCN hospitals and all CCN providers in the catchment areas of the VAMCs participating in the COMPACT Act.
5) Educate and train VHA staff to recognize what is in the "best medical interest" of the Veteran. Further empower leaders, clinicians, and administrators to align themselves with the Veteran's needs to build and sustain trusted relationships.
   a) Case management for Veterans seeking SUD treatment must consider all the treatment modalities and options that are necessary for full recovery, with no gaps in that care. A Veteran assessed at an elevated risk should never be discharged from a detox facility for a period of time while they wait to be admitted to MH RRTP and other appropriate programs, inside or outside VHA. These gaps can increase the probability of a relapse between treatments.
   b) VHA administrators should not have the authority to override a physician's recommended referral to a CCN provider under "best medical interest." Regulations and procedures need to be clear and precise that irrespective of the statutory wait time standard, if a physician recommends treatment within a shorter time frame and VHA cannot meet that time frame, the Veteran must be referred to a CCN provider of same services whenever a CCN provider can admit the Veteran before direct VHA care becomes available.
6) Veterans should be notified without delay of CCN eligibility in all appropriate circumstances when VHA is approaching a deadline to determine if VA care is available, including an explanation of how to request a Community Care referral and the process by which a Veteran can appeal a CCN denial decision. When a CCN referral is denied and the Veteran appeals the decision, the VA must provide a response outlining the justification for the denial and appeal instructions following the decision in a timely manner not to exceed 10 days from the date the appeal is submitted. When MH RRTP is considered as a treatment option for cases of mental illness or SUD, urgency is required to ensure the Veteran receives timely and appropriate access to care.
7) Require the VA Office of the Inspector General (OIG) to audit each VAMC's ability to advise Veterans on CCN eligibility, inform Veterans of their right and ability to seek CCN services, deliver CCN referrals in a timely manner and appropriately approve and coordinate CCN referrals for Veterans. The OIG will submit a report to Congress annually on its findings.

Again, on behalf of The Independence Fund, and all the Veterans we have helped access the care they deserve and earned, we appreciate the opportunity to testify before the Subcommittee. We hope the examples we provided shine a light on the exemplary work being done by many VAMCs across the country to offer timely and urgent service to struggling Veterans, and also highlight where there is inconsistency, miscommunication or failure to adhere to directives which hurt the people it is our privilege and duty to honor and serve.

Wounded Warrior Project
Statement of Jennifer Silva, Chief Program Officer on "Combatting a Crisis: Providing Veterans Access to Life Saving Substance Abuse Disorder Treatment"
April 18, 2023

Chairwoman Miller-Meeks, Ranking Member Brownley, and distinguished members of the House Committee on Veterans' Affairs Subcommittee on Health – thank you for inviting Wounded Warrior Project (WWP) to submit this written statement for the record of today's hearing on veterans' access to Department of Veterans Affairs (VA) substance use disorder (SUD) treatment.

For 20 years WWP has worked to fulfill our mission to honor and empower wounded warriors. In addition to our advocacy before Congress, we offer more than a dozen direct service programs focused on connection, independence, and wellness in every spectrum of a warrior's life. Our organization has grown alongside the warriors we serve and we remain committed to tailoring our programming to the evolving needs of a post-9/11 generation of warriors that has become increasingly diverse.

In this context, assisting warriors with their mental health challenges has consistently been our largest programming investment over the past several years. In Fiscal Year 2022, WWP spent more than $82 million in mental and brain health programs – an investment consistent with the fact that more than 7 in 10 respondents to our 2022 Annual Warrior Survey self-reported at least one mental health condition.[24] As diagnoses of post-traumatic stress disorder (PTSD), depression, and anxiety have consistently ranked among the top five most self-reported conditions across previous editions of our Annual Warrior Survey, our Mental Health Continuum of Support has developed over the last decade and now allows us to engage each individual based on their unique needs.[25] In Fiscal Year 2022 alone, WWP provided warriors and their family members with nearly 55,000 hours of treatment for mental health conditions, including PTSD, traumatic brain injury, SUD, and other mental health conditions.

Our specific focus on assisting warriors with substance abuse has followed a similar evolutionary path. In 2020, WWP recognized a gap in mental health services for veterans struggling with a substance use disorder and a co-morbid mental health disorder (e.g., PTSD). An increasing volume of veterans connected with our Mental Health Continuum of Support programs were sharing similar stories about their difficulty accessing clinical treatment.

---

[24] WWP's 2022 Annual Warrior Survey can be viewed at https://www.woundedwarriorproject.org/mission/annual-warrior-survey.

[25] More information on WWP's Mental Health Continuum of Support can be found at the end of the document.

Providers were telling veterans that their SUD had to be treated independently before receiving PTSD care, or vice versa. Delays in finding the appropriate care in a timely manner would not only fail to capitalize on the veterans' desire to change their life circumstances, but in some cases cause further damage to their mental and physical health along with declines in family and social relationships. Hearing these stories, WWP committed to investigating further and commissioned the RAND Corporation to conduct a landscape study on the most effective way to treat post-9/11 veterans with co-occurring mental health and substance use disorders.

The resulting report, *Improving Substance Use Care: Addressing Barriers to Expanding Integrated Treatment Options for Post-9/11 Veterans*,[26] has helped guide WWP's programming and advocacy before Congress. Data provided in WWP's 2019 Annual Warrior Survey, in combination with findings from the literature on SUDs and mental health disorders in veteran populations, revealed the high level of need for both substance use and mental health care among post-9/11 veterans. Among their key findings, RAND concluded that:

- Veterans screening positive for PTSD or depression are almost 20 percent more likely to screen positive for hazardous alcohol use or a potential SUD;
- Mental health treatment facilities typically specialize in treating one type of disorder or the other;
- Mental health treatment facilities often require veterans to abstain from substance use, but veterans may be using substances to manage their mental health symptoms;
- Veterans who receive substance use treatment alone may be at risk for failing to meet their treatment goals if their mental health symptoms are not addressed; and
- Integrated, evidence-based approaches that address both substance use disorders and mental health disorders concurrently and provide ongoing support for recovery can improve outcomes for this population, but it is critical that veterans are able to access programs and facilities that are equipped to treat the veteran population.

The RAND report includes a number of recommendations for improving options for and access to treatment for veterans with co-occurring SUDs and mental health disorders. One of these recommendations is to decrease barriers to accessing treatment.[27] They write, "given the difficulty of engaging the veteran population, it is essential to reduce barriers to care to help veterans not only initiate care but also to reduce dropout once enrolled."[28] The report also emphasizes the importance of ease of access to services and "limited delays in setting up initial and continuing care appointments."[29]

For these reasons, WWP has committed itself to ensuring that veterans who seek help are connected quickly to clinical programs that meet their needs. The Department of Veterans Affairs (VA) is a critical resource and partner for accomplishing those goals, and as discussed below, their collaboration with two key programs has helped lead to more successful outcomes for warriors who have engaged WWP for help. Our work has also spotlighted gaps and efficiencies that inform specific calls to action for this Subcommittee focused on accelerating

---

[26] Eric R. Pederson et al., RAND, Improving Substance Use Care: Addressing Barriers to Expanding Integrated Treatment Options for Post-9/11 Veterans (2020).

[27] *Id.* at 150.

[28] *Id.*

[29] *Id.* at 154.

access to care, addressing provider shortages, enhancing data reporting, and strengthening case management services.

Addressing Access Challenges Through WWP Programs

Currently when a warrior reaches out to WWP for mental health support, their first step to finding care is a conversation with our Triage team. The Triage team conducts screenings of a warrior's mental health history, provides the warrior with information about our various mental health offerings, and refers the warrior to the most appropriate mental health program within WWP or an external resource. In FY 22, our Triage team received 12,610 referrals to find warriors appropriate treatment, placed 10,634 referrals for mental health support (including 5,630 referrals to external outpatient care providers), and made their first connection with interested warriors an average of 1.04 days later. Warriors assessed as needing SUD treatment were most often either referred to WWP's Warrior Care Network or Complex Case Coordination (C3) program.

Warrior Care Network

Wounded Warrior Project's Warrior Care Network is a two-week intensive outpatient program where warriors are helped to minimize the interference of mental health issues in their everyday lives. WWP partners with four academic medical centers across the country to provide this treatment to help warriors manage their PTSD, TBI, SUDs, and other mental health conditions.

Since publication of WWP-commissioned RAND report on co-occurring SUD and mental health disorders, WWP has invested additional resources to ensure that the Warrior Care Network is providing this integrated treatment for veterans through our academic medical center partners. Warriors who complete the Warrior Care Network program have seen significant improvements in their PTSD and depression symptoms and improved functioning and quality of life. Most significant to today's hearing, treating mental health and SUD concurrently has led to reduced substance use habits. For those being treated as part of Warrior Care Network's SUD program, the pre-treatment average of 6.1 days of substance use per week was reduced to 1.6 days after treatment. After six months, warriors' substance use remained reduced at an average of 4.1 days of substance use per week.

While Warrior Care Network academic medical center partners provide veteran-centric comprehensive care, aggregate data, share best practices, and coordinate care in an unprecedented manner, partnership with VA has helped create a broad continuum of support that has been critical. In 2016, the VA and WWP created a first-of-its-kind partnership, signing a Memorandum of Understanding (MOU) aimed at ensuring continuity of care and successful discharge planning for Warriors receiving treatment from both WCN and VA. This partnership included providing VA staff to assist part time at each AMC, facilitating coordination of care and integrating the AMC care team.

The MOU and partnership were expanded and enhanced in 2018, establishing four full time VA Liaison positions, embedded at each AMC. The VA Liaisons are responsible for ensuring that medical records are seamlessly shared between VA and WCN, that warriors are fully registered with VA, and that they get follow up care appointments after WCN graduation at the

VA. In 2022, the VA renewed the MOU for a third time, continuing to fund one VA Liaison at each AMC site. Each VA liaison facilitates national referrals throughout the VA system as indicated for mental health or other needs. During 2022 alone, VA Liaisons served 708 warriors. Over the FY 18-22 period (beginning when VA Liaisons were assigned):

- 88% of veterans served by Warrior Care Network took advantage of connecting with a VA Liaison.
- 53% of veterans that met with a VA Liaison discharged from Warrior Care Network with a VA appointment scheduled.
- More than 3,000 referrals for VA care were opened. Among the most requested appointments were mental health care, VA benefits, and primary care.
- More than 19,000 hours of collaborative hours between VA Liaisons and academic medical center employees and veterans.

In sum, Warrior Care Network results and collaboration with VA has validated our belief that community-based, veteran-centric, intensive mental health and substance use care can lead to exceptional health improvements and increased engagement between veterans and VA when properly structured and managed.

Complex Case Coordination (C3)

Wounded Warrior Project's C3 team serves warriors with complex challenges that are often multi-faceted and require urgent action. They connect warriors to internal and external resources and treatment options to provide them with immediate assistance. When working with warriors, the C3 team assesses each of their unique needs and works with them to develop an individualized plan. They work to identify the resources that will best meet the warrior's needs and often act as a liaison between VA, the Department of Defense (DoD), and private community resources throughout the course of the warrior's treatment.

All facilities that the C3 team directs warriors to are carefully vetted by a WWP Clinical Psychologist for modality review while the C3 Director conducts on site vetting for a review of their operations. These facilities must participate in the VA Community Care Network or provide a specialty care need. C3 has established a menu of facilities that offer different types and modalities of care including PTSD, SUD, dual diagnosis, MST, grief, serious mental illness, and eating disorders. These facilities vary from inpatient, residential, partial hospitalization, intense outpatient, and treatment with residential capabilities.

The C3 team works a case in three phases. First, they work to stabilize the warrior, conducting an assessment and determining their needs. The second is to maintain the situation while they work to build an action plan, mobilize resources, and advocate for the warrior's needs. The third is the transition, where the team coordinates wrap around services and conducts follow-up. By pursuing these phases with nearly 1,200 warriors to date, the C3 team has developed significant history referring veterans to VA's Mental Health Residential Rehabilitation Treatment Programs (MH RRTPs) and provides the most significant perspectives on the access to care challenges facing warriors who pursue that care through VA.

Addressing Access Challenges Through Advocacy

As previously stated, WWP's most significant partner in meeting the needs of veterans with SUD and other mental health disorders is VA. Among its most intensive care options are its MH RRTPs, which provide residential treatment services to veterans with mental health issues, SUDs, medical concerns, or those dealing with homelessness or unemployment. There are currently 249 MH RRTPs throughout the country, and they are often an important resource for warriors experiencing co-occurring SUDs and mental health diagnoses. MH RRTPs offer a range of services and evidence-based psychotherapies.

Unfortunately, veteran access to MH RRTPs has been frustrated in several instances by the current access standard landscape. The VA MISSION Act (P.L. 115-182 § 104) required VA to establish access standards for community care and VA subsequently established these standards for primary care, mental health, non-institutional extended care, and specialty care.

However, VA did not include a specific access standard for residential care, and they do not consider MH RRTPs to fall within their access standards for mental health or specialty care.

Access Standards under VHA Directive 1162.02

Instead, VA uses VHA Directive 1162.02 ("Mental Health Residential Rehabilitation Treatment Program") to define the admission criteria for MH RRTPs and to establish when a veteran is eligible for residential care in the community. The Directive states that all admission decisions must be completed within 7 business days from the referral. Veterans requiring priority admission must be admitted within 72 hours. For all other veterans, they must be admitted as soon as possible after a decision has been made. If they cannot be admitted within 30 calendar days, they must be offered alternative residential treatment or another level of care that meets the veteran's needs and preferences. Alternative residential treatment can be a program in the community, another program within the VISN, or another program in another VISN.

Whenever there is a gap of greater than two weeks for any veteran accepted into a mental health RRTP, providers must maintain clinical contact with the veteran until the time of admission, and address any urgent mental health care needs that arise.[30] Under the Directive, this responsibility should generally fall to the Mental Health Treatment Coordinator (MHTC). The MHTC is responsible for ensuring a veteran's continuity of care while receiving mental health treatment. They are to be the veteran's Point of Contact, clinical resource, and member of the veteran's assigned outpatient general mental health team, except under certain circumstances. The MHTC is also supposed to be notified when a veteran is not accepted for care, and they are supposed to be included in the discharge and transition planning process.

Unfortunately, VA's admission goals seem aspirational when compared to its most recent admission data. According to a VA briefing provided to veteran service organizations in February 2023, only 38 percent of veterans assessed as needing priority MH RRTP admission in the first quarter of FY 23 were admitted within 72 hours. While 17 percent requested a later date, this leaves many veterans outside of the window required by the Directive. Similarly, data published by the Government Accountability Office in February 2023 showed that, in Fiscal

---

[30] *See* VHA Handbook 1160.01 ("Uniform Mental Health Services Handbook").

Year 2021, health care systems with mostly rural veterans had an average waiting time above 30 days for MH RRTP programs.[31] Health care systems with some (~27 days) or few rural veterans (~23 days) were only slightly faster.

Wounded Warrior Project's assistance for warriors seeking MH RRTP access, while positive in many instances, has shown similar shortcomings. The lack of a consistently applied access standard has essentially resulted in no true access standard for MH RRTP. Local policy variations have resulted in unpredictable referral decisions. Wait times are not uniformly calculated and can be impacted by inconsistent policies about completion of other, less intensive treatment options. More specifically, some VA facilities will require a veteran to exhaust all outpatient programs before considering them eligible for a MH RRTP program. For patients with co-occurring mental health and substance use disorders, some VA facilities will utilize partial treatments (e.g., SUD care only) while waiting for dual-diagnosis treatment (e.g., treatment for SUD and PTSD) beds to open, satisfying the access standard but not getting the veteran to the appropriate program more promptly. Transparent staffing challenges have limited communication and bed availability. Identifying alternative treatment options that would result in community – or even VA – referrals and faster access to care consistent with Directive access standards are not uniformly accepted. Consequently, some warriors will only pursue care after asking for assistance of a trained and passionate advocate like WWP, or even worse, decided to stop pursuing care altogether.

WWP Access Issues Validated by VA Office of the Inspector General (OIG)

In January 2023, the OIG released a report on noncompliance with community care referrals for MH RRTPs within the VA North Texas Health Care System.[32] The report found a number of instances where the VA North Texas Health Care System failed to follow VHA Directive 1162.02. Throughout most of fiscal years 2020 and 2021, veterans were put on waitlists for two to three months to receive care at the local VA North Texas domiciliary substance use disorder program (DOM SUD) and were not offered referrals for care in the community. Requests by the veterans for community care referrals were inappropriately denied.

The OIG specifically reviewed 15 VA North Texas DOM SUD consults placed for 10 patients as part of their investigation. Seven consults were closed when the patients were admitted within 30 days and two were closed when patients declined admission. Unfortunately, the remaining six consults ended after an average wait time of 79 days before the patient was offered a DOM SUD admission or after being removed from the pending bed placement list.

Although VA North Texas staff knew the wait time to admission for care was over 30 days, no community care options were offered to these patients.

The OIG report concludes that the VA North Texas chief, Patient Administration Services, misinterpreted VA policy on MH RRTP care and community care referrals and provided inaccurate information to staff and patients. The report goes on to say that "failure to discuss alternative resources or treatment options, including community residential care, may have

[31] GOV'T ACCOUNTABILITY OFF., VA MENTAL HEALTH: ADDITIONAL ACTION NEEDED TO ASSESS RURAL VETERANS' ACCESS TO INTENSIVE CARE 31 (Feb. 2023).

[32] OFF. OF INSP. GENERAL, U.S. DEP'T OF VET. AFFAIRS, NONCOMPLIANCE WITH COMMUNITY CARE REFERRALS FOR SUBSTANCE ABUSE RESIDENTIAL TREATMENT AT THE VA NORTH TEXAS HEALTH CARE SYSTEM (Jan. 2023).

contributed to patient's increased risk of negative outcomes due to delayed access to DOM SUD services."

This report found other instances of VA North Texas failing to follow VHA policy. The Bonham MH RRTP failed to follow VHA's minimum scheduling requirements to contact veterans four times to schedule a requested service before closing a consult. The OIG wrote that this "failure to adhere to VHA minimum scheduling requirements may hinder efficient patient scheduling and contribute to barriers to accessing DOM SUD services." VA North Texas also failed to follow the VHA requirement that staff assign a mental health treatment coordinator to patients that are either receiving outpatient mental health treatment, have been admitted to an inpatient mental health setting, or those that are waiting to receive a different level of care, such as those waiting for placement at an MH RRTP.

In their response, VA North Texas noted that this time period was during the peak of the COVID-19 pandemic and that VA North Texas had the highest COVID-19 census in the VA system for several months in 2020 and 2021. They also point out that some community care facilities were not accepting admissions during this time. VA North Texas argues that staff were doing the best they could with difficult circumstances and that while VA guidance was misinterpreted, very few patients were ultimately affected. While this may be true in this specific instance, WWP has seen a pattern of these types of issues reported at VA North Texas around the country.

Action in Progress

As WWP has consistently raised the problems with MH RRTP access over several months, we appreciate that Congress has taken important steps to address the mental health and substance use crisis amongst our veteran population in recent years. The Commander John Scott Hannon Veterans Mental Health Care Improvement Act (P.L. 116-171 § 201) required VA to develop a clinical provider treatment toolkit and accompanying training materials for comorbid mental health conditions, comorbid mental health and substance use disorders, and comorbid mental health and chronic pain. That toolkit is now publicly available on the VA website.

The Support the Resiliency of Our Nation's Great (STRONG) Veterans Act (P.L. 117-328, Div. V § 303) included provisions related to SUD and mental health. Section 503 requires VA to conduct a study on inpatient mental health and substance use care at VA, including if there are sufficient geographic offerings for inpatient mental health care, sufficient bed spaces, and wait times. The study must also include recommendations on new locations for RRTPs and where new beds can be added. Section 504 also requires a study on treatment at VA for co-occurring mental health and SUDs. The study must include information on the availability of treatment programs, geographic disparities in access to these programs, and average wait times. WWP is eager to see the results of these reports and use them to inform future advocacy.

Moreover, to the extent access issues are created by staffing shortages, WWP is grateful for recent congressional action to improve VA's mental health staffing capabilities. The *STRONG Veterans Act* (P.L. 117-328, Div. V) also includes provisions that will expand the Vet Center workforce (§ 102), create more paid trainee positions in mental health disciplines (§ 103), and offer more scholarship and loan repayment opportunities for those pursuing degrees or training in mental health fields (§ 104).

Recommendations for Future Action

While WWP applauds the work Congress and VA have already undertaken, there is much more work to be done. Based on the data we've outlined and our experiences attempting to place warriors into residential care for co-occurring mental health issues and SUDs, WWP provides the following recommendations:

VA Access Standards Must Ensure Prompt Access to Residential Mental Health and Substance Use Services

The access standards contemplated by the VA MISSION Act (P.L. 115-182 § 104) and memorialized in the Code of Federal Regulations (38 C.F.R. § 17.4040) do not, in practice, extend to mental or substance use disorder care provided in a residential setting. VA has maintained adherence to access standards for this type of care through VHA Directive 1162.02, which establishes a priority admission standard of 72 hours and, for all other cases, 30 days before a veteran must be offered (not necessarily provided) alternative residential treatment or another level of care that meets the veteran's needs and preferences at the time of screening.

Due to this approach, veterans seeking mental or substance use disorder care provided in a residential setting are not subject to the access standard protections assigned under law. VA is not required to inform these veterans of their expected wait time. See P.L. 117-328, Div. U, § 122. Veterans are not guaranteed the soonest possible starting time before a community referral must be made. See P.L. 117-328, Div. U, § 121; 38 U.S.C. § 1703(d)(4). The access standards used are not applicable to community care network providers who receive referrals for these veterans' care. See P.L. 117-328, Div. U, § 125; 38 U.S.C. § 1703B(f).

Most importantly, if appropriate community-based providers are identified and available to provide treatment, veterans waiting beyond VHA's policy-backed access standards have no dependable, consistent recourse to be referred for that care. VA has presented data suggesting that only 38% of veterans meeting priority admission criteria were admitted to VA within 72 hours, and that the average wait time before admission among all veterans receiving MH RRTP care was 24 days – just 6 days less than the 30-day access standard and among a population where 53% were admitted within 14 days (information on admissions within 30 days was not provided in the presentation).

At least two approaches show potential to address this problem. First, 38 U.S.C. § 1703(d)(1) can be amended to specifically include access standards for residential mental health or substance-use services.[33]10 Second, 38 U.S.C. § 1703B can be amended to ensure that residential mental health or substance-use services are included as part of the extended care service access standards that VA must prescribe. Either path would help provide certainty that access standards are not left to VA policy and carry the same opportunities and predictability that are extended to other medical services as part of the VA MISSION Act.

---

[33] *See, e.g.*, S.5348 (117th Congress).

Advance Policies that Promote a Stronger Mental Health and Substance Use Treatment Provider Base Across the United States

In January 2023, the U.S. Department of Health and Human Services' (HHS) Substance Abuse and Mental Health Services Administration (SAMHSA) released the results of its 2021 National Survey on Drug Use and Health (NSDUH), which contains fresh evidence of the extent of mental health and substance use challenges across the country.[34] Results from the survey show that while veterans may be at heightened risk for these health challenges and more likely to experience them, the broader national context must be considered to help adequately address access to care issues that exist and may continue to arise.

Among the findings most pertinent to today's hearing, 29.5 million people aged 12 or older showed alcohol use disorder, 24.0 million showed a drug use disorder, and 5.6 million showed an opioid use disorder.[35] These findings run parallel to findings that nearly 1 in 4 U.S. adults with a mental illness[36] and are particularly striking within the context that more than 150 million Americans live in a federally designated mental health professional shortage area.[37]

One way for Congress to act outside of the VA health system – but nevertheless helping veterans, particularly those in underserved areas – is to pass S. 462, the Mental Health Professionals Workforce Shortage Loan Repayment Act.[38] This bill would authorize the federal government to repay up to $250,000 in eligible student loan repayment for mental health professionals who work in mental health shortage areas. As written, this bill requires an annual commitment to full time employment in substance use disorder treatment. Although the STRONG Veterans Act enhanced and expanded VA's internal staffing capabilities, we believe that policies to help address a nationwide shortage of medical personnel will bring stronger assurance that mental health and substance use services are available to veterans regardless of whether it is initially pursued at VA.

Ensure More Consistent Reporting on the Relationship Between SUD and Veteran Suicide

According to VA's National Veteran Suicide Prevention Annual Report for 2022, the prevalence of alcohol use disorder among "Recent Veteran VHA Users" who died by suicide was 19.6%, cannabis use disorder 8.3%, and opioid use disorder 4.9%.[39] Overall, while suicide rates fell from 2019 through 2020 for those with any mental health or SUD diagnosis, suicide

---

[34] SUBST. ABUSE AND MENTAL HEALTH SVCS., KEY SUBSTANCE USE AND MENTAL HEALTH INDICATORS IN THE UNITED STATES: RESULTS FROM THE 2021 NATIONAL SURVEY ON DRUG USE AND HEALTH, *available at* https://www.samhsa.gov/data/sites/default/files/reports/rpt39443/2021NSDUHFFRRev010323.pdf.

[35] *Id.* at 32.

[36] *Id.* at 39.

[37] BUREAU OF HEALTH WORKFORCE, HEALTH RES. AND SERVS. ADMIN., U.S. DEP'T OF HEALTH AND HUMAN SERVS., DESIGNATED HEALTH PROFESSIONAL SHORTAGE AREAS STATISTICS, FIRST QUARTER OF FISCAL YEAR 2023 (Jan. 2023) (as of December 31, 2022).

[38] Federal regulations stipulate that, to be considered as having a shortage of providers, a designation must have a population-to-provide ratio that meets or exceeds a certain threshold. Mental health designations may qualify for designation based on the population to psychiatrist ratio, the population to core mental health provider ratio, or the population to both psychiatrist and core mental health provider ratio.

[39] Off. of Mental Health and Suicide Prevention, U.S. Dep't of Vet. Affairs, 2022 National Suicide Prevention Annual Report 27 (Sept. 2022).

rates rose for those with substance use disorders.[40] Insights like these are helpful for policymaking; the data above is particularly compelling for the subject of today's hearing. Yet even though access to mental health and substance use disorder services is a VHA priority and part of VA's National Strategy for Preventing Suicide, comparable data was not presented in the 2021 report. In 2020 and 2019, mental health and substance use disorder discussion covers periods dating back to 200518;[41] however, no comparable data can be found in the September 2018 report.

While we appreciate the earnest efforts of VA to report on veteran suicide data, WWP supports the laudable goal of more comprehensive and consistent annual reporting. The Not Just A Number Act (S. 928) would create several annual reporting requirements for VA, including an examination of trends in suicide rates or deaths among veterans who have a diagnosis of substance use disorder. In addition to creating expectations about consistent reporting on health data and trends, this legislation would go considerably further by looking at trends related to Veterans Benefits Administration usage that have not been addressed in prior annual reporting. In sum, passing this legislation would create more potential for VA and the broader veteran support community to make more informed decisions about where to focus resources to help prevent veteran suicide.

Make Case Management Services More Accessible

Wounded Warrior Project's approach to helping warriors find care for co-occurring SUD and mental health disorders has been successful thanks in part to strong case coordination and communication. As discussed previously, VA Liaisons co-located at Warrior Care Network's partner academic medical centers have been an indispensable tool in creating a stronger continuum of care for warrior patients. Between FY 2018 and FY 2022, that collaboration has resulted in over 9,000 cases consultations by VA staff at academic medical centers.

Similarly, our C3 program has also delivered more positive results for veterans on account of close collaboration with VA. Among nearly 1,200 veterans served though C3, 30 percent of those enrolled for care at VA stated the VA is not aware of their current mental health situation. Because C3 works to identify community-based providers that are in the Community Care Network, our advocacy on the veteran's behalf often results in significant communication with local VA mental health leaders once veteran permission is acquired. Subsequent VA- provided referrals for care result in lower out-of-pocket expenses for the veteran than what may have been sought independently (or without WWP assistance) and closer coordination of care before and after community-based treatment.

This positive engagement with VA can go even further when considering the typical presentation of a warrior who works with our C3 program. For example, 16 percent of warriors did not have an appointed primary care provider at VA before working with WWP and subsequently established a point of contact for current and ongoing referrals. 78 percent had been unemployed for 6 months or more and could surely benefit from more streamlined support

[40] *Id.*

[41] OFF. OF MENTAL HEALTH AND SUICIDE PREVENTION, U.S. DEP'T OF VET. AFFAIRS, 2020 NATIONAL SUICIDE PREVENTION ANNUAL REPORT 27-28 (Sept. 2020); OFF. OF MENTAL HEALTH AND SUICIDE PREVENTION, U.S. DEP'T OF VET. AFFAIRS, 2019 NATIONAL SUICIDE PREVENTION ANNUAL REPORT 12-13 (Sept. 2019).

from Veterans Benefits Administration programs like Veteran Readiness and Employment. An equivalent number of veterans also reported unstable housing as a barrier to care. Future care for other conditions would appear more likely as well given that these veterans often present with multiple medical diagnoses (1,149 clinical diagnoses among 422 warriors in a recent sample).

One program that may warrant closer inspection is VA's Mental Health Intensive Case Management program. These programs are required at Veterans Health Administration health care systems serving 1,500 or more veterans identified on the National Psychosis Registry.

Designed specifically to optimize the health status, quality of life, and community functioning of veterans diagnosed with serious mental illness who frequently utilize VA mental health inpatient and emergency services, perhaps a complementary program can be made available to veterans with less severe medical diagnoses.

Given how the veterans we serve often present with complex needs, inspiration for improvements to case management can be found in the Federal Recovery Coordination Program (FRCP) that previously assigned recovering Service members with recovery care coordinators responsible for overseeing and assisting the Service member in their course through the entire spectrum of care, management, transition, and rehabilitation services available from the federal government. The program also called for assignment of medical care managers and non-medical care managers who were responsible for, among other tasks, helping resolve problems involving financial, administrative, transitional, and other matters that arose during recovery and transition.

In 2018, the FRCP transformed into the Federal Recovery Consultant Office (FRCO) in response to the Presidential Executive Order, "Comprehensive Plan for Reorganizing the Executive Branch." While this shift may have created some efficiencies, WWP encourages a fresh assessment of whether the FRCO can serve as a similar hub for veterans seeking more assistance with complex cases involving SUD and/or mental health disorders. WWP's experience has shown that veterans are likely to benefit from a heightened level of support often present with co-occurring SUD and mental health disorders.

Conclusion

Wounded Warrior Project thanks the Subcommittee on Health and its distinguished members for inviting our organization to submit this statement. We are grateful for your attention and efforts towards addressing this critical issue of substance abuse amongst our nation's veterans. We look forward to continuing to work with you on these issues and are standing by to assist in any way we can towards our shared goals of serving those that have served this country.

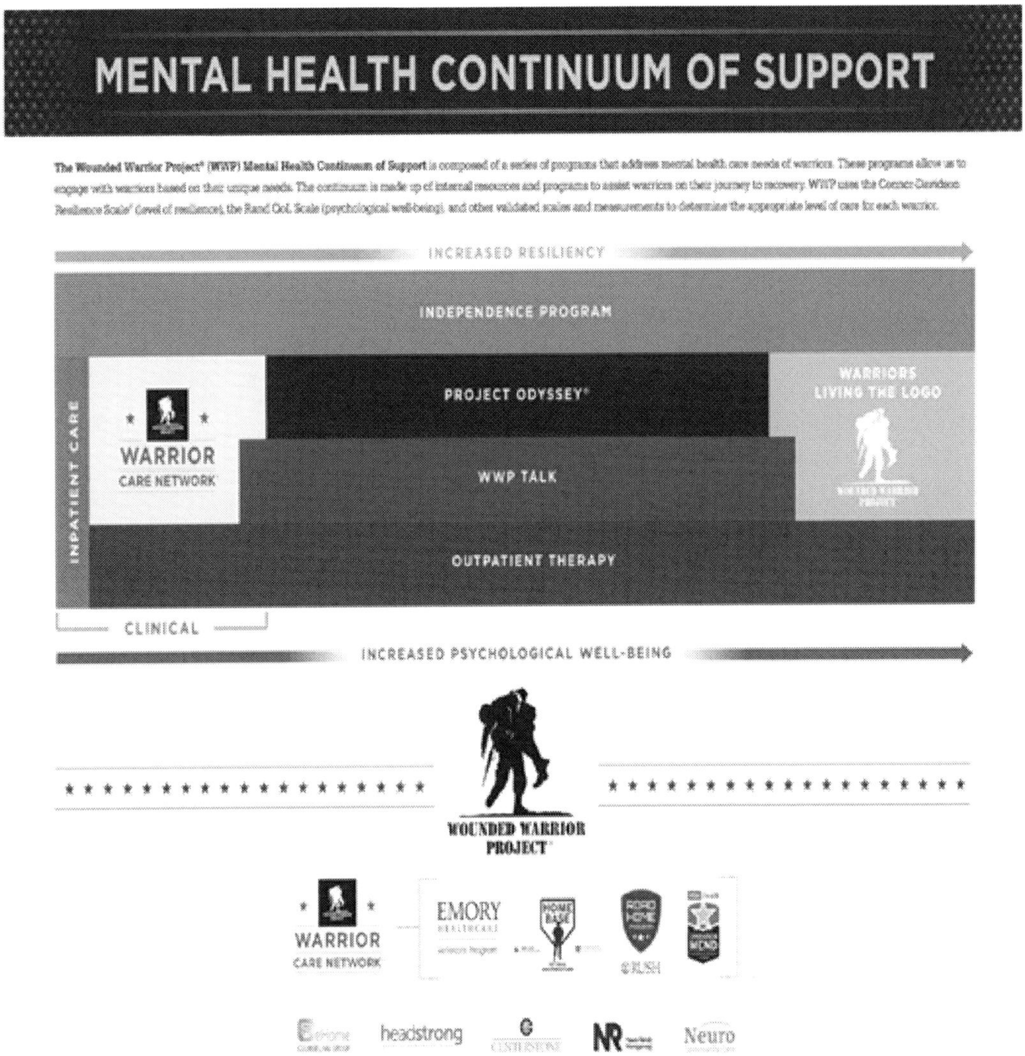
MENTAL HEALTH CONTINUUM OF SUPPORT
The Wounded Warrior Project® (WWP) Mental Health Continuum of Support is composed of a series of programs that address mental health care needs of warriors. These programs allow us to engage with warriors based on their unique needs. The continuum is made up of internal resources and programs to assist warriors on their journey to recovery. WWP uses the Connor-Davidson Resilience Scale (level of resilience), the Rand QoL Scale (psychological well-being), and other validated scales and measurements to determine the appropriate level of care for each warrior.
INCREASED RESILIENCY
INDEPENDENCE PROGRAM
INPATIENT CARE
WARRIOR CARE NETWORK
PROJECT ODYSSEY®
WARRIORS LIVING THE LOGO
WWP TALK
OUTPATIENT THERAPY
CLINICAL
INCREASED PSYCHOLOGICAL WELL-BEING
WOUNDED WARRIOR PROJECT®
WARRIOR CARE NETWORK
EMORY HEALTHCARE
HOME BASE
ROAD HOME
RUSH
headstrong
Neuro

The continuum of support doesn't define an exact, prescriptive path to recovery, rather the individual needs of each warrior to determine the order and frequency of appropriate program engagement. For example, a warrior in acute psychological distress may be referred to a number of clinical intervention programs. Another warrior with less severe mental health issues may participate in only one or two programs. Subsequently, any warrior who has a setback may be re-evaluated and referred back to one or more programs for additional care. The goal is to provide the appropriate amount of care a warrior may need to get to his or her highest possible level of resilience, psychological well-being, and healing.

INPATIENT CARE
Clinical Intervention

Inpatient care is reserved for warriors in severe psychological distress who have exhausted all other resources. WWP may be able to fund inpatient services in order to stabilize warriors so that they can be engaged with other mental health programs in the continuum. The goal is to sustain and facilitate movement in the continuum through other programs.

WARRIOR CARE NETWORK
Clinical Intervention

To accelerate the development of advanced models of mental health care, WWP partners with four world-renowned academic medical centers to form Warrior Care Network®, leveraging our collective commitment and expertise. The Warrior Care Network treatment model delivers a year's worth of mental health care during a two- to three-week intensive outpatient program (IOP). This unique veteran-centric approach increases access to treatment and improves outcomes. Warrior Care Network provides a path to long-term wellness, improving the way warriors are treated today and for generations to come.

PROJECT ODYSSEY
Engagement Intervention

Project Odyssey is a 12-week mental health program that uses adventure-based learning to help warriors manage and overcome their invisible wounds, enhance their resiliency skills, and empower them to live productive and fulfilling lives. Based on their unique needs, warriors can participate in an all-male, all-female, or couples Project Odyssey. The program starts with a five-day mental health workshop, where warriors are challenged to step outside the comfort of their everyday routines. This opens them up to new experiences that help develop their coping and communication skills. After the workshop, participants work together with WWP to stay engaged, achieve their personal goals, and make lifelong positive changes.

★ PROGRAMS WITH MULTIPLE STAGES OF ENGAGEMENT ★

Within the continuum of support there are additional programs/resources that can be engaged at nearly any point in the continuum. These are WWP Talk and outpatient therapy. The Independence Program, which also encompasses multiple stages of engagement, is a unique component of the continuum. The resources provided by the Independence Program allow the most severely wounded warriors the ability to lead a full life at home instead of a long-term facility.

OUTPATIENT THERAPY • *Engagement and Clinical Intervention*

An additional clinical resource available to warriors across the stages of the continuum is outpatient therapy. Here WWP funds external partners to provide individual, family, or couples therapy delivered by a culturally competent therapist in the closest geographic location to the warriors as possible. With multiple funded clinical partners, warriors are able to engage in traditional outpatient sessions or, if in a remote location, engage in virtual therapy.

WWP TALK • *Engagement and Coordination Intervention*

WWP Talk is a telephonic emotional support program that breaks down the barriers of isolation and helps both warriors and family members plan an individualized path toward their personal growth. Participants work one-on-one with a dedicated team member during weekly emotional-support calls. Together, they set tangible goals and develop skills that lead to positive changes, like increased resilience and improved psychological well-being.

INDEPENDENCE PROGRAM
Engagement, Coordination, and Clinical Intervention

The Independence Program provides long-term support to catastrophically wounded warriors living with injuries such as: a moderate to severe brain injury, spinal cord injury, or neurological condition that impacts independence. The program is designed to support warriors who, without high-touch services, would struggle to live day to day due to the severity of their injuries. The Independence Program increases access to community services, provides rehabilitation through alternative therapies, and empowers warriors to achieve goals leading to a more independent life. Because every journey is different, we work as a team with warriors, their family members, and their caregivers to set goals to live a fulfilling life, at home, with their loved ones.

★ LIVING THE LOGO ★

WOUNDED WARRIOR PROJECT

The WWP logo is much more than a trademark – it is what we see as the ultimate goal for all warriors engaged with the continuum of support to achieve. It is the collective goal of the continuum of support (through resources and teammates) to empower warriors to make it to this final phase and live our logo. The logo, one warrior carrying another warrior, represents a peer assisting a fellow veteran – in essence, carrying him through the recovery process until he can walk of his own accord (through heightened resiliency and psychological well-being). Eventually, as resiliency reaches the highest levels in the continuum, warriors are empowered to help carry fellow veterans, essentially becoming force multipliers as they are engaged as peer mentors.

Thomas Sauer Miramar Health April 18, 2023

Testimony before the House Veterans Affairs Committee, Subcommittee on Health

Chair Miller-Meeks, Ranking Member Brownley, and members of the Subcommittee:

I am honored to testify before you today. My name is Tom Sauer, and I'm a Navy and Marine Corps Veteran, having spent the better part of my adult life wearing the cloth of our nation. I'm a former enlisted Marine infantryman, a 2006 Naval Academy graduate, and a former Navy Explosive Ordnance Disposal officer. Today, however, I'm the owner and CEO of Miramar

Health, a Veteran-owned and operated Community Care Provider for intensive substance use disorder (SUD) and mental health treatment, exclusively for America's Veterans.

Mental health and addiction treatment are deep passions of mine, because depression and addiction killed my dad. Five days before I graduated from high school, and three weeks before I shipped out for the Marines in 1999, a methamphetamine overdose took his life after decades of struggle, just like so many millions of Americans suffering from our country's disastrous mental health and addiction crisis.

Thanks to recent legislation, thousands of veterans have enhanced access to life-saving mental healthcare and addiction treatment within the VA's Community Care Network (CCN). We've provided intensive, custom-tailored, world-class mental health and addiction treatment for nearly 250 Veterans from a dozen VA Medical Centers across the Western United States, typically for 30, 60, and sometimes 90+ days. This treatment is for our veterans who are truly suffering, in crisis, and often near death from suicide or overdose resulting from America's disastrous mental health and addiction crisis.

In three and a half years, we've grown from one small clinic with six employees, to eight residential facilities and one large outpatient facility. These facilities are staffed by nearly 100 phenomenal physicians, nurses, psychologists, therapists, medical technicians, case managers, and support staff, many of whom are Veterans themselves. I could not be any prouder of them.

I didn't come all the way out here to tell you this just so I could pat myself on the back, but rather to simply convey the sincerity of our intentions and to lay out how important this challenge is. Miramar believes in our partnership with the VA by bridging both capability and capacity gaps within certain VAMCs and in being an advocate to Veterans in need, all while providing them with the highest quality care.

In other words, we do not consider ourselves to be just another government contractor. We are partners and teammates with the VA, and we're here asking for your help to ensure our nation's Veterans receive the lifesaving care they need and deserve by strengthening that partnership.

The overwhelming majority of front-line, boots-on-the-ground VA personnel we directly interact with are fantastic, dedicated, and lifesaving public servants. There are many who, in my mind, deserve medals and parades for saving the lives of Veterans.

I am here today to advocate for veterans in need to access care ANYWHERE, IMMEDIATELY, and we can figure out the paperwork later. The current VA policy of having 30 days to find a bed in a given region does not meet the URGENT LEVEL of this CRISIS.

Specifically, we've encountered several occasions where, despite community care being available for a Veteran in crisis, they're either put onto waiting lists for up to 30 days before receiving care, when they don't have 30 minutes without becoming a very real risk to suicide or overdose. I have first-hand knowledge of these suicides and overdose deaths since I've owned Miramar, so I understand the devastation this policy can cause.

We believe this issue could be rather easily corrected through a legislative carve-out for Community Care eligibility, as with Urgent Care, when it comes to urgent and emergency mental health and addiction treatment.

This could be done by clarifying and ensuring the COMPACT Act is being implemented as intended and that Veterans are aware of this option for receiving care.

We urge you to ensure that our veterans have access to the care they need when they need it through the Community Care Network.

We appreciate your consideration of this matter, and we are willing to work with you to address these issues and ensure that our guys and gals get the care they so desperately need.

Thank you, Chair and members of the Subcommittee. Each of you, your staffers, and the committee's staff are champions for America's Veterans, so I am exceptionally grateful to you and your commitment to serving them, and that you are holding this important hearing today.

In conclusion, thank you for addressing the issues we raised today. Veterans' lives depend on it. Thank you again for the opportunity to appear, and I look forward to answering your questions.

Prepared Statement of Brendan Dowling

Good morning, Chair Miller-Meeks, Ranking Member Brownley, and distinguished members of the subcommittee.

My name is Brendan Dowling, and I am currently Miramar Health's Veteran Outreach Manager.

I am formerly a Navy SEAL that served in multiple military campaigns for the Global War on Terror from 2001–2014. My service spanned across numerous deployments in multiple combat zones.

Since last summer, I have had the pleasure of visiting over 141 VA facilities that provide medical, clinical, counseling, or VBA services to Veterans across the Western US.

This includes 94 VHA facilities; 18 Medical Centers, 74 Community Based Outpatient Clinic's, and 35 Veteran Centers.

I look forward to answering any questions you may have.

Statement for the Record

Prepared Statement of Cohen Veterans Network

Cohen Veterans Network

Cohen Veterans Network
72 Cummings Point Road
Stamford, CT 06902

Cohen Veterans Network
Statement of Dr Anthony Hassan
Chief Executive Officer
On
"Combatting a Crisis: Providing Veterans Access to Life Saving Substance Abuse Disorder Treatment"
April 18, 2023

Dear Chairwoman Miller-Meeks, Ranking Member Brownley, and distinguished Subcommittee Members,

On behalf of the 50,000 veterans and family members that we have served in our network of 24 outpatient mental health clinics across 15 states, thank you for the invitation to submit a statement for the record to the Subcommittee on Health, Committee on Veterans' Affairs Legislative Hearing. We appreciate the opportunity to address the importance of access to outpatient mental health care, especially substance use disorder treatment for our veterans. Effective early intervention is vital in prevention of chronic and severe behavioral health conditions and related alcohol and substance use comorbidities which may develop as a consequence of escalating biopsychosocial challenges and attempts to self-medicate in its absence. Moreover, it is instrumental in managing risk for subsequent suicidal behaviors and overdose which unfortunately, are increasingly endemic within our veteran population.

Cohen Veterans Network, Inc. (CVN) is a not-for-profit philanthropic organization [501(c)(3)] founded in 2016. CVN is focused on delivering mental health services for post-9/11 veterans, service members, and their families. Cohen Military Family Clinics are committed to improving mental health outcomes through a network of customized, outpatient clinics in high-need communities, in which trained clinicians deliver client-centered, evidence-based care. Additionally, CVN is committed to removing barriers to care and advancing the field of mental health.

CVN provides accessible outpatient behavioral health care for veterans and their family members. Services are provided without regard to the clients' ability to pay or characterization of discharge. Family is defined broadly, including veteran's spouses but also parents, siblings, adult children, and others as defined by the veteran. The CVN model is client centered, evidence based, and targeted. Core services include psychotherapy using evidence-based protocols and industry best practices, medication management, and case management.

Evidence based protocols and practices are utilized to address mental health adjustment and family issues which may be contributing factors in the veteran's care. Approximately 53% of CVN clients are veterans or active-duty military members with 47% family members including adults and children. Top presenting problems include family concerns, anxiety, adjustment disorders, depression, and posttraumatic stress disorder (PTSD). All clients receive a comprehensive screening including the Columbia Suicide Severity Rating Scale (CSSRS) and a full biopsychosocial assessment prior to beginning treatment. CVN conducts comprehensive screening for alcohol and substance misuse, abuse, and dependence as they are frequent co-occurring conditions for individuals seeking mental health treatment. Given the complex needs presented by many veterans, medication management and case

Cohen Veterans Network

Cohen Veterans Network
72 Cummings Point Road
Stamford, CT 06902

management are readily available to all clients seen in our clinics. This extra support is vital to decrease self-management, link veterans to more support and guide them through healing and recovery.

The Criticality of Accessible Upstream Intervention for Veteran's Coping with Mental Health Issues

The US is currently facing a national crisis in mental health and mental healthcare, however rates of mental health disorders among post 9-11 veterans remain significantly higher still. Suicide risk for both male and female veterans are dramatically above those of their civilian counterparts. In the VAs (Veterans Affairs) 2022 annual report the rate was cited as 57.3% above the rate for non-veteran adults. Furthermore, research indicates that current substance use disorders (SUDs) signal increased suicide risk among veterans especially among women, and that co-occurring psychiatric disorders partially explained associations between SUDs and suicide.[1] Alcohol and Substance use disorders (AUD/SUD) have been reported to occur at a rate of approximately 11% in veterans seeking care from the VHA (Veterans Health Administration) and onset of SUDs can emerge secondary to and comorbid with other mental health problems such as post-traumatic stress disorder (PTSD) and depression.[2] Comorbidity of SUD (substance use disorder) among those with PTSD has been reported between 35-50% and these patients have been found to have greater drug use severity and worse treatment outcomes.[3] Additionally marital and family issues have been identified as significant factors among veteran families due to a range of military specific challenges including frequent relocations and deployments over the course of a military career with spouses reporting higher rates of mental health issues including depression than their civilian counterparts.

Women veterans report the highest rates of PTSD among post 9-11 veterans and per VA data, one in three women veterans have experienced military sexual trauma (MST). The incidence of lifetime SUD is significantly higher for women veterans with a history of sexual assault. Moreover, needs assessments suggest that their unique service needs may not be ideally met within the VA, and many are unaware of or fail to take advantage of their VA benefits based on their failure to identify as veterans

Access and Eligibility Within the VA

Challenges related to access and wait times within the Veterans Health Administration have been well established but perhaps more germane to the current discussion is the rates at which veterans receive care through the VA. Based on the agencies own estimates about two thirds of veterans receive their

---

[1] Bohnert, K. M., Ilgen, M. A., Louzon, S., McCarthy, J. F., and Katz, I. R. (2017) Substance use disorders and the risk of suicide mortality among men and women in the US Veterans Health Administration. *Addiction*, 112: 1193– 1201. doi: 10.1111/add.13774.

[2] Teeters, J. B., Lancaster, C. L., Brown, D. G., & Back, S. E. (2017). Substance use disorders in military veterans: prevalence and treatment challenges. *Substance abuse and rehabilitation*, *8*, 69–77. https://doi.org/10.2147/SAR.S116720

[3] Boden, M.T., Kimerling, R., Jacobs-Lentz, J., Bowman, D., Weaver, C., Carney, D., Walser, R. and Trafton, J.A. (2012), Seeking Safety treatment for male veterans with a substance use disorder and post-traumatic stress disorder symptomatology. Addiction, 107: 578-586. https://doi.org/10.1111/j.1360-0443.2011.03658.x

Cohen Veterans Network

Cohen Veterans Network
72 Cummings Point Road
Stamford, CT 06902

healthcare outside this system. This is due to a multitude of factors including not only wait times but also eligibility, awareness, and preference. As a result of this a robust network of accessible and culturally competent services is necessary to serve these veterans who are unlikely to be seen within the VA. Current VA access standards require a veteran to be seen within 30 days but may seldom be met. VA uses VHA Directive 1162.02 ("Mental Health Residential Rehabilitation Treatment Program") to define the admission criteria for MH RRTPs and to establish when a veteran is eligible for residential care in the community. This Directive states that all admission decisions must be completed within 7 business days of the referral. Veterans requiring priority admission must be admitted within 72 hours. In all other cases, the veteran must be admitted as soon as possible after the decision has been made. If a veteran cannot be admitted within 30 calendar days, alternative residential treatment or another level of care that meets the veteran's needs and preferences must be offered. Alternative residential treatment can be a program in the community or another program within the VA. In cases where there is a gap of two weeks or more for a veteran accepted into a mental health RRTP, clinical contact must be maintained until the time of admission, and urgent mental health care needs that arise must be addressed. The MHTC is responsible for ensuring a veteran's continuity of care while receiving mental health treatment.

Given these limitations and the relatively small proportion of veterans who receive their care through the VA, the case is easily made that other community providers and Veteran Service Organizations play a key role in meeting the needs for essential services for mental health and SUD care. Accessible community-based care may function as a stopgap or interim resource or an alternative to VHA where access is insufficient, or services are unavailable. In recognition of these realities funding and coordinating with these services becomes imperative. Additionally restrictive policies related to duration of services or payment to these community agencies needs to be addressed in light of the need for robust partnership vs. competition in providing desperately needed care in an expeditious, deliberate, and coordinated manner.

How CVN Services Address Upstream Drivers of Low-Density High-Cost Residential Care

At CVN we have diagnosed and managed over 1,659 veterans with AUD/SUD since 2018. Early and upstream intervention for depression, anxiety and post-traumatic stress pave demonstrable impact on the trajectory of veterans through the care system. Comorbidities with other mental health disorders in veterans treated at CVN were identified at elevated levels with approximately 78% of SUD diagnoses occurring in conjunction with 1 or more comorbid disorders, including depression (47%), anxiety (26%) and PTSD (46%). Evidence based interventions to address symptoms and enhance quality of life, reduce subsequent levels of care required, hospitalizations and emergency department visits. Early outpatient mental health intervention, especially in conjunction with case management services may prevent development of severe symptoms, build coping skills, and address marital and family conflict reducing risk of suicide, as well as further health and mental health crises, overdose and even homelessness among veteran populations.

CVN provides focused intervention through episodes of care averaging 8-12 sessions over a typical course of 120-180 days with rates of remission and clinically significant change which rival those reported in comparable samples based on an independent validation study. Few veterans who receive care require referral to a higher level of care and average improvements on quality of life (QLES-SF) and Dyadic Adjustment are considerable. Wait times for care vary across clinics with a goal of < 14

Cohen Veterans
Network

Cohen Veterans Network
72 Cummings Point Road
Stamford, CT 06902

days and a typical wait time of under 30 days to receive biopsychosocial assessment with subsequent initiation of therapy within 7-10 days thereafter. CVNs goals are not only to save lives but to change lives. Early intervention is critical for success and is robustly supported by the business case as compared with higher levels of care which are associated with the increased severity and chronicity of symptoms and disorders which develop when these issues are not identified and treated at an early stage.

On the issue of SUDs, the VA would be well served to enhance its existing Community Care Network (CCN) to ensure that access standards are met and that veterans in crisis are not being maintained on waiting lists or managed at levels of care inadequate to their assessed treatment needs. With the standard set for 72 hours for priority admission to residential/inpatient SUD care, the VHA will need additional purchased care options in most if not all localities on a continuous or recurring basis and the standard should not be violated to accommodate patients in VA direct care to improve VA metrics at any level. Embracing community partnerships and ensuring effective coordination of care must guide the future direction in terms of SUD/AUD treatment for the benefit of veterans and their families.

At CVN we are committed to doing our part to address veteran mental health needs and supporting the larger effort currently undertaken by the VHA in conjunction with our partner veteran serving organizations (VSOs) to assure effective and timely care is being provided to veterans experiencing SUD/AUD. Our 24 clinics will continue to support their communities by addressing relational and adjustment challenges and common comorbidities which predispose veterans to or lead to more significant mental health concerns concomitant with greater disruptions in functioning and requiring higher levels of care

Looking forward, CVN will continue to strongly support the existing CVN-VAMC partnerships and do our utmost to foster new ones. We are eager to continue to work with VA, VHA as part of the VA Community Care Network to continue to expand the support available to veterans to treat the comorbidities which frequently occur with substance abuse disorders and to improve veterans' quality of life. CVN thanks Chairwoman Miller-Meeks and the other distinguished members of the Subcommittee on Health for their tireless and essential life-saving efforts on behalf of our US veterans. We look forward to continuing to work with you on these vital issues.

Cohen Veterans
Network

Cohen Veterans Network
72 Cummings Point Road
Stamford, CT 06902

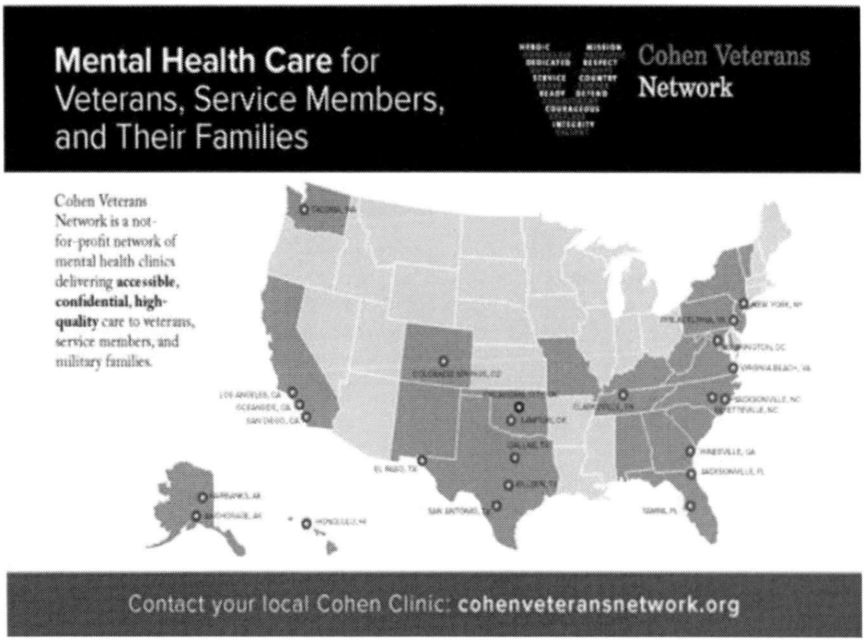

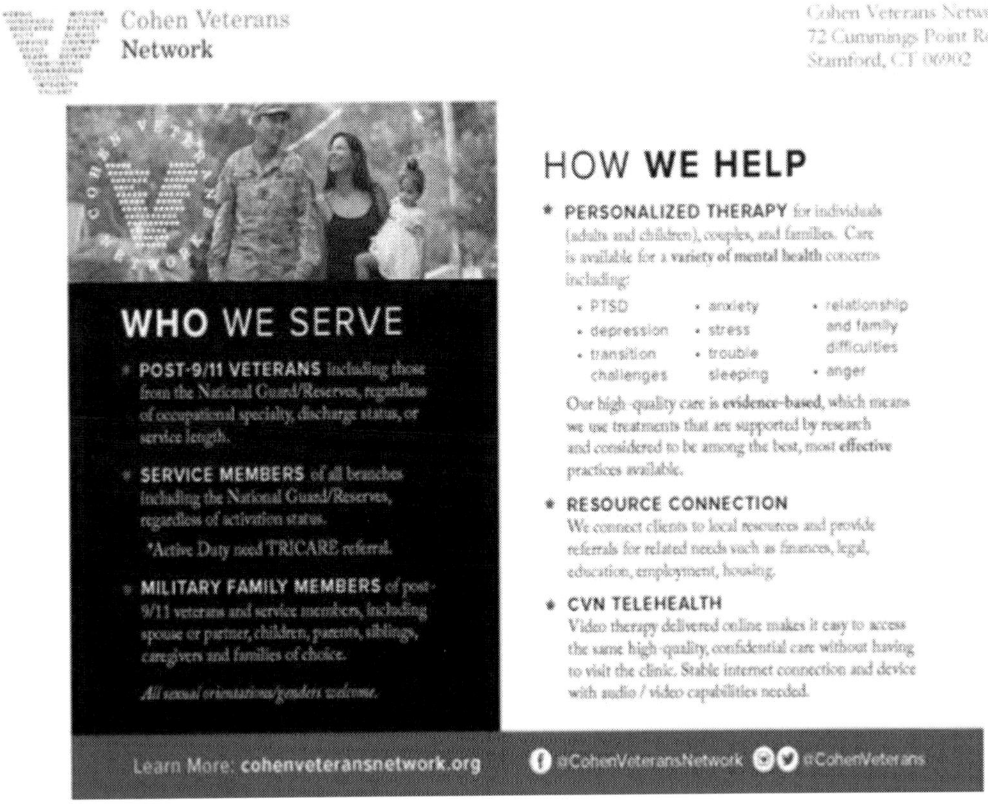
Cohen Veterans Network
Cohen Veterans Network
72 Cummings Point Road
Stamford, CT 06902
WHO WE SERVE
POST-9/11 VETERANS including those from the National Guard/Reserves, regardless of occupational specialty, discharge status, or service length.
SERVICE MEMBERS of all branches including the National Guard/Reserves, regardless of activation status.
*Active Duty need TRICARE referral.
MILITARY FAMILY MEMBERS of post-9/11 veterans and service members, including spouse or partner, children, parents, siblings, caregivers and families of choice.
All sexual orientations/genders welcome.
HOW WE HELP
PERSONALIZED THERAPY for individuals (adults and children), couples, and families. Care is available for a variety of mental health concerns including:
PTSD
depression
transition challenges
anxiety
stress
trouble sleeping
relationship and family difficulties
anger
Our high-quality care is evidence-based, which means we use treatments that are supported by research and considered to be among the best, most effective practices available.
RESOURCE CONNECTION
We connect clients to local resources and provide referrals for related needs such as finances, legal, education, employment, housing.
CVN TELEHEALTH
Video therapy delivered online makes it easy to access the same high-quality, confidential care without having to visit the clinic. Stable internet connection and device with audio / video capabilities needed.
Learn More: cohenveteransnetwork.org
@CohenVeteransNetwork
@CohenVeterans

Chapter 2

Connections to Care: Improving Substance Use Disorder Care for Veterans in Rural America and Beyond*

Committee on Veterans' Affairs

Wednesday, June 14, 2023
U.S. Senate, Committee on Veterans' Affairs,
Washington, DC.

The Committee met, pursuant to notice, at 3 p.m., in Room SR– 418, Russell Senate Office Building, Hon. Jon Tester, Chairman of the Committee, presiding.

Present: Senators Tester, Brown, Blumenthal, Manchin, Sinema, Hassan, Moran, Boozman, Cassidy, Tillis, Sullivan, and Tuberville.

Opening Statement of Chairman Jon Tester

Chairman TESTER. I want to call this hearing to order. Good afternoon. I want to thank the panelists here. We got another panel after this one. I want to thank them for being here, too.

And I want to thank my friend, Senator Tuberville, for filling in for Senator Moran, at least for the first part of this Committee.

Senator TUBERVILLE. Yes.

Chairman TESTER. Many veterans deal with the invisible wounds of war. For some, that may mean challenges with their mental health. For others, they may turn to substances in order to cope with the burdens that they bear. And for many, these are linked. According to the latest data, about 1.1 million veterans suffer from both substance abuse/use disorder and mental health conditions.

Today, we have gathered leaders from the Department of Veterans Affairs as well as researchers, advocates, and oversight officials to discuss how we can improve veterans' access to high quality treatment for SUD.

We know barriers exist, whether it be stigma, wait times, or finding the right treatment option, and for veterans in rural communities, like so many veterans in Montana, it can be even

---

* This is an edited, reformatted and augmented version of Hearing Before the Committee on Veterans' Affairs United States Senate, Publication no. S. HRG. 118–193, dated June 14, 2023.

In: Supporting Our Veterans
Editor: Gina P. Sharpe
ISBN: 979-8-89530-504-1

harder to access care. Rural areas often have shortages of healthcare professionals, and the VA is no stranger to that challenge. Almost 70 percent of primary care health professionals' shortage areas across this country are in rural or partially rural areas, and a recent study found that 136 hospitals in rural communities closed between 2010 and 2021.

Improving access to care for rural veterans by purchasing care from community care may not be the answer because rural areas are relatively underserved generally. You cannot buy it if it ain't there.

That is why it is so important to bolster the VA's workforce. I am proud to say that through resources Congress has provided VA has added some 1,100 positions nationwide since FY '22 to improve SUD care veterans. That is good work, and they need to be thanked for that.

VA provides coordinated care to veterans with an understanding of the unique life experiences and conditions that the veterans face. However, there is work to be done to ensure all veterans have timely access to that care. I have heard numerous issues with veterans not being able to readily access VA's residential care for mental health and SUD, the RRTP program. That is why I included a provision in my STRONG Veterans Act enacted last December to study RRTP wait times and availability to better inform the development of additional RRTP sites and bed spaces.

Building off that effort, I will be introducing legislation very soon to make community care really work for veterans, and that includes being able to access residential SUD and mental health care in the community when that care is needed. For veterans who need this level of care, there is no time to waste, and we need to ensure they are given all the options available.

I want to thank you all for being here today. I look forward to your testimony. I look forward to the discussion. With that, I will turn it over to Senator Tuberville for his opening statement.

Opening Statement of Senator Tommy Tuberville

Senator TUBERVILLE. Thank you, Mr. Chairman, and thanks for the witnesses being here today to discuss this very important topic and a top priority of mine, which is veterans' access to substance use treatment.

On behalf of Ranking Member Moran, I would like to give a special welcome to Chelsey Simoni who is here with us today. She is Co-Founder and Executive Director of HunterSeven Foundation. Ms. Simoni is an Army veteran, flight medic, clinical nurse researcher, and advance practice provider. She continues to serve her country by advocating for her fellow veterans to get the care that they deserve.

We are here this afternoon to determine if the VA is meeting the needs of veterans, specifically veterans who reside in rural and highly rural areas, when they need treatment for substance use disorders. The VA continues to claim suicide prevention is their top clinical priority. Therefore, ensuring veterans have prompt access to high quality treatment for mental health conditions and addictions is critical in achieving our shared goal of combatting veteran suicide.

As overdose deaths are increasing across America and especially in our rural areas, so is the need for high quality mental health care and addiction treatment. That is why I continue to wonder why the VA will not use the tools and authorities Congress has given them to save the lives of veterans who are most at risk. When veterans make the decision to seek treatment for their mental health conditions or addictions, VA must ensure that they are met with high quality care that provides veterans with timely access choices and no red tape.

I look forward to hearing from each of the witnesses today on this important topic, Mr. Chairman.

Chairman TESTER. Thank you, Senator Tuberville.

Now, for our first panel. And I want to thank you all for having names that I should be able to pronounce. Dr. Erica Scavella, Assistant Under Secretary for Health for Clinical Services at the Department of Veterans Affairs, she is accompanied by Dr. Tamara Camel—Dr. Tamara Campbell, I guess I was wrong, Executive Director of the VA Office of Mental Health and Suicide Prevention, and Dr. Bradley V. Watts, Director of the Veterans Health Resource Center at the VA's Office of Rural Health. I thank all three of you for being here.

Dr. Scavella, the floor is yours.

Panel I: Statement of Erica Scavella Accompanied by Tamara Campbell and Bradley V. Watts

Dr. SCAVELLA. Thank you. Good afternoon, Chairman Tester, Ranking Member Tuberville, and distinguished Members of the Committee. Thank you for the opportunity today to discuss VA's substance use disorder treatment programs in rural America. Accompanying me today are Dr. Tamara Campbell, the Executive Director of the Office of Mental Health and Suicide Prevention, and Dr. Bradley Watts, Director, Veterans Rural Health Resource Center.

For the past decade, there has been an increase in morbidity and mortality from substance use disorders as powerful and illicit drugs have become more widespread. For fiscal years 2018 through 2022, the number of veterans diagnosed with a substance use disorder and receiving treatment in VA increased from 522,000 to over 550,000.

VA is committed to ensuring all veterans have access to treatment for substance use disorder regardless of where they live. Core characteristics of substance use disorder services include timely same-day triage, a no-wrong-door approach, concurrent treatment for coccurring needs, and veteran-centered and individualized treatment based on the needs and the preferences of veterans.

Over the last decade, VHA has worked to mitigate risk factors associated with overdose and suicide among veterans related to opioids and stimulants, including launching a national Opioid Safety Initiative and Stimulant Safety Initiative. Beyond treatment for substance use disorder, VA provides primary and secondary prevention specific to opioid use disorder in addition to efforts specific to the risks associated with substance use in general. As an integrated healthcare system, VA is uniquely positioned to address the needs of veterans diagnosed with substance use disorder.

Current policy requires facilities to provide access to the comprehensive continuum of care of substance use disorder treatment services ranging from early intervention and harm reduction services through intensive outpatient and, when needed, residential or inpatient treatment. Current policy also requires facilities to provide same-day outpatient access to veterans with emergent substance use treatment needs. This care can be provided in person or via telehealth in several settings, to include our general mental health clinics, our Primary Care-Mental Health Integration clinics, and substance use disorder specialty clinics.

VHA national policy explicitly states that veterans cannot be denied care due to their use of a substance. Further, both national and the VA DoD Clinical Practice Guideline for the Management of Substance Use Disorders define expectations that veterans be retained in care and that programs do not use criteria that would automatically discharge them from treatment.

VHA offers comprehensive care in Mental Health Residential Rehabilitation Treatment Programs, or MH RRTPs, to veterans with co-occurring mental health, substance use, medical, and psycho-social needs. Today, more than 70 domiciliary substance use disorder programs are in operation, with over 1,700 beds. We are focused on specifically providing intensive residential substance use disorder treatment.

VHA recognizes the importance of timely access to the Mental Health Residential Rehabilitation Treatment Programs for veterans and requires this intensive level of care to be available to them. We will continue to review our policies and address concerns from many stakeholders related to the concerns you mentioned.

Veterans living in rural communities often face unique characteristics that limit their access to health care. Barriers such as long distances to clinical facilities and a shortage of qualified providers can put rural veterans and their families at risk. To overcome these challenges and reach rural veterans with critical health care needs, VA has expanded access through telehealth programs and leveraging the skills of our existing clinicians. This includes the development and ongoing expansion of Clinical Resource Hubs, which are a network of VA centers in large urban settings that are skilled in delivering their services to veterans in rural areas at medical centers, VA Community Care Clinics, and in the home through the telehealth services.

In conclusion, we appreciate the Committee's continued support with this shared mission. Nothing is more important to VA than supporting the health and well-being of the Nation's veterans and their families. VA has employed broad evidence-based strategies to address the opioid epidemic. This critical work saves lives.

My colleagues and I are prepared to respond to any questions you may have and look forward to working with you on some remaining barriers that make it challenging for us to meet this mission. We are committed to providing world-class care to our Nation's veterans. Thank you.

[The prepared statement of Dr. Scavella appears on page 43 of the Appendix.]

Senator TESTER. Thank you, Dr. Scavella. To the second, I might add, on that testimony.

So I will start out with a few questions that I have. I come from a State that is pretty darn rural. In fact, in some departments, the whole State is considered a rural State. Even our most populated areas are considered rural.

We have a treatment facility at Fort Harrison. It is a 24-bed— by the way, Fort Harrison is a long ways from Plentywood, Mon- tana. Okay? And so it is our State capital. It is where we have our VA hospital. And they have a 24-bed residential treatment program for veterans' mental health, eight beds for SUD, eight beds for co- occurring SUD, and then eight beds for PTSD.

I have got two questions. The first question is: What makes VA unique and able to provide residential care for veterans that have comorbidities like SUD and PTSD?

And then the second question is: How common is it—because in my world there is not a lot of treatment centers out there. There is just not a lot of treatment centers. So how common is it in rural America that the only choice they have is the VA for a veteran that has these issues?

Dr. SCAVELLA. Thank you, Chairman Tester, for that question. So to answer your first question related to why VA is uniquely able to provide the care to the veterans with these substance use disorder diagnoses and other co-occurring comorbidities, the first is that we are the largest integrated healthcare system in the United States. We provide comprehensive care for our veterans from primary care through pain management, general mental health, as well as substance use disorder. And so we treat the whole patient, and we are able to see that due to the fact that we have an integrated record. We can communicate with our colleagues to provide that care. So that is one of the reasons why we are certain that we can communicate internally, do warm handoffs when required to pass patients' information along, to make sure we are providing that care.

The second question that you asked, which is related to the availability of services in rural locations, you recounted your statistics in your State very well. We know that we have challenges, but we do have facilities in Montana specifically for substance use disorder.

And our commitment is from the time of identified need to make sure that we are bringing those veterans in if they need inpatient or residential services, to start that referral and to get the care provided as soon as possible, preferably on the same day but within 72 hours if it is for priority needs.

Chairman TESTER. Okay.

Dr. SCAVELLA. Yes.

Chairman TESTER. So I talked to you about the distances. So when you are referring to community care, oftentimes you have no choice. Oftentimes, it is a long ways away. What role does that figure in your decision-making, distance from home?

Dr. SCAVELLA. So distance from home is important to us to consider. The average patient may have to drive an average of 185 miles or greater to get the residential inpatient—the residential services that we would like to provide to them. So distance is a consideration.

What we want to do is provide the soonest care possible in the best way possible. If we can keep them within the VA system to provide that care, we will. If distance is prohibitive, and/or the time between the appointment referral and the time that the appointment is going to be given, we can make a referral to the commu nity, and we do that through some of the authorities provided in legislation.

Chairman TESTER. Okay. So what is the wait time for RRTP, typically?

Dr. SCAVELLA. Thank you for that question, Chairman Tester. The first question that you are asking about the wait times, we have a goal of getting our patients in within 72 hours if it is for a priority care. If it is for routine residential care, the goal is 30 days. We are able to meet that need in over 50 percent of our patients, but if there is a concern voiced by the veteran or the family, we can work with our community partners.

I am going to turn it to Dr. Watts to see if there is anything he would like to add to that answer.

Chairman TESTER. Sure.

Dr. WATTS. I think, as you indicated, the challenge is often that there are not community resources available for the most vulnerable rural veterans even if we do want to make those referrals. So the action could end up causing the veteran to need to travel many hundreds of miles in order to achieve that care in a timely way. So it is often a sense of tradeoff between those two.

Chairman TESTER. Okay. So before I turn it over to Senator Tuberville, you said 50 percent of the time you are hitting the 72. Fifty percent you are hitting the 30 days for routine, too, or are you making the 30 days more often than that?

Dr. SCAVELLA. Our average time, Senator Tester, for the referrals is between eight to 20 days when we look at our data, so we are hitting that. However, we are also being very aggressive with making sure that we are staying engaged with those patients, making sure that if something changes that we are able to adjust our plan. If something changes in the acuity of that veteran, their situation changes, we can make those adjustments.

And again, I will turn it over to Dr. Campbell to see if there is anything she would like to add to that answer.

Dr. CAMPBELL. Thank you again for that question. I just want to reiterate that many of our veterans choose to stay within VA, and so if they choose to stay within VA, we will keep them in VA and engage them in other forms of treatments. We have stepped care models. So we may be engaging them in telehealth services or out-patient treatments while they are waiting for residential care because they have chosen, or they choose, to stay within VA.

Chairman TESTER. Okay. Thank you. Senator Tuberville.

Senator TUBERVILLE. Thank you, Mr. Chairman.

Dr. Scavella, is that how you pronounce it? Scavella? I know people mispronounce my name all the time, too.

Chairman TESTER. Never.

Senator TUBERVILLE. Never, right? Doctor—and this is for all three of you. I would like to kind of get to the bottom of this. I just recently reviewed a memo issued on May 24, 2021, signed by the Assistant Under Secretary of Clinical Services, which recommends all VA medical centers establish syringe service programs, also known as clean needle exchanges, for veterans enrolled in VA health care experiencing substance use disorders.

Now Federal law prohibits taxpayer funds to be used to purchase needles or syringes for the injection of illegal drugs. Why do we believe that the VA is above this? I do not understand that. Doctor, could you start out? And if anybody has got any—just all we are looking for is information.

Dr. SCAVELLA. So thank you for that question, Senator Tuberville. One of the things that we understand from looking at the research is that veterans who participate in a syringe exchange program, or people in general, are more likely to seek care from the entity providing those services for their substance use disorder. So in addition to reducing the passing, the contracting of other infectious diseases through those syringes, we also know that there is a greater likelihood that they are going to look toward us, look toward that entity to get overall help with their substance use disorder.

I will turn it over to Dr. Campbell for some additional.

Senator TUBERVILLE. Okay.

Dr. CAMPBELL. Just to reiterate—and thank you again for that question—our job is for the protection of veterans and also for the protection of the public. So the comorbid and co-medical issues that present with IV drug use, HIV and hepatitis C, we are able to help reduce that with this program.

Senator TUBERVILLE. Dr. Watts, you got anything to add to this?

Dr. WATTS. Nothing to add.

Senator TUBERVILLE. Okay. I just do not know who authorized this, number one. I know if Secretary McDonough did it, he is not a doctor, and so you know, it is very concerning to me that we are giving out needles, you know, for drugs and when it is illegal. You know?

So what authority does the Assistant Under Secretary of Clinical Services have to issue guidance to every VA medical center given the priority VA has had on care and pain management? You know, why is the memo not signed by the Secretary himself? He did not even sign this. I mean, do you know? Do you have any follow up on that?

Dr. SCAVELLA. So thank you for the question, Senator Tuberville. That memo was drafted, as you stated, in May 2021 through the authority that the Assistant Under Secretary for Health for Clinical Services had, which is to oversee the clinical care provided as a chief medical officer for the Department of Veterans Affairs.

Senator TUBERVILLE. Ms. Campbell, do you know anything about that?

Dr. CAMPBELL. Just to add that within the Federal guidelines within the hospital we provided them within our hospital setting.

Senator TUBERVILLE. Yes. Dr. Scavella, I wonder why the Secretary did not sign this himself. Do you know?

Dr. SCAVELLA. Senator Tuberville, I cannot answer that question. Senator TUBERVILLE. Okay.

Dr. SCAVELLA. I do not know.

Senator TUBERVILLE. I will ask him myself, but it is pretty concerning.

Do you know who is administering this program at facility level? Do you know who has the authority?

Dr. SCAVELLA. Thank you. I will ask my colleague, Dr. Campbell, to provide an answer to that question. Thank you.

Dr. CAMPBELL. So each facility—thank you. Each facility certainly has a ‘‘quad member,’’ medical director, as you know, chief of staff, and the SUD coordinator or manager over that program would assist in overseeing it.

Senator TUBERVILLE. Is this person also in charge of care management plans; do you know that?

Dr. CAMPBELL. So they would have a team, a multidisciplinary team, sir, to help them with the planning, with the entire care team planning for this.

Senator TUBERVILLE. All right. Is the VA managing data surrounding these programs; Dr. Scavella; do you know? Do we have data on where this is headed?

Dr. SCAVELLA. So we do have some data on outcomes related to our veterans and their ability to successfully engage with us for substance use disorder. We know through all of our multidisciplinary care plans related to substance use disorder that we have reduced the number of veterans who are starting opioids for the first time, that are taking opioids in combination with other medications such as benzodiazepines. We also know that we are seeing fewer deaths from accidental and intentional overdoses. So there are some improvements with the overall comprehensive substance use disorder program that we are very proud of as far as ensuring that our veterans are improving.

Senator TUBERVILLE. Do you know if we are handing—if we are just handing out syringes to newly—I guess new patients from the VA that come in first off? And are we just handing out needles, or are we putting them in some kind of detox plan?

Dr. SCAVELLA. So thank you for that question, Senator Tuberville. We would be bringing our patients in for comprehensive care. It would not be provided in a vacuum. But I will rely on my colleague, Dr. Campbell, to add some details to that answer.

Dr. CAMPBELL. Thank you again. Dr. Scavella is absolutely correct. It is an entire team that works with these patients. They are not in isolation. And that team includes—medical practitioners are included in that team, and we emphasize certainly the biopsycho- social approach to treatment.

Senator TUBERVILLE. Well, just a quick statement on it, I think this is pretty concerning when we are really not following the law here, and I hate that we fall back on an easy plan when we should be really, really helping these veterans because we got a huge prob- lem. You know, the fact that the VA is the country's largest integrated healthcare system and it is administering a clean needle exchange program when they should be creating treatment plans for veterans experiencing substance use disorders, to me, it is not very common sense and it is really—you know, I do not think we are doing the veterans—I do not think we are doing them right.

So I think, to me, it is poor use of taxpayer money and again it is really a disservice, you know, when we have got all these veterans out there and a lot of them have huge problems, that we do not treat the problem immediately and we are just kicking the can down the road in some of these situations.

So hopefully—and I am going to write a letter to Secretary McDonough and get some answers from him. It is pretty concerning that, you know, we just do not make it—we do not want to make it easy on ourselves. We want to make it tougher, you know, to make sure that we give good health care.

Dr. Watts, I am sorry I did not have a question for you, but if you have got anything to add to that.

Dr. WATTS. Nothing to add, thank you.

Senator TUBERVILLE. Okay. Thank you, Mr. Chairman. Chairman TESTER. Do you guys want to comment on the statement as far as treatment plans and furnishing needles? Is there a treatment plan involved before needles are furnished?

Dr. SCAVELLA. So thank you for that question, Chairman Tester. As Dr. Campbell stated, veterans would be engaged in a comprehensive care program to identify all of the underlying comorbidities including mental health concerns, serious mental illness, also pain management, to work on a comprehensive plan to reduce the use of substances and reduce the substance use disorder in that veteran. So, yes, those veterans would be engaged in a comprehensive care plan with very specific goals in place.

We would also be using incentives to encourage them to change their behavior. And, we are providing comprehensive care for veterans before they get into a situation where they are using substances and identifying risky behavior very early on, if possible, but then when they are in a situation where they need assistance with substance use disorder, we are providing comprehensive care.

Chairman TESTER. Thank you for the clarification. Senator Brown.

Senator Sherrod Brown

Senator BROWN. Thank you, Mr. Chairman. Thank you. As some on this Committee know because I have mentioned it fairly ad nauseam, I have been doing roundtables. And Senator Tester has written, also by many others on this Committee, the PACT Act. I have done roundtables in almost half of Ohio's counties now, and what I hear—I will do it at a VFW or a Legion or a DAV hall, and I will hear over and over the difficulty of transition from the military to civilian life and hear generally the most—many people I talk to, many former soldiers, marines, or sailors will say that their commanding officers and the military does not really care that much about that safe, that easier, handoff to the point that veterans organizations and the VA do not know where these veterans, these recently become veterans, live.

So, Dr. Campbell, one question to you and then a comment. And thank you, Mr. Chairman, for your time. Talk about the VHA proactive outreach to servicemembers transitioning back to civilian life, especially on mental health and potential substance use disorders.

Dr. CAMPBELL. Thank you for that question, Senator Brown. So we have strong collaborations with the Department of Defense and interagency collaborations through our Domestic Policy Council. We are involved with the Transition Assistance Program, where we are interfacing with the Department of Defense, with those veterans who are going to be discharged. We know that that first year is a vulnerable year, and so we provide them with resources regarding the benefits that they have as well as all the services that can be provided, not just mental health services but medical services as well.

Senator BROWN. I hope that—thank you, Dr. Campbell. I hope that suggests that the VA continues to work with us on the Adam Lambert Improving Servicemember Transition to Reduce Veteran Suicide Act. It is important that we do more there, and I am hopeful that you will continue to work with us on that.

Dr. CAMPBELL. Absolutely, sir. We have very strong suicide prevention outreach workers at every VAMC, and we are leveraging our Governor's Challenge as well as Mayor's Challenge to help us. Senator BROWN. I understand you are doing that at the VA and you work for the VA, but do you believe we are finding those men and women returning home, or the VA is finding them, local veterans organizations are finding them? Ohio has one in each—at least one in each—county, veterans service officers in all 88 counties, who work for veterans. Are these entities finding these veterans when they are coming home?

Dr. CAMPBELL. We are certainly collaborating with them. We know we can do a better job. We have quarterly meetings with the VSOs, and so we are leveraging every opportunity we have to find them.

Senator BROWN. Is it better than it was 10 years ago?

Dr. CAMPBELL. We are trending better than it was 10 years ago.

Senator BROWN. Okay, one comment. I want to quickly mention the Chillicothe VA, southern Ohio. The Secretary has come out at my request, seems perhaps unusually interested in that. It serves—it is the only rural VAMC in Ohio. It is important in Appalachia. The past year, my office has worked with community leaders and local VA staff to ensure that the facility is resourced in a way that continues to serve Ohio veterans.

During the Trump administration, it looked like it was slated for closure. Secretary McDonough and all of you and my office were working with the union, in essence, saved it, but there still is not the attention paid. I do not think it is as dedicated to the future of this facility as the veterans in southeast Ohio. And it is mostly AFSCME members, I am sorry, AFGE members and AFSCME are believing it should be.

It is essential that access to treatment for substance use disorders, particularly including inpatient treatment, remain available for local veterans. So I just want to say VA must listen better than it has to Chillicothe, to me, to those advocates, that this VA, which is I think probably the biggest employer in town, as it often is in smaller communities, but most importantly, a very, very, very important focal point for serving veterans. Just wanted to let you know that, how important that is, and remind you.

Dr. CAMPBELL. Yes, sir. Thank you.

Chairman TESTER. Senator Tillis, if you are ready. If not, I will go to Blumenthal.

Senator TILLIS. I am ready.

Chairman TESTER. You are up.

Senator Thom Tillis

Senator TILLIS. Thank you all for being here. I know that when we talk about veteran suicide we always, I think appropriately, point out how many of those who are committing suicide have no connection to the VA. What do we know about the population of veterans who have substance abuse problems? I know it is hard to know what you do not know or take a roll by asking everybody that is absent to raise their hands, but do we have any data that would give us an idea of just how many, how big the problem is, and what the ratios are between people who have a connection to the VA and do not?

Dr. SCAVELLA. So, Senator Tillis, thank you for that question. We know that we are actively treating approximately 6.2 million of our veterans of the 9 million that are enrolled, and we know that there is approximately another 9 million that are not enrolled. We know that within our system for this most recent fiscal year that we have approximately 550,000 that are dealing with substance use disorder. So if we extrapolate those numbers to the population that is not coming in, it may be around the same number since we are essentially touching half.

We do—as we previously stated, we have lots of outreach that we are doing to try to make sure we are meeting veterans where they are, working with our community partners to bring them in to service, and also just letting them know that we are here for them when they are ready to come in.

Specific to data that is outside of our catchment area, I can check with my colleagues, but I do not believe we have that readily available, but we would be happy to get that to you.

Senator TILLIS. The reason I ask the question is that we have to find more ways to make more connections and I believe that we are in a time-sensitive, unique position to do that as a result of the Camp Lejeune Toxics Act. I do not know if you all have noticed, but there is a few of those annoying ads that come on about every 30 seconds on whatever TV outlet you are watching. And there has been some debate here about capping legal fees and doing those kind of things for people that are signing up for law firms.

One of the things that I wanted to do was to simply put out— and we are going to file a bill. I am going to talk with members about co-sponsorship. But, something I have told them to call the Patriot Bill of Rights, and that is simply an informed disclosure before you sign a retainer with an attorney who is going to help you with a case for Camp Lejeune, to say: Did you know that you could call your—did you know you could call this 1–800 number to the Department of Navy? If you are not connected to the VA, here is the number for the VA. Here is the number of your Congressmen and Senators who do casework all the time and prevent you from having to pay legal fees. And then here are these Veterans Service Organizations that are building expertise around this area, who can also provide you help at a far lower cost than the legal fees. Have them fully understand all the tools that many of them would not have.

But just imagine, even if they decide to sign the retainer, if we can just get them to make the call and get connected, what benefit that has for the population. And we have got a free sort of oppor tunity here to increase awareness because the trial lawyers are trying to go out there and sign everybody. Why wouldn't we want to formally or fully inform them and potentially create a relationship that does not exist today?

I mean, we could have hundreds of thousands of veterans make a contact they have never made before. We can save their life. We can determine whether or not they have substance abuse problems and actually get them into care that you all do an extraordinary job of.

So I am hoping we are going to speak with more Members about it, but it seems like it ends the debate of capping legal fees. It gives us an opportunity to touch a number of veterans who for the first time that they may ever be connected is through a law firm that is trying to make money, and hopefully, get a benefit for the veteran.

But it seems to me to be a fairly sensible approach. What is wrong with my idea?

Dr. SCAVELLA. Senator——

Senator TILLIS. I am not trying to poison the well by positioning it as a sensible approach, but——

Dr. SCAVELLA. Yes, I will say that since this is the first time that any of the three of us on this panel have heard about this and since the Secretary has not had an opportunity to weigh in, we would be happy to review——

Senator TILLIS. We are going to send the text over to you. It is literally as simple as I have described it, so I will be very interested to see what the Department's position is on the bill fairly soon here. Thank you all.

Thank you, Mr. Chair.

Dr. SCAVELLA. Thank you.

Chairman TESTER. Senator Blumenthal.

Senator Richard Blumenthal

Senator BLUMENTHAL. Thank you, Mr. Chairman. You know, I have believed for some time that one of the challenges is outreach, whether it is through the media or person-to-person contact.

In Connecticut, we have a partnership between the Connecticut VA health system and a group that is called Connecticut Harm Reduction Alliance run by a very able young man named Mark Jenkins, and they have established what is called a Rover Program since RVs, literally, recreational vehicles, provide harm reduction supplies to communities. I have gone around with some of them, and they are stocked with all the stuff that is necessary to provide what people suffering from substance disorder need. And the program in Connecticut has been tremendously successful, now has over 35 of these rovers serving 26 communities, and it plans to expand nationally.

As I mentioned, outreach partnership with the VA—the VA cannot operate in isolation. It has to seek partnerships with community groups like the Connecticut Harm Reduction Alliance. What plans do you have to try to seek to provide more access to substance use disorder treatment programs in the non-VA community?

Dr. SCAVELLA. So thank you for that question, Senator Blumenthal. We clearly understand within the Department of Vet erans Affairs that substance use disorder, especially considering opioid use disorder, is a whole-of-government and whole-of-nation approach that is required. We do need to continue to leverage those community partnerships, as Dr. Campbell stated earlier, to make sure that we are reaching veterans where they are, especially if they are not engaged in our care.

We do have several programs in place to address veterans who may be at risk, to include our Overdose Education and Naloxone Distribution program, to make sure that we are providing tools and education, to give both veterans and their families and caregivers the signs and symptoms to look for if someone is potentially getting close to overdosing, and then giving the tool, the naloxone, to actually do the reversal. So that is one of the things that we are doing. We are also engaged with many different community partnerships, to include the Governor's Challenge and others, to really identify veterans who may be at risk. The Hannon Act provided for the ability to engage with veterans within the first year of post-separation from the Department of Defense. So we are leveraging that as well, making sure that we are reaching those veterans where they are, participating in their TAP classes, to make sure that we are giving them the tools that they need to engage with us, perhaps not immediately but hopefully when they think of it and realize that they have that benefit and they are entitled to that care.

Senator BLUMENTHAL. I may have missed it in your testimony, but do we have—you know, we use these figures, 21 veterans everyday commit suicide. Is there an accurate, up-to-date number?

Dr. SCAVELLA. Senator Blumenthal, I am going to turn that over to Dr. Campbell, but we do have some updates on that number.

Dr. CAMPBELL. So thank you for that very important question. We all know one suicide is one too many, and so we really are leveraging everything we can. That number has trended downward to 16.8 according to the last annual report, and we continue to review those numbers daily.

Senator BLUMENTHAL. According to which report?

Dr. CAMPBELL. The last annual suicide——

Senator BLUMENTHAL. Oh, the last annual report.

Dr. CAMPBELL. Yes, sir.

Senator BLUMENTHAL. And how do you—what data do you—how do you access data on veteran suicide? What kind of data is available?

Dr. CAMPBELL. Sure. Thank you for that question. So we work with the Centers for Disease Control and World Health Organization, and we use scientific methodology utilizing their definitions of what a suicide is to develop that report and to look at those numbers.

Senator BLUMENTHAL. And did they have—how did they define suicide? In other words, is there a definition of suicide?

Dr. CAMPBELL. So that——

Senator BLUMENTHAL. Substance use disorder taken to a certain level can constitute a form of self-destruction?

Dr. CAMPBELL. That definition certainly is determined by the coroner's office, and they look at each individual case and determine that.

Senator BLUMENTHAL. Thank you. My time is expired, but I will want perhaps to follow up on this issue. Thanks.

Chairman TESTER. And there will be opportunities for questions for the record, Senator Blumenthal.

That concludes our first panel. You got off lucky because there usually is more people than that here, but there is a vote going on right now. Thank you guys for your testimony. I appreciate it very much. You are certainly welcome to stay for the second panel if you choose.

And now I will introduce the second panel. I would like to welcome Dr. Julie Kroviak, Principal Deputy Assistant Inspector General in the Office of Healthcare Inspections at the VA's Office of Inspector General. Then we have Dr. Jonathan Cantor, who is Policy Researcher at the RAND Corporation. Then we have Naomi Mathis, who is Associate National Legislative Director of the Disabled American Veterans, and we have Chelsey Simoni, Co-Founder and Executive Director of the HunterSeven Foundation.

Dr. Kroviak, you have the floor.

Panel II: Statement of Julie Kroviak

Dr. KROVIAK. Thank you, Chairman Tester and Committee members. I appreciate this opportunity to discuss the OIG's oversight of VHA's substance use disorder treatment programs.

The OIG's Office of Healthcare Inspections reviews the quality and safety of health care provided across VHA and communicates these findings through public reports. The majority of our healthcare inspection staff have significant experience providing direct clinical care to veterans, and such experience adds unique insight to our oversight work. This is particularly true of mental health teams staffed with board-certified psychiatrists, psychologists, licensed clinical social workers, some of whom are combat veterans. These team members have cared for veterans facing the very issues we are discussing today.

VHA faces significant challenges in meeting the needs of individuals with substance use disorders, and rural settings can pose additional obstacles in addressing these patients' needs. In that veterans with substance use disorders often have additional mental health diagnoses that place them at higher risk for suicide, seamless and timely care coordination is critical. The Committee's focus on rural veterans is appreciated as veterans living in highly rural areas are 65 percent more likely to die from suicide than those residing in urban settings, an unsettling statistic that VHA faces in addressing their top clinical priority, to reduce veteran suicide.

Our oversight is much broader than just major medical centers. We reach out into rural communities with our VISN and CHIP reviews that analyze VA rural facilities, including the most highly rural CBOCs, and our Vet Center reviews will review the Mobile Vet Centers, important outreach units for many of our rural communities.

To meet the increasing demand for services, including mental health and substance use disorder treatment, VHA depends on community care. The OIG has identified persistent administrative errors and communication failures among VHA, its third-party administrators, and community care providers, as well as between the care providers and their patients. These failures amplify risks for patients with high-risk mental health issues and complex disease. My written statement details two reports that provide insight into the complexity of coordinating care for patients with substance use disorder at two distinct stages of treatment needs.

Earlier this year, we substantiated the allegation that in 2020 and 2021 North Texas staff did not follow VHA policy requiring that patients be offered alternative options for residential substance use disorder treatment within VA or the community when the wait time for this service exceeded 30 days. This practice not only potentially delayed the treatment for these veterans but also has the potential to fracture trust between patients and the healthcare system upon which they rely.

The second report describes the mismanagement of a patient at the Tomah VA, a rural facility in Wisconsin, who was suffering from acute alcohol withdrawal and subsequently died at another VA hospital. We found failures in the clinical management of this veteran that likely contributed to their death. Assessments and stabilization efforts for patients at risk for life-threatening consequences of alcohol withdrawal leave no room for error, especially in rural settings when transfers to higher level care must be anticipated early.

To improve the quality of administrative and clinical practices in rural facilities and across the system, VHA frontline staff need policies and guidelines that are clear, standardized, and current. For example, just last month, our office published an advisory memo alerting the Under Secretary for Health that VHA's Mental Health Handbook had not been recertified as required by 2013. Handbooks support frontline clinical decision-making, and such direction must be clear, accurate, and current. Standardizing the oversight of frontline performance can also support consistency and accountability.

Additionally, while it is important for VHA staff to inform veterans of all care options available for their needs, ignoring that the current community care framework does not adequately address critical gaps in coordination may further increase the risk to patients. Our office has published reports related to community care, detailing delays in diagnosis and treatment, lack of or miscommunication between providers, and significant quality of care concerns.

The OIG will continue to provide meaningful oversight to support and improve the quality of health care provided to our Nation's veterans. We also recognize the need to enhance and adapt our work to best support this dynamic healthcare system. We remain grateful for the participation and cooperation of VHA staff across the country and for their commitment to caring for those who have served.

Chairman Tester, this concludes my statement. I would be happy to take any questions you may have.

[The prepared statement of Dr. Kroviak appears on page 53 of the Appendix.]

Chairman TESTER. Thank you, Dr. Kroviak.

Next up we have the policy researcher from the Rand Corporation, Dr. Jonathan Cantor.

Statement of Jonathan Cantor

Dr. CANTOR. Chairman Tester and Members of the Committee, I want to thank you for your invitation to testify today on what is a pressing and urgent public health problem. My name is

Dr. Jonathan Cantor, and I am a policy researcher at the nonprofit and nonpartisan RAND Corporation. I have conducted extensive research on the geographic availability and accessibility of substance use disorder treatment for veterans, military servicemembers, and the civilian population.

In my testimony, I will discuss three main issues: first, the complexity of substance use disorder treatment for veterans given the frequent existence of co-occurring mental health disorders. Second, a brief overview of the geographic accessibility of substance use disorder treatment for veterans. Third, why it is difficult to assess disparities in access.

And then finally, I have a few recommendations to enhance data collection and reporting to improve our understanding of the geographic availability and accessibility of substance use disorder treatment for veterans.

In 2020, around 12 percent of veterans 18 years or older had a substance use disorder, and approximately 1.1 million veterans suffered from both a substance use disorder and mental illness. Less than 10 percent of veterans with a substance use disorder in 2020 received any treatment.

There are a multitude of reasons for why a veteran would not receive the necessary care. First, some veterans who use substances do so to self-medicate their post-traumatic stress disorder symptoms. Second, many veterans fear seeking mental health or substance use disorder treatment because it could negatively affect their career advancement. Third, co-occurring disorders often go unidentified. A practitioner may identify a substance use disorder or a mental health disorder but not necessarily both. Fourth, the appropriate treatment for an individual with a substance use disorder and co-occurring mental health disorder is more complex than treating one or the other alone.

A key determinant for whether an individual receives substance use disorder treatment is how far they have to travel for care. To date, there have been very few studies that have examined distance to substance use disorder treatment as a barrier to care for a national sample of veterans.

In 2019, the Wounded Warrior Project partnered with RAND researchers to understand geographic accessibility of co-occurring substance use disorder and mental health treatment. Our calculations indicated that, on average, Wounded Warrior Project alumni were around a 10-minute drive time from the nearest substance use disorder or mental health treatment facility with a co-occurring program. In contrast, for these veterans, the closest VA medical center with a co-occurring program was around a 60-minute drive time from where the veteran lived.

Our results were encouraging. Most Wounded Warrior Project alumni veterans were able to access treatment programs for co-occurring substance use disorder and mental health disorders within 60 minutes.

Almost one-quarter of U.S. veterans reside in rural communities. There is a concern that it is more difficult for rural veterans to receive care given they must travel farther than veterans that live in urban settings. The geographic accessibility of substance use disorder care could also vary based on the race and gender of the veteran.

Our study did not focus on these potential disparities because there are extensive data challenges in quantifying these differences. Such analyses should require at least detailed data on the addresses or the ZIP codes of the veteran, as well as data on their race, ethnicity, age, sexual orientation, and gender. Finally, and perhaps most challenging, the data would need to include whether the veteran suffered from substance use disorder only or substance use disorders and mental health disorders.

Drawing on my research and existing work, I provide several recommendations in my written testimony. I want to highlight two.

First, the Substance Abuse and Mental Health Service Administration's Behavioral Health Treatment Locator could include additional information on specific treatment approaches available for veterans.

Second, either the Substance Abuse and Mental Health Service Administration or VA should consider conducting regular audit studies among non-VA facilities to get a more accurate understanding of the forms of treatment offered, approximate wait times to the next appointment, and total capacity of the facilities for substance use disorder treatment, and they should vary the calls based on the sociodemographic characteristics of the veteran.

Far too many Americans, especially veterans, fail to receive treatment for substance use disorder each year. I am confident that we can increase the number of veterans who receive treatment and reduce the number of drug overdoses. However, that will require an infusion of funding to improve current data collection systems and ensure that veterans can access the information necessary to make treatment decisions.

Thank you for your time, and I am happy to answer your questions.

[The prepared statement of Dr. Cantor appears on page 64 of the Appendix.]

Chairman TESTER. Thank you for your statement, Dr. Cantor. Next, we have Naomi Mathis, Associate National Legislative Director of the Disabled American Veterans. Naomi?

Statement of Naomi Mathis

Ms. MATHIS. Chairman Tester, Ranking Member Moran, and Members of the Committee, DAV is grateful for the opportunity to appear before you today to address concerns with access to the VA substance use disorder treatment program.

DAV members are injured and ill, service-disabled, wartime veterans that utilize the VA healthcare system at extremely high rates, which many depend on as their sole source of health care. Our one million-plus members live throughout the country and provide us with an insight into their unique struggles with access to care.

Our written testimony provides our entire position. However, I will focus on the challenges, barriers, and our recommendations.

First, rural veterans face issues accessing health care similar to those faced by the general population, including a lack of transportation. In rural communities, distance to a healthcare facility, time, cost of fuel, and access to transportation are all exacerbated and known barriers to care. Veterans who lack access to public transportation or are no longer able to drive because of age, health, or driving restrictions rely on family, friends, or community service organizations.

To help such veterans, DAV operates a fleet of vehicles around the country to provide free transportation to VA medical facilities for injured and ill veterans. While this program is highly successful and beneficial for the veterans we serve, we continue to face administrative challenges with expediting volunteer driver examinations. Specifically, there is a breakdown in the onboarding process for our volunteer drivers.

For example, our transportation coordinator in Montana told us they had 30 applications for volunteer drivers. However, by the time VA completed the onboarding process, a year and a half later, only two applicants remained interested in volunteering. During my recent trip to New Hampshire, our coordinators there expressed similar concerns. By contrast, we are hearing of other facilities that can onboard in as little as 3 days.

We recommend VA standardize and expedite the volunteer driver onboarding process VHA-wide.

Next, the Philippines is the only foreign country in which there is a VA outpatient clinic to serve eligible veterans. In October 2022, we began receiving complaints from our members who indicated VA Manilla had completely stopped dispensing controlled medications, including those undergoing mental health and substance use disorder treatments. Options faced by this population of veterans are to either stop the medication, utilize the community, travel to Guam or to the United States whenever a refill is needed.

Guam, American Samoa, Puerto Rico, U.S. Virgin Islands, and the Northern Mariana Islands face even greater challenges due to limited or poor infrastructure. Veterans living in these areas often have to take commercial aircraft, which are not disability-friendly, to get to medical appointments or fill prescriptions. Not one of the VA OCONUS has a specialty SUD program.

We recommend VA conduct a needs assessment to determine if adding substance use disorder programming for outside community—outside CONUS communities is warranted.

Mr. Chairman, an additional barrier facing veterans residing outside of the United States is the Beneficiary Travel Self-Service System, which was designed to automate the travel reimbursement claims process. However, there continue to be complaints regarding the slow processing of payments and improper payments made to beneficiaries. VA must fix and modernize this system in consultation with stakeholders on the Beneficiary Travel Self-Service System.

Lastly, as we celebrate the 75th anniversary of the integration of women into the Armed Forces, we must remember that women veterans are the fastest growing cohort in the VA system. Therefore, VA must continue to accommodate this growing population and their gender-specific needs.

As a combat woman veteran, I experience longer wait times for specialty care at VA than my male counterparts, including mental health care. VA reports fewer than half of all residential facilities have separate dorm space for women veterans and only 13 programs have gender-specific services for women veterans compared to 27 programs exclusive to men. I will note that none of them are located in rural areas.

Additionally, women veterans with substance use disorder who experience longer wait times for treatment could have an increased risk of suicide. This may be due to VA's lower capacity to address women's needs.

We recommend VA conduct a nationwide analysis to determine if expanding gender-specific substance use disorder inpatient care is warranted.

This concludes my testimony, and I look forward to any questions you and the Committee may have.

[The prepared statement of Ms. Mathis appears on page 76 of the Appendix.]

Senator Jerry Moran

Senator MORAN [presiding]. Thank you very much.

Now, Ms. Simoni, we look to you for your testimony. Ms. Simoni is the Co-Founder and Executive Director of the HunterSeven Foundation.

Statement of Chelsey Simoni

Ms. SIMONI. Senator Moran, Senator Hassan, thank you so much for sitting here and listening today. This story is very personal to me as it is a lived experience, so I appreciate it.

Today, I speak before the Committee as a licensed healthcare provider with advanced medical degrees, including public health and epidemiology as well as specialty certifications. I have spent over 15,000 hours working in emergency medicine, long- and short- term substance use settings, and military veteran-specific mental health clinics. I have published in numerous academic journals and presented at conferences nationwide.

However, I speak to the Committee today as a sister of a combat- wounded marine losing his battle with addiction, as the child of an alcoholic mother and heroin-addicted father. I speak today as a disabled Army veteran dealing with constant, debilitating pain and the uninterrupted emotional burden I face daily. The testimony I share today is, unfortunately, entirely true.

By 14, I had a job, I skipped school, and I never got my homework done. I got into fights and did everything I was not supposed to do, so I failed my freshman year of high school.

At 15 years old, I lost my oldest brother to an overdose. My mother told me my 24-year-old brother planned to enter substance abuse treatment the following Monday. He did not make it. He had shot up the night before with friends of my father's, and he had fallen asleep and began to choke on his throw-up. Instead of calling 911 and keeping him awake, those he was with had moved his body into the hallway where he choked on his vomit and died.

Shortly after his death, I was expelled from school. My behavior was self-destructive, and I lacked structure and discipline. It was difficult to talk about my situation at home with those who did not understand, especially those who had just thought I was a bad kid but never figured out to ask why.

By 16, in 2007, my youngest brother had signed up to serve as an infantryman in the Marine Corps. We wrote each other often. And while he was in boot camp at Parris Island, he loved it. He loved every single minute of it. And I had just graduated high school when my brother told me he was going to be deployed as one of the first marines into Marjah, Afghanistan, under President Obama's surge to disrupt Taliban forces. He spent 7 months in southern Afghanistan.

While he was deployed, I would sit at night and watch the evening news and keep to myself in the loop about what was going on in the war. Every time I heard an unnamed marine casualty occurred, my heart sank. It was almost daily. In total, 68 marines were killed in action during that 7-month deployment, and 694 marines were wounded in action. In turn, I enlisted in the Army.

In August 2011, he redeployed to Sangin, Afghanistan, for 8 months. Thirty marines had been killed in action while 582 marines were wounded in action. Of those wounded marines was my brother. While he was on—while he had lost men he considered brothers and witnessed his closest friend suffer near-death amputations from hidden explosive devices and others who had been physically ripped apart by RPK machine gun rounds, my brother felt lucky. He had sustained outrageous blast injuries from explosions and rocket-propelled grenades, one blast so severe that an MRAP vehicle had flipped over on top of him, throwing him from the turret, causing him to break four ribs, fracture his skull and sections of his lower back.

He came home, but the physical pain was mute compared to the emotional guilt and moral injury he tried so hard to hide. Over the next year, he struggled with pain, physical, depression, and guilt overwhelmed his life. What began as a short-term Vicodin prescription for pain management became a full-blown addiction where he would steal fentanyl patches from the regiment's Navy corpsmen. He had kept his habit under the radar until a random drug test had found opioids in his system. Sixteen days later, he was dis- charged under other than honorable conditions for illicit drug use, and he was homeless, jobless, emotionally and physically unstable, and addicted. He was too embarrassed to seek help and suffered in silence.

Around the same time, I suffered a severe spinal cord injury while serving in the Army. I remember the electrifying pain. It was like no pain I had ever experienced before, but my adrenalin was high, and the mission made the pain seem nonexistent. It was not until later that evening I lost control of my bladder, and pins and needles drove up my leg, causing debilitating painful paralysis.

At 21 years old, I was told my injury led to the discs in my lower back partially paralyzing my spinal cord and I needed surgery. My military career was placed on hold, but that was not the case for the rest of my team.

In the months leading up to the major surgery I was scheduled for, I was given more than 300 pills of the mild opiate, hydrocodone-acetaminophen, better known as Vicodin. I was told to take them every six hours for pain. In case the Vicodin was not working, I was given 100 pills of tramadol, a synthetic opioid that reduces the pain felt through the central nervous system. To lessen the right-sided leg numbness and severe neuropathy and muscle spasms, I was given 100 pills of Flexeril. My anxiety was front and center, so I was given 30 pills of Lorazepam, the anti-anxiety benzodiazepine to take as needed for anxiety.

Two weeks later, I received a call that one of my closest friends that I had known since I was 14 was killed in Dawlat Shah, Afghanistan. I felt hopeless, motionless, and stuck in time, and I could not move. The pain had gotten worse. And the more pills I took, the pain I had was less and less, and as time went on everything became easier to deal with or at least what I thought.

I went through a three-hour surgery and was on the road to recovery. The first few nights were hell. I had severe nightmares, dreams I would never wish on anyone. I would wake up covered in sweat and unable to move, and the pain worsened. I was given 60 pills of oxycodone-acetaminophen, also known as Percocet, and was told to stop taking the Vicodin as it may have been an adverse reaction.

I could not swallow the pills without vomiting, worsening my post-operative pain. I was sent home with an eight-ounce bottle of Oxydose, liquid oxycodone. It helped with the pain. Eventually, it subsided as I healed.

I felt great. Looking back, I cannot remember a time in my life where I felt that relaxed or carefree. I could sleep. My mind stopped overthinking, and my heart stopped racing. I was not sad, and I was not worried about the future. I was enjoying the present. And when I started to feel myself come back to reality, I grabbed the medicine bottle, and I would take another sip.

Like most 21-year-olds, I did not have a way to measure the amount I was taking, instead, relying on my balance to let me know if I had taken enough. I do not remember much besides laying in bed, thinking, isn't life great. I loved how I felt in those moments. It was an unmatched feeling.

I took medication not for the physical pain but to cover my emotional pain, which worked very well until it almost killed me. Late one night, I was laying in bed, and I had drank too much. I laid back and felt a sudden sickness. I went to get up and felt my legs get weak. Using the side of my bed, I slowly slid to the ground, and I do not remember much afterward as I woke up a few minutes later covered in vomit. I cried as I knew what had happened.

The next day, I knew I had to get rid of it, which was not easy, but what kept me motivated was returning to uniform and being with my team again. There is a reasonable probability that this is what kept me alive today. To this day, I know I cannot take Percocet as I enjoy it too much.

While dealing with my situation, my brother battled something similar. He figured out his steps, and he ended up staying with my aunt on her couch. He was addicted to prescription opiates. When those ran out and he could not get more, he turned to heroin.

He was alone one night and had shot up heroin, and it was discovered later that it had traces of fentanyl. He passed out on her couch, and when our aunt found him he was covered in vomit and not breathing. She called 911 and began CPR. His lips were dusky and cold. He was given Narcan, intubated, and rushed to the emergency department where the medical team worked to save his life. The doctor said it was a miracle he was alive.

While my brother faced his battles, I received medical clearance to remain in the Army despite having a life-changing surgery. My provider told me that the chances of another injury occurring were highly likely. As mentioned and as predicted, years later, I suffered a reinjury, this time equally as painful, but I could still move and manage. For me, long story short, my career was over.

It was always—it will always be the most dangerous time in any servicemember's life when you are leaving a tight-knit group and leaving a feeling of belonging and reintegrating into a society that could not care less about you, your service, your situation, or your struggles. There is no team or tribe that you can turn to or fall back on. There is no safety net or mirroring experience in a fellow veteran for you to voice your feelings on.

I went to bed as a servicemember and woke up the following day as a civilian. My pain had become increasingly worse. My temper was short, and my frustration grew.

I woke up one morning my senior year of college, and it was like a trap door falling underneath me. I had a commemorative military pistol from my unit, a Sig Sauer P250 .45 ACP under my bed, and I laid down on my bedroom floor, looking up at the ceiling, with my pistol in my right hand. I pointed the gun toward myself and put the barrel in my mouth. I can still remember the cold feeling and taste of steel.

The only reason I am still here today is twofold. I could not kill myself in my grandparents' house, and I reached out to somebody who served in the military, and I said to them, I am not okay, and got the help I received.

In short, I invite you to read the remaining of my testimony as this is something very personal to me, and I appreciate the time. I know I went over, so thank you very much.

[The prepared statement of Ms. Simoni appears on page 84 of the Appendix.]

Senator MORAN. Ms. Simoni, thank you very much.

Senator Margaret Wood Hassan

Senator HASSAN. Thank you, Ranking Member Moran.

And, Ms. Simoni, thank you so much for your testimony. Just a couple of things, I was Governor of New Hampshire as we began to see what had been an increasingly bad opioid and heroin epidemic turn to a fentanyl epidemic. The thing that gives me hope and the thing that has made some progress possible although we have much more work to do, as your testimony indicates, is thatpeople like you have spoken up about their experience, about the fact that opioids, and particularly this new class of opioids and fentanyl, is extraordinarily addictive and that we have to treat substance use disorder as the disorder that it is.

And we have a lot of work to go, both to help people get into recovery and stay in recovery and recognize that sometimes relapses happen, right, and treat it like an illness that way. We also have to go after the unbelievably insidious cartels that are trying to drive up demand for this drug that is so cheap for them to make and easy for them to transport.

I also want to thank you for talking about the difficulty of the transition period for servicemembers because what I hear from especially servicewomen and women veterans in New Hampshire is how difficult this period is and how alone people, veterans feel, especially women veterans, especially women veterans in rural areas. So I thank you for giving voice to that. I thank you for being brave enough to do it. And I know that everybody on this Committee, both sides of the dais, want to work with you and veterans throughout the country to make progress on these issues and to make sure that veterans understand how deeply we appreciate your service.

With that, I am going to turn to a couple of questions to Dr. Cantor just because I want to—what I want to do is not only recognize the problem but talk about what is working and what is not and what we still need to do.

And with that, Dr. Cantor, as we are talking about veterans and particularly veterans who fall through the cracks as they transition out of service, or as they are dealing with substance use disorder, or whether they are dealing with mental health challenges, we now have the 988 Suicide and Crisis Lifeline that veterans in crisis can call, and they can be connected to the Veterans Crisis Hotline for help just by pressing option 1. What impact has 988 had on connecting veterans to the Veterans Crisis Hotline?

Dr. CANTOR. Thank you for the question. I do not know of any specific research at present that has discussed or looked at the linkage between the 988 lifeline to the veterans crisis line as of yet.

Senator HASSAN. Okay. Is it an area that you think we need data about and explore, yes?

Dr. CANTOR. Yes, I would agree with you.

Senator HASSAN. Okay. And I want—part of my reason for asking the question is just so that any veterans who may follow this hearing know that now this crisis hotline is there and the wait times are relative—you know, I think they are averaging about 40 seconds, if I have got my data correct, and that there is this option for people. And so I hope veterans will take advantage of this.

The other thing I would want veterans watching to know is that there are a couple of programs, the Buddy Check program, our Solid Start program, that are really intended to lift up Veterans Service Organizations as they reach out to their peers to provide support.

I also, Dr. Cantor, wanted to talk about telehealth. My colleagues and I have worked together on a bipartisan basis to expand access to opioid treatment. Last year, we passed into law the Mainstreaming Addiction Treatment Act, which I led with Senator Murkowski. That removed unnecessary barriers for doctors to prescribe lifesaving medication-assisted treatment for people struggling with opioids, including veterans.

However, veterans in rural areas may still have limited access to in-person healthcare providers to initiate and monitor substance use disorder treatment. So we are going now from about 150,000 docs nationally who could prescribe buprenorphine to opioid addiction to 1.8 million now that we have removed this barrier, but we still have to be able to get people in front of a doctor to get that treatment.

So, Dr. Cantor, can you discuss the role of telehealth in expanding veterans' access to lifesaving medication-assisted treatment?

Dr. CANTOR. Thank you for the question. I think since the COVID–19 pandemic there has been this drastic increase in telehealth availability.

Senator HASSAN. Yep.

Dr. CANTOR. And I think that it is an outstanding question. There has been some research that has examined the telehealth utilization rates.

Senator HASSAN. Yep.

Dr. CANTOR. I think it is still under review as to whether or not the effect of the quality of care that veterans receive differs between inpatient and telehealth.

Senator HASSAN. Yep.

Dr. CANTOR. And I think without that being answered first I think we just need more information, data.

Senator HASSAN. Yes. Well, one of the things that I am trying to drill down on here is if you have veterans in a rural area who do not have a primary care doctor in the area or a doc who is expert in treating substance use disorder. We need to get people in front of a doctor and begin that relationship.

I am going to continue, Mr. Chair, to push for telehealth resources when it comes to treating opioid abuse disorder because if we are expecting people to drive hours for this kind of treatment I think it is going to be an effective denial of access to them. Thank you for letting me go over.

Senator MORAN. A Kansan can relate to what you say. Senator Cassidy.

Senator Bill Cassidy

Senator CASSIDY. Thank you all. I have been pulled every which way, so if I sound like I am asking something which others have already asked, I apologize because I probably am.

Ms. Simoni, your statement that military veteran care should be less about the VA and more about the veterans themselves, what a powerful statement. And we know, oftentimes, it becomes the other way around; it becomes more about the institution than it is about the veteran. So can you just say what should we be doing to make sure that the VA provides the services that veterans need, when they need it, in a location which is convenient?

Ms. SIMONI. Sure. I appreciate that. Yes, I have noticed from being a veteran myself and utilizing the VA, but also being a healthcare provider, that we start to come to these hearings and we hear more about the actual—you know, the VA more, less aboutthe veteran. And so you know, for a lot of these veterans, Post-9/ 11 specifically, less than 40 percent are enrolled in VA care.

So when you look at the rural health aspect and you look at somebody who is (a) suicidal or has a dual diagnosis of, you know, TBI, chronic pain, mental health disorder, you have got to look at it holistically. You can treat one thing. You can treat substance use the day of, sure, within 48 hours, but if you do not have something to back that with—you know, physical pain, such as myself, or emotional pain. I was discharged honorably but medically retired. I was without my team.

So mental health is lacking. You know, polytrauma, substance use, dual diagnosis, we have nothing to do that with.

So when a veteran comes to me and says, I am in crisis, I know my time is limited. If that veteran is addicted to substances and they are wanting treatment, you have to meet the veteran where they are at. You cannot expect them to drive hours away or wait days, hours. Hours is too much. It takes 10 minutes from the time you have a thought of suicide to the action itself. Ten minutes. That is a short amount of time.

And if you cannot help a veteran when they say, I am ready— because you can spin your wheels and you can say, hey, you know, we have treatment available, but if they are not ready, if they are not committed, they are not going to do it.

You know, you have to bring health care to them. And with all due respect, as somebody who has telehealth and virtual care, I can tell you right now as a provider that is not the right route to go for substance use because you cannot physically assess that patient. You cannot physically determine if they have injection marks on their arms. You cannot see if they are currently struggling. You cannot see below, my legs, where I cannot stop moving my legs.

So we need to meet the veteran where they are at, and it does not matter the extent of how that is. You just make sure you get it done. You know? And that is—these are people I served with. If I have to stay awake 24 hours a day and make sure that they are okay and they do not kill themselves, I will do that because——

Senator CASSIDY. So as a doc who greatly knows the advantage of being in the room with somebody to give me information, I can totally relate.

Dr. Cantor, you kind of put the statistics on this, that your testimony is showing that less than 10 percent of veterans with a substance use disorder in 2020 received any treatment and a key determinant is whether an individual receiving SUD, how far they have to travel.

Now Ms. Simoni, a health provider, finds telehealth as a poor substitute for in-person health. Any comments on that?

Dr. CANTOR. I think that we just basically need more research in terms of the quality of care for telehealth, and I have already stated that previously. I think that there is not enough known currently in terms of actually to determine whether or not one provides better care versus the other. I just think we need more information.

But to your point about veterans in general, about not receiving care, I think it is a persistent issue across the healthcare system; it is not just veterans. A large, significant proportion of the countrydoes not receive care for substance use disorder as well. So I would not just say it is just a veterans' issue in terms of the lack of care. Senator CASSIDY. So is the issue specific—we know about the deaths from despair and how that is often centered in men, and now increasingly in women, who do not attend college or do not graduate from college, et cetera. So are we talking about a veteran issue, or are we talking about a demographic issue because you mentioned how it is true whether you are a vet or not? So again, is this peculiar to veterans, or they are just part of that same demographic?

Dr. CANTOR. I think it is a systemwide issue. I think veterans have unique challenges in terms of both receiving treatment and then comorbidities when frequently having mental health issues along with substance use disorder. So they are a very unique population, but in terms of actual capacity and delivery of care, I think it is a systemwide problem.

Senator CASSIDY. It seems like that a veteran would have more options for care because the veteran still has the VA plus a more traditional healthcare system. So is that not a correct analysis?

Dr. CANTOR. I think it is just that mostly that most folks who need care do not actually receive it.

Senator CASSIDY. I am a little frustrated on this, sorry. Are they not receiving it because they do not seek it because they are too much into their addiction and they do not want to get out of their addiction or because they do not have access to the resource even if they want to get out of their addiction?

Dr. CANTOR. For veteran-specific or just people in general?

Senator CASSIDY. Well, let us just stay with veterans.

Dr. CANTOR. I think it is a combination of both, that there is a lack of knowledge in terms of where they can receive care and it is difficult to navigate the actual system and the fact that whether or not there are numerous barriers about care, but I do not want to just oversimplify any one individual person's decision as to whether or not to seek care.

Senator CASSIDY. Yes, but unless we have some sort of—I am not simplifying an individual.

Dr. CANTOR. Yes.

Senator CASSIDY. But unless we have some sort of—kind of—you know, we actually feel like, you know, 40 percent of people just do not want care. They are in their addiction. They would rather be an addict than actually go seek care. I worked in an inner city hospital, and frankly, that is kind of what I found sometimes. But we need to have numbers behind that because we are being asked to apply resources, but unless you have a sense of what the need is and the particulars of it—so anyway, that is—anyway, okay. I yield.

Senator MORAN. Thank you, Doctor. Senator Manchin.

Senator Joe Manchin III

Senator MANCHIN. Thank you, Mr. Chairman, and thank all of you. I appreciate very much you all being here.

Dr. Kroviak, according to the U.S. Census, we are the third most rural State in America, West Virginia. We do not have one city or one town over 50,000 population. So we are a State of towns and about 1,800,000 people.

But with that being said, how do you all determine what a rural veteran is? What is your determination of rural veterans?

Dr. KROVIAK. So in our oversight work, we would look to VHA's definition of rurality. So they have highly rural and rural locations that are based on data. I believe it is with HUD and—I am blank- ing on the other. But they have a system in place that we follow when we conduct our oversight work.

Senator MANCHIN. Yes, if you could get back to me on that——

Dr. KROVIAK. Absolutely.

VHA Response: The Veterans Health Administration (VHA) relies on standard definitions of rurality developed by the U.S. Department of Agriculture Economic Research Service (USDA-ERS). The USDA-ERS uses a framework for determining rurality called the Rural-Urban Commuting Area Codes, or RUCA codes. The RUCA codes consider population density, urbanization, and daily commuting to classify geographic areas. RUCA is based on U.S. Census data and the 2006–2010 American Community Survey (ACS) and can be applied to either counties or census tracts. The VHA uses RUCA codes to group Veterans into Urban, Rural, and Highly Rural based on their residential address that is mapped to a census tract and its corresponding RUCA value assigned for rurality.

RUCA includes primary classification codes numbered from one to ten, with one being an urban area and ten including the most rural. Generally, a Veteran is considered rural or highly rural if their residence is in a census tract with a RUCA code between two and ten. USDA-ERS is due to update the RUCA data using 2016–2020 ACS data in Fiscal Year 2024.

OIG Response: The VA OIG does not make our own determination of which VHA facilities are considered rural. Rather, we follow VA's definitions. We have provided Senator Manchin's staff a link to VA's website where they explain their methodology. Because the definition of rurality is managed by VA, we have also connected the Senator's staff with the appropriate contacts at VA to provide any additional information that is needed.

Senator MANCHIN [continuing]. Because my whole State should be. I have four different veteran hospitals and some clinics.

Also, I was going to ask you on services. I understand we are having a hard time. Basically, in a very rural area, we have the mobile. We have a mobile VA clinic. Are they able to treat for substance abuse?

Dr. KROVIAK. So there are Mobile Vet Centers that do not provide treatment but can serve to set veterans up with clinical support for detox, withdrawal, more intense services as well as long- term substance abuse treatment.

Senator MANCHIN. I mean, I am saying if they are far away from a center and they need services and they cannot get to the centers on a frequent basis because of transportation, is the mobile service available to them?

Dr. KROVIAK. So I would have to get back to you on whether the mobile services can actually offer intensive—the intensive treatment you are describing.

VHA Response: Readjustment Counseling Service (RCS) maintains a fleet of 84 Mobile Vet Centers (MVCs) to extend focused outreach, direct services, and referral services to communities that do not meet the requirements for a "brick-and-mortar" Vet Center. In many cases, these communities are distant from existing services and are considered rural or highly rural. Each MVC includes a confidential counseling space for direct service provision, as well as a state-of-the-art satellite communications package that includes fully encrypted teleconferencing equipment; access to all relevant Veterans Affairs (VA) information technology systems; and connectivity to emergency response systems.

MVCs are placed at parent Vet Centers with close access to rural communities, major military installations, and used as demand developers in areas with unmet needs. MVCs are easily moved to meet the demands across the country, whether it be to support an event or a long-term solution to unmet demand. RCS utilizes MVCs in these communities while often seeking to establish a Vet Center Community Access Points (CAPs). RCS staff work with local partners to establish CAPs by using donated office space for face-to-face appointments to occur in the communities where the need exists. Services are provided anywhere from once a month to several days per week. These partners are often Veterans Service Organizations, community providers, and local governments. Additionally, virtual services are available for all Vet Center clients, and would be available to support those who are unable to attend in person.

OIG Response: The programs and services that can assist rural veterans with accessing intensive substance use disorder treatment are managed by VA. We have therefore connected Senator Manchin's staff with the appropriate contacts at VA to assist in providing additional information on their capabilities.

Senator MANCHIN. One final thing from the clinics, I was at—we have some problems, as you know, in some of the deaths that we had in one of our hospitals. But I was there talking about substance abuse, and I had one of the nurses who was very straight- forward, and she says, well, if you all did not call and raise so much Cain with us about because we will not give veterans their drugs they want, because if we do not give it to them they would call and berate that service, that that hospital is poor and give them poor ratings, which brought more scrutiny. Are you familiar with all of this?

Dr. KROVIAK. So I understand the concern they are finding. I am not familiar with the specific statistics.

Senator MANCHIN. Do you know if that has been changed?

Dr. KROVIAK. If the——

Senator MANCHIN. I understand we put a piece of legislation that changed you could not—you cannot complain about the disbursement of drugs because I can tell you a lot of the veterans knew exactly. They knew more than the pharmacists knew about what drugs they wanted and why they wanted them, and they were determined to get those drugs. And if they did not, they would call their representatives, Senators or Congress people, and complain they were getting poor service, and we found it mostly over drug dispensation.

Do you have a—I can see you want to say something.

Dr. KROVIAK. If I could just add, though, it is a fair concern. The pendulum has swung dramatically, and veterans who are on a chronic opioid or any type of chronic pain treatment, to aggressively taper is not an appropriate form of management.

Senator MANCHIN. We are not saying, aggressively. Some of these nurses know better than what anybody else knows.

Dr. KROVIAK. No question.

Senator MANCHIN. They are not able to do their job, but I am hoping that has reversed. Does anybody up there know about what I am talking about? Have you heard? Chelsey, do you want to talk?

Ms. SIMONI. Yes, I have heard about it, and I have experienced it, and it is twofold like you mentioned.

Senator MANCHIN. Tell me which way it is going.

Ms. SIMONI. Well, so it is not always the veteran that is seeking the drugs. You know, I mean, it is an interesting move, but I bring this as one month of pills from the VA that I did not ask for, that the providers thought I needed. And I said to them, if I take all these, I probably will not wake up.

This is one month, and so with all due respect, trazodone to help me sleep, ropinirole and——

Senator MANCHIN. Is that on a daily basis?

Ms. SIMONI. This is on a daily basis.

Senator MANCHIN. Oh, someone take a picture of this.

Ms. SIMONI. But this is—so it is not always the veteran that is asking for these.

Senator MANCHIN. So it is basically being prescribed to them.

Ms. SIMONI. We are not looking at it from a holistic perspective.

Senator MANCHIN. You got to be kidding me. This is——

Ms. SIMONI. Oh, there is two more. There is two more.

Senator MANCHIN. Put them all out there. Yes, please, get this.

Ms. SIMONI. And so if I take these together, there is a good chance I will not wake up. And thankfully, as a healthcare provider, I know I cannot take this with this and that with that. But these are all my pills, and so——

Senator MANCHIN. Have you talked—I mean, knowing that you have the medical expertise, have you talked to the providers why they did this?

Ms. SIMONI. When I said to the provider—I went to the VA two months ago, and I said, my back is getting worse. My spine is collapsing on itself.

Senator MANCHIN. Right, right.

Ms. SIMONI. I am 32 years old.

Go to physical therapy. Here is some more gabapentin. This should help with the numbness.

I said, that does not work. I have been doing this for 10 years. What else can I do?

Oh, you can have a spinal fusion.

So I cannot walk. I said, this is not—that does not work for me. I cannot sleep. I cannot stop tossing and turning, and it is solely based on an injury.

And so if this is not an addiction in the making—and this is recent. This is one month. If this is not an addiction in the making, I do not know what is, and this is why it is critical to see patients in person.

Senator MANCHIN. Well, this is what I was saying, too. I have been told basically—and I have talked to a lot of our servicemembers who have been deployed, and they are able to get anything they want, any concoction they want, just to get through the day.

Ms. SIMONI. Except if they want alternative treatment, respectfully.

Senator MANCHIN. It is the same, isn't it? Mr. Chairman, we have got to do something.

Senator MORAN. Thank you, Senator Manchin. Senator Sullivan.

Senator Dan Sullivan

Senator SULLIVAN. Thank you, Mr. Chairman. And, boy, Ms. Simoni, that is some serious—
—

Senator MANCHIN. I teed it up for you.

Senator SULLIVAN [continuing]. Drugs you got there. You know, we have had hearings on this. I want to commend Senator Manchin. He has done a lot in this area, on this topic.

Dr. Kroviak, that was not one of the questions I was going to ask, but is there a concern from the IG's Office about these kind of prescriptions that could lead to a dangerous situation?

Dr. KROVIAK. That is catastrophic care coordination like I have never seen, and it is a huge concern when multiple providers are involved. Usually we see the greatest concern between VHA and the community. When that information is not being shared real time, dangerous concoctions can happen like this, and patients might be completely unaware.

Senator SULLIVAN. So are those all from the VA?

Ms. SIMONI. Yes, sir.

Senator MORAN. How many providers? Does that come from more than one, obviously, more than one provider?

Ms. SIMONI. Neurology, mental health, and that is it. Two.

Senator SULLIVAN. From the same VA? Which VA is that?

Ms. SIMONI. New England VA Healthcare System. It is in the New England VA Healthcare System.

Dr. KROVIAK. So there is a misstep in medication reconciliation, and I obviously do not know the specifics of your care, but that sounds like a big gap in medication reconciliation.

Senator SULLIVAN. Yes, you might want to look into that. Right? We do not want anyone from that system or any system, or any of our veterans, dying of a drug overdose that is induced by too many pills. That is outrageous.

Let me turn to the topic at hand, Dr. Kroviak, and—by the way, I want to thank all the witnesses. A lot of you are veterans and are caring for veterans. It is not easy. So all four of you I actually appreciate very much. I read all your backgrounds. Impressive what you have done and your concern, so thank you to all the witnesses here.

Do we have a sense—just going back to some basic issues—on wait times with regard to the VA, and is there a significant difference between urban and rural areas in terms of wait times?

Dr. KROVIAK. So we do look at those in rural versus urban. We do see somewhat of an increase in rural if you look at fiscal year '22. It is not—I think some of the mental health differences for referrals were seven or eight days' difference, and I can get those exact numbers that our office drew from VA data. But it is measurable in terms of when you compare rural to urban, that rural has a longer wait time, especially for specialty care.

Senator SULLIVAN. Okay. You know, I come from a State with more vets per capita than any State in the country, and our very rural State, Alaska, we do not even have one full-service VA hospital in the State.

And one of the issues that my State has experienced, particularly with regard to rural providers, is the lack of experience in terms of the providers themselves. And so can you speak to that? Are there recruitment efforts that are being made with regard to trying to get more experienced providers in our rural areas? Maybe this is an issue beyond Alaska.

And what can we do about it? Is there pay scales that we can provide? Are there incentives that we can provide to make sure we are getting high quality providers to people in rural Alaska? It should not matter on your ZIP code how good your VA or private care provider is.

Dr. KROVIAK. So I appreciate the question. Unfortunately, in oversight, we have no role in determining VA's hiring or retention and recruiting activities. So that would be better directed to them. But if I could just say, we do understand the quality concerns that you are describing, particularly again when you go out into the community, that clinical information sharing opportunities are lost or so delayed that I cannot tell you what type of quality of care is happening outside of the VA, and I am very concerned they cannot either. So your concerns about the caliber or the credentialing, the experience of the providers they are hiring, in VA as well as in the community, is definitely warranted.

Senator SULLIVAN. Let me ask one final question, and I will throw it out for all the witnesses. Senator Cassidy, Dr. Cassidy, was talking about this issue of the prevalence of substance abuse in the veteran population, and then beyond just the veteran population, Dr. Cantor, he was a having a discussion with you.

But it also certainly seems like it is a younger generation issue. Is that a trend that you are seeing, any of you, in your experience, that these substance abuse issues are hitting a younger demographic, and if so, why? And if not, then maybe that is not an area of focus. Anyone on that? No one knows whether—go ahead.

Ms. SIMONI. I can speak on behalf of civilian. Every—I work 40 hours a week in the ER, doing three on, four off, and I see roughly, at Mass General Hospital, 10 overdoses a week in just my practice alone in individuals under the age 35.

Senator SULLIVAN. So it is a younger demographic.

Ms. SIMONI. From my practice and personal experience, yes.

Senator SULLIVAN. Anyone—Dr. Cantor, have you seen this as a broad demographic trend, or you do not have the data on it?

Dr. CANTOR. I do not have the data on that.

Senator SULLIVAN. Anyone else? Dr. Kroviak?

Dr. KROVIAK. I do not have the data, but if you are targeting an age group, we are doing work now in that high risk transition period from active duty to civilian, or to veteran, when you will find typically a younger age. And we are doing work now looking specifically at ensuring that those diagnosed during active duty with opioid use disorder, that that information is translated into the VA record. We are seeing there are a lot of gaps in even ensuring that once the diagnosis is made in active duty that veterans are being recorded as having that diagnosis and immediately getting treatment and support for it. So it does softly hit your age target that you were describing.

Senator SULLIVAN. Okay, good. Thank you. Thank you, Mr. Chairman.

Senator MORAN. Thank you, Senator.

Maybe for Dr. Kroviak or anyone, so are there statistics that— let me preface what I am going to say. So 2014, we saw an inability of the VA within their hospital system to meet the needs of veterans. That is when we saw and learned about the fake waiting lists, the fake appointment lists, and we responded; Congress responded with CHOICE in 2014. So for 10 years, we have been trying to figure out how we can get the Department of Veterans Affairs to provide health care in more locations by using community care.

Community care existed before CHOICE. My view is that CHOICE was implemented by the Department of Veterans Affairs in which it needed more, greater restrictions in our language to make sure that community care was actually provided. We had to encourage the Department to use that option.

So we passed MISSION, giving some pretty specific directions and outlines in which the circumstances—and again, only in the circumstance in which a veteran wants to have community care. And still, we find that the gaps continue.

My interest in this, I mean, is broad across the country—the deaths in the hospital in Arizona, et cetera—but it is also very local for me. I represent a State—a congressional district at the time that is the size of the State of Illinois. There is no VA hospital, and it is hours to drive for almost every veteran to a VA hospital.

And so we have tried legislatively to encourage, force, require when the choice was the veteran's to receive care in the community.

Any inspector general reports that demonstrate any success in those efforts? Are things getting better? Do we still have problems in the utilization of community care?

I have legislation that we are going to, I hope, mark up soon that will require you to make those analyses so that we can determine whether or not the efforts that we have undertaken over a decade are making a difference. Any commentary?

Dr. KROVIAK. Your question is massive; I mean, it really is. I am a bit biased as a former provider in the VA. What CHOICE did not solve, what MISSION has not solved is when you are engaging with the community, reliably getting that clinical information back, so VA and the community provider are on the same page at the same time to manage the veteran's care.

It gets so much worse when there is complexity introduced. So if there is a mental health diagnosis, if there is a cancer that requires multidisciplinary specialties to get involved, the coordination is enormously difficult, and it remains so.

And technology is likely the ultimate solution, but we are not there yet to where the EHRs can interface, to have that real-time connection going.

Every report the Office of Healthcare Inspection writes touches on some form of care coordination gaps, failures, and they are usually highlighted in that community care collaboration setting. Sountil there is a way to ensure that a primary care provide in the VA who sends their patient out to the community for that dermatology or cardiology referral, until they can know in real time how that patient is being managed, you have no assessment of the quality.

Senator MORAN. What is the current capability?

Dr. KROVIAK. It depends on the part of the country. You know, there are HIEs, but our understanding is very few community providers participate in the Health Information Exchanges. We are still especially in some rural communities relying on faxes, and those faxes get sent to a space in a facility where already a stressed staff in terms of number have to just scan those records in, and we do not even find there is uniformity in the scanning. So the record might be there for the provider to look at, but they have no idea how to find it, what is the naming convention. It is a dangerous relationship right now.

Senator MORAN. And are there other reasons? Perhaps you are suggesting that a provider within the VA would be reluctant to make the referral because the lack of communication between——

Dr. KROVIAK. I do not want to imply that they would delay care intentionally for their patient, but when we do hear stories where the veteran is choosing to stay, I can, you know, honestly say, I get it, where they are choosing to wait for the VA provider as opposed to being sent into the community. But I do not want to suggest that we have anything that VA providers are scared to send their patients so they do not because that is something we have not looked at.

Senator MORAN. I would tell you that, anecdotally, so many times I have—mostly what I know about what is going on in veterans' lives is the conversations I have with veterans. No offense to RAND or to the Inspector General.

Dr. KROVIAK. None taken.

Senator MORAN. I should read your reports more frequently, but veterans are willing, usually, to have a conversation. And so often it is that, I am seeking community care, but I cannot get the referral from the Department of Veterans Affairs.

So there seems to me to be some bias if it is based upon a concern about medical care, but it is certainly a slow process——

Dr. KROVIAK. Yes.

Senator MORAN [continuing]. By which the VA will make the decision when someone asks, when a veteran asks for community care.

And what I have heard in the time that I have been here in front of this panel is that there is no time to spare. And so a system that is designed to save lives and improve one's well-being, particularly, I suppose, it could be other things than mental health and drug addiction, but certainly in those circumstances we need a system in which a referral is made quickly.

I understand that in many communities across Kansas and the country there are not enough providers in mental health and substance abuse services to make those referrals to. It is a shortage across the board. But I want—it is a goal of mine—to make sure there are no artificial, unnecessary impediments, or no bias against a veteran who chooses or needs care quickly or needs care becauseof geography, that the VA is not making those referrals in a timely, medically necessary fashion.

Dr. KROVIAK. Again, that is a huge undertaking, and I really appreciate the concern. Even if you take it out of this one aspect of community care you are looking at, this is a massive system, and it has a lot of policies and practices in place. And getting frontline staff to consistently apply those rules is difficult, especially when you do not have standardization across the board that builds in that accountability.

In my oral testimony, I highlighted incredibly dated handbooks and guidelines for clinical practice. So we cannot fix the interface of EHR today, but things that we can do in the immediate term is update the policies and practices, clinical and administrative, give the front line a chance to practice the rules consistently, and then standardize some type of structure at whatever level, maybe even looking at the VISN, to make sure those rules are being carried out. That is an immediate or a near immediate solution that will at least get you more comfortable that the staff is offering the veteran, based on the wait times, care that they need and the opportunity they have to get care outside the VA.

Senator MORAN. Well, it is another experience, and as an Inspector General you would not, I do not think, find this surprising. So many times, I mean, I bring a case to the Department of Veterans Affairs, and nationally, here in Washington, DC, I am told that this is the policy and if it was not the policy we have now fixed the policy. But that is—well, let me be more precise. It is often the case that that is not what the person in the VISN or in the hospital or in the community outpatient clinic—that is not what they know the policy to be.

So I am often told, here is the policy. Senator Moran, we have got the policy that you want. But that is not close to what——

Dr. KROVIAK. The SOP, the local business rule, might be completely different. So the frontline staff is being honest; here is what I do because I am told to do this. And they are being honest when they are delivering the policy. And when they conflict, who loses? The veteran.

Senator MORAN. Yes. I am not off this topic. I mean, I am off this topic for the moment, but I am not off this topic generally.

Let me highlight how grateful I am to Ms. Simoni for what is a very difficult testimony to provide. I appreciate you sharing your personal and family story.

You indicated in your testimony that the data you shared with the Committee also notes many examples of where care offered by the VA has fallen short for many of your fellow veterans. Would you expand on what you are telling us?

Ms. SIMONI. Of course. You know, you are the Senator of Kansas. So I mean, a perfect example, you know, in terms of community care——

Senator MORAN. You have got something else in your bag?

Ms. SIMONI. No, no. I wish. I usually have a lot of—no. You know, it brings me back to the fact I deal mostly with oncology and veterans with terminal cancers, and you know, SOP goes out the window when time is on the clock. And I mean, I say that in the most humble way possible, but year to date, we have lost—only the ones that I know of, that I have physically cared for—119 Post-9/ 11 veterans from cancer.

And so two years ago, we had a veteran who was in the Kansas VA healthcare system. He was on this third diagnosis of terminal cancer, and the VA said to him, there is nothing more we can do. And being he was only 34 years old, with three kids, I did not accept that. I said, let me try. Let me call. Let me do something.

And so we finally got him care down at MD Anderson, and when he requested through his provider who writes the order or the allowance for community care, his provider says, that is not evidence- based. You cannot go there. I am not writing that order.

And we fought for two weeks, and as two weeks goes by, time is running out. Finally, I said, I will pay for it myself because you can always make more money but you cannot save a life once it is gone. And myself and my co-worker, Matt, reached out to your office, and you had him squared away, like squared away instantly. And it saved his life, and he is still alive today, which is incredible because he was given a terminal diagnosis two years ago.

So this is something we face every day. And I mean it in the most humbling way possible; I do not have time. My patients, my veterans, the people I served with, myself, my brother, we do not have time to wait for processes to be implemented or systemic problems to be fixed. These are—time is running out.

Twenty-four hours in a day. Time is running out. Every single 24—every hour that goes, that time matters. And if I have to pay for it myself, I will because you can always make more money but you cannot save a life once it is gone.

Senator MORAN. That was not the answer I was soliciting, but I appreciate the fact that you took extra—greater willingness to go another step to make a difference.

It is also a good reminder. And I make the same mistake. I talk about the MISSION Act in terms of geography, which is a huge component to people for substance abuse and mental health issues and suicide and just general care. But the MISSION Act is also designed to get expertise that may not exist within the VA, perhaps such as oncology, that can also serve a veteran if that is, again, his or her choice.

You know, Ms. Simoni, that I recently introduced the Veterans' HEALTH Act that aims to address some of the issues that we are talking about today. Would you share with me, so I can repeat it when we have a debate and conversation about this legislation, why your organization decided to endorse that legislation?

Ms. SIMONI. Absolutely.

Senator MORAN. Please do. Please tell me why your organization endorsed that legislation.

Ms. SIMONI. Oh, sure. So I have bad hearing.

Senator MORAN. My wife tells me I am a terrible communicator.

Ms. SIMONI. I just—I cannot hear that well. So our organization supported that legislation because, you know, at the end of the day, like I said, it is not about if we vote Democrat, Republican, you know, whether veterans—whatever it may be. This is about the veteran.

And so the HEALTH Act I found very interesting because it allows us to get the veteran care where they are at. And for a lot of these rare cancer cases—and a lot of these are rare cancers that we deal with. Substance use. Like I mentioned, it is dual diagnoses and polytrauma. It has to be looked at holistically.

And so a lot of my patients end up dying because they do not receive unique veteran-specific care, and I believe that your HEALTH Act can make a big difference in that. I believe that they will be able to receive care at some of the best hospitals in the country, such as MD Anderson, such as Moffitt, such as Dana-Farber, more quickly, more adequately, more holistically, and at the end of the day, that is all that matters to me and our organization.

Senator MORAN. Thank you.

Ms. Mathis, your written testimony included a recommendation to the VA to increase the number of Clinical Resource Hubs to better aid veterans who live in areas that experience bandwidth problems. We have been talking about technology, and we have been talking about telemedicine, telehealth.

My staff and I are proponents of this initiative of the Office of Rural Health and routinely ask the VA if they are requesting adequate funding for Clinical Resource Hubs or could benefit from additional hubs. In addition to serving on this Committee, I am an appropriator as well.

Can you share with us DAV's recommendations on how many additional Clinical Resource Hubs VA could use to serve VA's rural and highly rural veteran population?

Ms. MATHIS. Thank you for that question, Senator. I do not have the data as far as how many they need. That would be a VA data- driven kind of answer.

But I will say that in rural communities, as you know, they do have bandwidth issues. And if a veteran cannot get to the technology that is supposed to help them because they do not have the capacity to do so, then how is technology supposed to be helping that veteran?

So the Clinical Resource Hubs are really beneficial for the rural veteran to be able to get the quality care that VA provides, and so they do have efforts such as the Virtual Living Room where you can go to, say, your local DAV chapter and have a private conversation with your provider using these Clinical Resource Hubs or these Virtual Living Rooms as well.

Senator MORAN. I want to hear what you had to say, but I also thought of another issue.

Ms. MATHIS. Sure.

Senator MORAN. I could not hear either. So related to these topics, ATLAS pods was something that was touted—we have one in Kansas, in Emporia—in which mental health services were to be provided so that a veteran who did not have access to the technology or the broadband width to receive and send signals to a provider could go to a central location within the community. In this case, a Veterans Service Organization worked with a private company to put in the pod. The VA has paused the implementation of that.

Do disabled American veterans know about that program? Anything that you want to share with me or just I will use this as an opportunity to remind myself and the VA that pause has been going now for months.

Ms. MATHIS. I do not know about that program, but I am very interested to hear about it.

Senator MORAN. Okay. Do you think it could have merit?

Ms. MATHIS. I do not—I do not know.

Senator MORAN. Do not know.

Ms. MATHIS. I would have to look at it.

Senator MORAN. Okay. Anyone else? [No response.]

Senator MORAN. Thank you very much, all, for your testimony. I want to thank you, I do thank you, for being here.

We will continue to make certain that we do everything we can to see that veterans receive high quality care, particularly as it relates in this hearing to mental health and substance abuse disorders, and I am grateful for the care and compassion that each of you has shown for those who served our country.

One reason I was late, incidentally, is today is the 248th anniversary of the Army, and so we were cutting cake. I chair the Army Caucus, and I was responsible for helping cut the cake. But I am glad I made it to hear the testimony that I did and have the conversations with you.

We will keep the record open for a week in case my colleagues and I have questions that you can then reply to the record, and for today, the hearing is adjourned. Thank you.

[Whereupon, at 4:48 p.m., the hearing was adjourned.]

Appendix

Prepared Statements

Statement of Erica Scavella, M.D. FACP, FACHE Assistant Under Secretary for Health for Clinical Services, Chief Medical Officer Veterans Health Administration (VHA) Department of Veterans Affairs (VA) Before the Senate Committee on Veterans' Affairs "Connections to Care: Improving Substance Use Disorder Care for Veterans in Rural America and Beyond" June 14, 2023

Good morning, Chairman Tester, Ranking Member Moran, and distinguished Members of the Committee. Thank you for the opportunity today to discuss VA's substance use disorder (SUD) treatment programs in rural America. Accompanying me today is Dr. Tamara Campbell, Executive Director, Office of Mental Health and Suicide Prevention, and Dr. Bradley Watts, Director, Veterans Rural Health Resource Center.

There has been an upsurge in morbidity and mortality from SUDs over the past 10 years as powerful and hazardous illicit drugs have become more widespread in the United States. From fiscal year (FY) 2018 to FY 2022, the number of Veterans diagnosed with a SUD (which includes alcohol use disorder) and receiving treatment in VHA increased from 522,544 to 550,412.

Due to the complexity of SUD, no single remedy, no clinical or law enforcement intervention alone, nor any single agency, VA or otherwise, will suffice in meeting our nation's challenges with substance use and the associated overdose epidemic.

Therefore, VA is working alongside the White House's Office of National Drug Control Policy (ONDCP) and other Federal agencies to implement an evidence-based, comprehensive strategy to address the Nation's challenges with SUD and the threat they pose to the well-being of the American people. VA embraces its role in helping to fulfill the National Drug Control Strategy and is grateful for the support VA has received from Congress in implementing programs to ensure that Veterans receive the highest quality SUD prevention and treatment services they need and deserve. Treatment for rural Veterans with SUD occur in the context of VA's overall efforts to treat Veterans experiencing substance use concerns. Enterprise-wide efforts are focused on ensuring the needs of all Veterans with SUD are met with no wrong door to accessing care and focused attention to ensure application of those efforts to rural Veterans.

To reduce the burden of SUD in the Veteran population, it is important to use broad-based national preventative and treatment strategies. To achieve its goals, VA uses both whole-of-Government and whole-of-Nation approaches. These are exemplified by VA's interagency collaborations. As an illustration, the Department of Defense (DoD) and VA collaborated to produce clinical practice guidelines for the management of SUDs. To meet the needs of Veterans with or at risk of SUD, VA also collaborates closely with several other Departments and agencies, including the Departments of Health and Human Services, Energy, Justice, and Housing and Urban Development. VA's efforts in coordination with other Federal agencies support the priorities defined by the National Drug Control Strategy. In alignment with the Strategy and the President's Unity Agenda's priority to address the overdose crisis, VA is working to expand access to evidence-based treatment for SUDs and enhancing evidence-based harm reduction efforts aimed at reducing overdose fatalities. VA offers a comprehensive continuum of specialty SUD services for Veterans founded in the evidence. Our VA/DoD Clinical Practice Guidelines,[1] updated in FY 2021, provide the foundation for evidence-based treatment within VA and have positioned VA to respond to emerging drug use trends.

Overview of SUD Treatment at VA

Rates of substance use, types of substances used, and treatment for SUD vary geographically. VA is committed to ensuring Veterans have access to treatment for SUD regardless of where they live. Using the Census Bureau's Rural-Urban Community Area (RUCA) coding system that designates census tracts as urban, rural, highly rural, or unknown, we assigned patients these applicable codes based on their home address. Consequently, of the over 550,000 Veterans currently receiving SUD care from VHA (8.5% of all patients who received care from VHA), we determined that VA treated a total of 124,275 rurally-located Veterans with alcohol use disorder (AUD) and 66,439 rurally-located Veterans with drug use disorders through the second quarter of FY 2023 (Note: a Veteran may be counted in both data points). Of those

[1] https://www.healthquality.va.gov/guidelines/MH/sud/.

Veterans with drug use disorders, 18,880 were treated for opioid use disorder (OUD), 20,581 were treated for stimulant use disorder, and 38,465 were treated for cannabis use disorder.

Over the last decade, VHA has worked to mitigate risk factors associated with opioids and stimulants use among Veterans, including by launching a national Opioid Safety Initiative a decade ago and a national Stimulant Safety Initiative last year. In addition, VA provides comprehensive services for the treatment of SUD, including screening and brief intervention for alcohol use disorder; outpatient and intensive outpatient SUD specialty services; pharmacotherapy for OUD, including office-based buprenorphine, extended-release injectable naltrexone and Opioid Treatment Programs that provide methadone; evidence-based treatments for stimulant use disorder; SUD residential treatment programs; and withdrawal management. Peer specialists also are being embedded across the continuum to support Veterans in recovery and treatment for SUD within primary and specialty care settings, pain management clinics, emergency departments, and general mental health clinics. Beyond treatment for SUD, VA provides both primary and secondary prevention specific to OUD in addition to efforts specific to risks associated with substance use in general.

As an integrated health care system, VA is uniquely situated to address the needs of Veterans diagnosed with SUD by providing support to address co-occurring medical, mental health and psychosocial needs, including support for employment and housing.

Also, VA is incorporating data from both VA medical records and from public sources that, when combined, characterize communities in terms of social and environmental determinants of health. Oak Ridge National Laboratory is assisting VA with analyzing these data into predictive models for targeted prevention programs so we can better identify Veterans with the greatest challenges to recovery and get them the additional support they need. Through collaborations with the Lawrence Berkeley, Los Alamos, and Sandia National Labs, VA is making better use of medical record information to identify high-risk VA patient populations. Through work with JJR Solutions in Dayton, Ohio, a service-disabled Veteran-owned small business, VA has found that provider education sessions on opioid safety practices lead to more effective treatment for Veterans in primary care and reduction in overdoses.

Current policy, grounded in the latest evidence, requires facilities provide access to a comprehensive continuum of SUD treatment services ranging from early intervention and harm reduction services through intensive outpatient and, when needed, residential or inpatient treatment for SUD. In addition, current policy requires facilities provide same day outpatient access for Veterans with emergent substance use treatment needs. This care may be provided in person or via telehealth in several settings including general mental health, primary care mental health integration clinics, and SUD specialty clinics. Core characteristics of SUD services include timely same day triage, a no wrong door approach, concurrent treatment for co-occurring needs and Veteran-centered and individualized treatment based on the needs and preferences of the Veteran.

VHA national policy explicitly states that Veterans cannot be denied access to care due to their use of a substance. Further, both national policy and the VA/DoD Clinical Practice Guideline for Management of Substance Use Disorders define expectations that Veterans be retained in care and that programs do not use criteria that would require automatic discharge from treatment due to substance use. Over the last several years, there has been significant emphasis on engagement in care with a focus on meeting Veterans where they are in their recovery. Meeting people where they are is the underlying principle in harm reduction.

In addition, VHA continues to improve service delivery and efficiency by integrating services for mental health disorders, including SUD, into primary care settings. VHA-enrolled Veterans from all service eras have primary care teams (Patient Aligned Care Teams, or PACTs) with co-located mental health staff to identify and address potential mental health and substance use treatment needs. Secondary prevention services include diagnosis and assessment of possible SUD in patients presenting with medical problems that suggest elevated risk of SUD. While most Veterans with SUD are treated in outpatient programs, providers in these outpatient treatment settings are expected to collaborate with colleagues in inpatient and residential SUD care settings to coordinate Veterans' transitions across these levels of SUD care. Such efforts are necessary for helping ensure continuity of SUD care that is consistent with a chronic disease model of care and responsive to changes in Veterans' clinical status.

Considering the frequent co-occurrence of SUDs with posttraumatic stress disorder (PTSD), VHA also has assigned a SUD specialist to each of its hospital-level PTSD services or teams. The SUD-PTSD specialist is an integral member of the PTSD clinical services team and works to integrate SUD care with all other aspects of PTSD- related care. Among the specialists' responsibilities are identification and treatment of Veterans with co-occurring SUD and PTSD. Specialists also promote preventive services for Veterans with PTSD who are at risk for developing a SUD.

VHA provides two types of 24-hour care to patients with severe or complex SUD. These include inpatient withdrawal management and stabilization in numerous medical and general mental health units, equivalent to Level 4, Medically Managed Intensive Inpatient Treatment as specified by the American Society of Addiction Medicine Patient Placement Criteria (https://www.asam.org/asam-criteria/about-the-asam-criteria), and provision of care in Mental Health Residential Rehabilitation Treatment Programs (MH RRTP) otherwise referred to as Domiciliary SUD beds. VHA offers care in MH RRTPs to Veterans with complex, co-occurring mental health, substance use, medical, and psychosocial needs. Specialty Domiciliary SUD programs provide treatment equivalent to Level 3.7, Medically Monitored Intensive Inpatient Services, as specified by the American Society of Addiction Medicine Patient Placement Criteria. Today, more than 70 Domiciliary SUD programs are in operation with more than 1,700 beds focused specifically on intensive, medically monitored residential SUD treatment. In addition to those MH RRTPs formally designated as Domiciliary SUD programs, additional SUD specialized services are offered through tracks in other MH RRTPs, and most Veterans served (more than 95%) by MH RRTPs are diagnosed with a SUD. Several new Domiciliary SUD programs are under development with the number of programs expected to grow over the next few years.

Programs to end homelessness among Veterans are encouraged to have SUD specialists as a part of their multidisciplinary teams. There are SUD specialists working in the Department of Housing and Urban Development – VA Supportive Housing, Grant and Per Diem and the Health Care for Homeless Veterans programs; however, the use of SUD specialists can vary locally based on site-specific needs. These specialists emphasize early identification of SUDs as a risk for maintaining permanent housing, promote engagement or re-engagement in SUD specialty care programs, provide evidence-based SUD treatment services, and link Veterans to specialty SUD treatment when such Veterans need more intensive SUD treatment services. In 2022, VHA supported the expansion of VA case managers integrated with existing homeless program staff to assist Supported Services for Veteran Families (SSVF) grantees with engaging

Veterans experiencing SUD concerns into VA services, including but not limited to SUD specialty care or residential treatment when needed.

VHA's existing infrastructure within the Homeless Program Office provides a foundation by which HPO can quickly direct resources, through grants, to community providers with the intent of rapidly engaging or re-engaging Veterans with SUD services specific to their treatment needs. Because people experiencing unstable housing or homelessness are at high risk of overdose, VHA has been working to place Veterans experiencing homelessness into permanent housing.

Treatment for Alcohol Misuse

Within VA, patients with at-risk alcohol use or mildly severe SUDs may be treated with evidence-based brief interventions or medical management in primary care or general mental health. For those with more severe impairment, specialty SUD treatment programs provide intensive services, including withdrawal management, evidence-based psychosocial treatments, SUD medication, case management and relapse prevention provided in outpatient, intensive outpatient, and residential settings of care.

VA has developed services specifically focused on engagement in care for vulnerable Veteran populations. VA efforts include universal screening for at-risk alcohol use, urine drug screening for at-risk Veterans, the provision of peer support services, integration of SUD treatment within homeless programs, and collaboration with Veterans' courts and the work of our re-entry specialists to engage Veterans with SUD involved with the legal system.

Treatment for Opioid Use Disorder

With national initiatives like Stepped Care for OUD, Train the Trainer, and the Psychotropic Drug Safety Initiative, VA emphasizes access to evidence-based treatments for SUDs. These initiatives aim to increase access to both evidence-based pharmacotherapies and evidence-based psychotherapies for SUD. According to the National Survey on Drug Use and Health conducted by the Substance Abuse and Mental Health Services Administration, only 22% of the general population with OUD received medication for OUD in 2021. In calendar year 2022, VA more than doubled that rate, with over 47 percent of patients with OUD having received medications for OUD from VA within the last 12 months ending March 31, 2023. Appropriate use of medications approved by the Food and Drug Administration for OUD can lower the risk of illicit opioid use, overdose, suicide, and other mortalities.

Treatment for Stimulant and Cannabis Use Disorders

In 2022, VA provided psychosocial or behavioral therapy for SUD to almost 172,000 Veterans. VA is using national training initiatives to ensure that these treatments are as effective as possible, expanding access to strong, evidence-based cognitive behavioral therapies and contingency management programs. Notably, contingency management is the most effective evidence-based treatment for stimulant use disorder and has shown success in treating cannabis use disorder, two SUDs that are increasingly common in the VHA patient population. More than 6,200 Veterans have received contingency management treatment since 2011. Over 90% of the nearly 80,000 urine samples that those Veterans submitted tested negative for the target drugs, which are frequently stimulants and occasionally cannabis (THC). For Veterans with AUD, VA offers both evidence-based medications as well as evidence-based psychotherapies, separately or in combination depending on the shared decision-making between Veterans and their treatment providers. VA recognizes that not all Veterans with SUD will embrace abstinence among their recovery goals.

Harm Reduction

SUD, like hypertension or diabetes, is a chronic, relapsing condition; even Veterans who are striving to abstain from substances may not always be consistently successful. Because any exposure to substances can be fatal for individuals with SUD, VA provides Veterans with evidence-based interventions to protect them from harms, like overdose or infectious diseases like human immunodeficiency virus (HIV) and hepatitis, that could otherwise lead to their death. In just the past year, VHA equipped over 70,000 Veterans with naloxone to reverse potentially fatal opioid overdoses.

Furthermore, over 1 million naloxone prescriptions have been provided to Veterans since 2014, when we launched our Overdose Education and Naloxone Distribution (OEND) initiative. This initiative has led to more than 3,700 overdose reversals. As part of this effort, VA uses data-driven modeling to identify Veterans at high risk of overdose and conducts clinical case reviews to inform their customized treatment plans. We appreciate Congress' support, which has been critical for the success of VA's overdose prevention efforts by allowing VA to provide naloxone at no cost to Veterans at high risk for overdose.

VA has also aligned its policies and operations with interventions in the National Drug Control Strategy related to harms related to bloodborne infections spread through contaminated injection equipment, particularly HIV infection and chronic hepatitis C virus infection. VA pioneered integrated care for SUD patients with these life-threatening conditions, with cure rates among Veterans with alcohol, substance use, and mental health disorders that are similar to cure rates in those without these conditions.[2]

Education and Training

Overall, in support of its comprehensive approach to the treatment of SUD, VA has developed a wide array of substance use education programs for Veterans and providers in its efforts to expand SUD education and outreach. The programs are being implemented across the Department and can be classified as follows:

---

[2] Belperio PS, Chartier M, Ross DB, Alaigh P, Shulkin D. Curing Hepatitis C Virus Infection: Best Practices From the U.S. Department of Veterans Affairs. Ann Intern Med. 2017 Oct 3;167(7):499-504.

- Initiatives to educate primary care practitioners on the diagnosis and treatment of AUDs.
- Harm reduction approaches to reduce negative consequences of substance use.
- Programs developed for Veterans and Veterans' families.
- Clinician training and consultation programs to improve their knowledge, skills, and abilities to treat Veterans with SUD.
- SUD training programs for trainees participating in clinical training with VA.

In addition, VA is supporting SUD training for our future workforce and is implementing novel harm reduction approaches, including the development of mobile and internet-based applications. Beginning with the President's Budget for FY 2022, VA has requested support to directly respond to national priorities defined in the National Drug Control Strategy. The plan directly addressed the unique needs of Veterans with substance use concerns within the context of broader national priorities.

SUD Treatment Programs for Rural Veterans

To expand access to SUD treatment for Veterans, including those who reside in rural areas, who may not seek treatment in specialty care settings, VHA continues to invest in a complement of team members to increase access to evidence-based treatment for SUD both within and outside specialty SUD care. One of the essential interprofessional care team providers is the Clinical Pharmacist Practitioner (CPP). The CPP serves as the medication expert delivering comprehensive medication management (CMM) to Veterans using a patient-centered, collaborative approach in conjunction with all members of the health care team.

In delivering CMM care, the CPP focuses on ensuring medications are assessed for appropriateness, effectiveness, and safety given the patient's clinical status, comorbidities, other medications, and patient's ability to adhere to a medication regimen. CPPs improve VHA's ability to accomplish the quintuple aim of better care, reduced health care costs, improved patient experience, provider well-being, and health equity; CPPs have demonstrated positive impacts on access, Veteran engagement, treatment retention, and telehealth care delivery. CPPs provide risk mitigation strategies, perform screening, and deliver brief interventions, referrals, and treatment.

The CPP is part of the solution for the unmet need in OUD and AUD treatment, especially for rural Veterans.

Starting in FY 2020, as part of a rural health initiative, VA hired 64 CPPs across 52 rural facilities to support VHA's strategy to provide the best care in a timely manner. These CPPs ensure Veterans have access to a medication expert providing CMM services to 43,262 Veterans over 129,078 patient care encounters with over 68% of the visits delivered using telehealth modalities. To scale best practices and drive innovation, this project delivered system-wide training focused on SUD screening, care, and treatment with a whole health focus to 266 CPPs across the system. As a result of the training, there has been a 52% increase in CPPs delivering overall SUD care, 53% increase in CPPs providing AUD care, and a 97% increase in the number of CPPs providing OUD care since FY 2018. To continue improving SUD access to rural Veterans, VA has provided funding to 24 facilities to hire 30 new CPPs in

Primary Care Mental Health Integration and Behavioral Health Integrated Programs teams, which will include a provision of SUD care within their practice, including AUD, OUD, and stimulant use disorder in the fourth quarter of FY 2023. Priority will be placed on specific populations to decrease SUD disparities.

Veterans living in rural communities often face unique challenges that limit their access to health care. Barriers such as long distances to clinical facilities and a shortage of qualified providers can put rural Veterans and their families at risk. Rural Veterans have a 20% greater risk of suicide than their urban counterparts.[3] At the same time, rural areas have fewer mental health care providers than their urban counterparts.[4] To overcome these challenges and reach rural Veterans with critical health care needs, VA has expanded access through telehealth programs. This includes the development and ongoing expansion of Clinical Resource Hubs (CRH) – a network of VA centers in large, urban settings that are skilled in delivering their services to Veterans in rural areas at medical centers, VA community clinics, and in the home through telehealth technology.

Utilization of Telehealth for SUD Treatment

During the pandemic, VA was able to ensure continued access to SUD treatment to Veterans in rural areas through expanded use of telehealth. This was facilitated by pandemic prescribing flexibilities under Federal law that improved access to OUD pharmacotherapy (e.g., Buprenorphine) through virtual modalities in the absence of a prior in-person medical evaluation.

While the Drug Enforcement Administration (DEA) and the U.S. Department of Health and Human Services (HHS) have extended pandemic prescribing authorities while modernizing national telehealth regulations, not all States have. Variable restrictions in State rules may be barriers to rural Veterans getting SUD treatment through telemedicine, including for some of our most rural and vulnerable Veterans. This is a significant concern, which is why VA has endorsed a legislative proposal in the FY 2024 budget request (Maintaining Consistent Access to Critical Treatments Through Telehealth) to ensure VA providers can furnish clinically appropriate telehealth care to every Veteran they treat, regardless of where the patient is or resides or where the provider is licensed or located.

Despite telehealth challenges, the rates of SUD treatment and risk mitigation efforts are comparable between urban and rurally located Veterans based on the SUD treatment metrics that VA monitors. This includes the percentage of Veterans with OUD who receive life-saving medication for OUD, the percentage of Veterans with OUD and stimulant use disorder who received naloxone, and the percentage of Veterans with an overdose who receive an interdisciplinary team case risk review.

---

[3] McCarthy, J.F., Blow, F.C., Ignacio, R.V., Ilgen, M.A., Austin, K.L., & Valenstein, M. (2012). Suicide among patients in the Veterans Affairs health system: Rural–urban differences in rates, risks, and methods. American Journal of Public Health,102(S1), S111-S117. doi: 10.2105/AJPH.2011.300463.

[4] Varia, S.G., Ebin, J., & Stout, E.R. (2014). Suicide prevention in rural communities: Perspectives from a Community of Practice. Journal of Rural Mental Health, 38(2), 109.

FY 2024 President's Budget Expands Access to Treatment for Substance Use Disorders (SUD)

President Biden's FY 2024 Budget proposes continued support for VA initiatives started during FY 2022, with over 1,100 additional staff awarded enterprise-wide to help meet VA's SUD treatment priorities, including:

- Stepped Care to expand access to evidence-based treatment for SUD in settings outside specialty SUD Care;
- SUD Residential Treatment to reduce wait times and improve the quality of SUD care with expansion of staff and programs;
- SUD Telehealth to expand access to evidence-based SUD treatment through telehealth;
- Homeless Program SUD Treatment Coordinators to engage Veterans with SUD into VA SUD outpatient and residential services;
- Supported Employment Specialists to expand access to employment opportunities for Veterans in recovery; and
- SUD Peer Specialists to increase engagement and retention in evidence-based SUD treatment.

As of May 31, 2023, over 61% of the more than 1,100 positions have been filled or are in the final steps of the hiring process. VA continues to respond to emerging illicit drug threats to ensure the needs of Veterans experiencing substance use concerns are met. During FY 2024, VA plans to establish program management leads for harm reduction at each facility and will work collaboratively to develop policy and national tools to support implementation of targeted harm reduction strategies throughout VHA by addressing critical issues such as stigma and the need for technical assistance for the field to support implementation of emerging treatment approaches.

The VHA Office of Rural Health also continues to invest in research and innovation focused on meeting the needs of rural Veterans experiencing SUD. These projects, often proposed by rural VA medical centers, seek to understand opportunities and develop novel solutions in the rural SUD space. Examples include a telehospitalist-led pilot for inpatient management of AUD, a project developing a telehealth model to improve treatment access for rural Veterans with SUD, collaborative pain care for rural patients with OUD and other SUDs using telehealth technologies, and research to understand drivers of mental health services utilization at remote locations. These are ongoing projects without final results, but each will contribute to the future treatment options for rural residing Veterans experiencing SUD.

Conclusion

We appreciate the Committee's continued support in this shared mission. Nothing is more important to VA than supporting the health and well-being of the Nation's Veterans and their families. VA has employed broad, evidence-based strategies to address the opioid epidemic, including patient and provider education, pain management and access to non-pharmacological modalities, risk mitigation strategies, and addiction treatment for Veterans with SUD. This critical work saves lives. My colleagues and I are prepared to respond to any questions you may have.

Statement of Julie Kroviak, MD Principal Deputy Assistant Inspector General for the Office of Healthcare Inspections, Office of Inspector General, Department of Veterans Affairs Before the U.S. Senate Committee on Veterans' Affairs Hearing on Connections to Care: Improving Substance Use Disorder Care for Veterans in Rural America and Beyond June 14, 2023

Chairman Tester, Ranking Member Moran, and Committee Members, thank you for the opportunity to discuss the Office of Inspector General's (OIG) oversight of the Veterans Health Administration's (VHA) substance use disorder treatment programs in rural locations. The OIG's Office of Healthcare Inspections reviews the quality and safety of health care provided across VHA and communicates the findings through a variety of public reports. These include results from hotline inspections, national reviews, proactive comprehensive healthcare inspections, vet center inspections, and Veterans Integrated Service Network (VISN) reviews. For each of these reports, OIG clinical review teams provide recommendations for improving processes or further reducing risks to the veterans who entrust their health care to VA.

VHA faces significant challenges in meeting the complex needs of individuals with substance use disorders, and rural settings can pose additional obstacles in addressing those patients' needs. With more than three million veterans in rural and highly rural areas enrolled in VHA, the need for innovative and immediate healthcare access solutions for those veterans with substance use disorders is urgent.[5]

The devastating effects of substance use disorders on veterans, their families and caregivers, and communities cannot be overstated. Veterans with substance use disorders often have co-occurring mental health conditions that can place them at higher risk for suicide. Veterans living in highly rural areas are also 65 percent more likely to die from suicide that those residing in urban settings.[6] Given that VHA's top clinical priority is to reduce veteran suicide, timely access to evidence-based substance use disorder treatment programs is imperative to addressing the clinical needs of these high-risk patients.

The OIG reports highlighted in this testimony help to identify VHA challenges specific to providing veterans access to community care and coordination for high-risk patients. The risks to patient safety and care when either is deficient are significant and will only grow as VHA increases its reliance on community care providers. Recent OIG-collected data shows that in fiscal year (FY) 2022, more than 237,000 veterans enrolled at rural facilities have been referred for community care, including 7,400 for mental health treatment. The findings and recommendations in the highlighted reports that follow help underscore the need for (1) timely access to appropriate care, (2) oversight of VHA staff adherence to community care referral

[5] VHA Office of Health Equity (OHE), "Access to Care among Rural Veterans" (fact sheet), March 10, 2020.
[6] VHA OHE, "Access to Care among Rural Veterans" (fact sheet), March 10, 2020.

guidelines, and (3) care coordination and clinical information exchange between VHA and community care providers.

Our reports focus on issues relevant to leaders across the system in all settings—urban and rural. However, because of the inherent challenges of rural healthcare delivery, and the burdens these communities face in providing outreach and treatment to patients with mental health and substance use disorders, VHA and rural facility leaders must pay special attention when conducting risk assessments for these conditions. This statement focuses on a report involving a region of Texas to introduce key VHA requirements related to referrals for residential treatment for substance use. It also details a report that found substantial errors in the management of the care of a veteran undergoing alcohol withdrawal at the Tomah VA Medical Center, one of VA's rural facilities. While the findings from these reports are specific to one facility, they are intended to be reviewed and assessed across the system.

Noncompliance with Community Care Referrals for Substance Abuse Residential Treatment at the VA North Texas Health Care System

In August 2021, the OIG hotline received allegations that staff for the domiciliary substance use disorder treatment program (DOM SUD) at the VA North Texas Health Care System (VA North Texas) placed patients on waitlists for two to three months and failed to offer non-VA community residential care referrals for substance use disorder treatment.[7] The complainant also alleged that VA North Texas staff denied patients' requests for community residential care referrals, whereas patients from the Central Texas Veterans Health Care System in the same region (VISN 17), received community residential care treatment. During the OIG staff's review of the allegations [including examining 15 VA North Texas DOM SUD consults (referrals) and electronic health records for 10 patients], the team identified additional concerns related to compliance with required scheduling procedures and the assignment of mental health treatment coordinators to patients awaiting admission. To understand the context for the resulting report's findings, it is important to consider VHA's program goals and requirements.

Background

Mental health residential rehabilitation treatment programs (MH RRTPs) provide 24-hour treatment and rehabilitative services to patients with a range of needs and include domiciliary substance use disorder programs. MH RRTP is an umbrella term for a diverse group of residential programs that serve patients experiencing homelessness, substance use disorders, posttraumatic stress disorder, as well as other medical and mental health conditions. To be eligible for an MH RRTP referral, veterans must need a higher level of care than an outpatient program can provide but not be at imminent risk to themselves and others, and not meet criteria for a medical or acute mental health admission. VHA requires that each facility provide access to care at MH RRTPs through service agreements with other VA facilities or through referral to non-VA community residential care facilities.

---

[7] VA OIG, *Noncompliance with Community Care Referrals for Substance Abuse Residential Treatment at the VA North Texas Health Care System*, January 31, 2023.

The VA North Texas system includes a 40-bed DOM SUD at the Dallas VA Medical Center and a 69- bed DOM SUD at the Sam Rayburn Memorial Veterans Center in Bonham, Texas. The Central Texas VA system is in Temple, Texas, and has a 169-bed general domiciliary that offers substance use disorder treatment as a "track."

According to VHA's requirements, patients referred to MH RRTPs must be screened within seven business days by a team that includes a licensed mental health professional and a medical provider to determine whether admission is appropriate. If accepted, the patient must receive a tentative admission date and a point of contact at the MH RRTP.[8] So VHA can track admission wait times, the patient must be added to the pending bed placement list.[9] Since 2018, VHA has required staff to include information in the patient's electronic health record to improve tracking of program wait times and capacity.[10]

Community Care Program Eligibility Criteria

The MISSION Act mandated changes to VHA's community care program.[11] Those changes led to VHA's Office of Community Care issuing implementation guidance stating that "wait time and drive time access standards are only applicable to primary care, specialty care, and non-institutional extended care services." The guidance further said MH RRTPs "are considered institutional extended care services" and do not follow the same wait-time standards.[12] When MH RRTP care is not available withinVA facilities for an eligible patient who "elects to receive care in the community," VHA will authorize community residential care. Further, for MH RRTP admission wait times greater than 30 calendar days, facility staff must offer the patient alternative care that addresses the patient's needs and preferences, including a referral to community residential care or another VHA program. Additionally, facility staff should discuss outpatient care options with the patient while the patient awaits MH RRTP admission. It is important to note that the COVID-19 pandemic put additional stresses on VHA and that the Texas facilities were not alone in facing long wait times. In February 2021, VHA estimated that 3,500 patients nationally were pending admission with an average wait time of more than 150 days. At that time, VHA required MH RRTP staff to provide alternatives, including community residential care, if unable to admit patients within 30 days.[13]

---

[8] VHA Directive 1162.02, *Mental Health Residential Rehabilitation Treatment Program*, July 15, 2019. Tentative admission date refers to the MH RRTP staff's expected date of bed availability.

[9] VHA Directive 1002, *Bed Management Solution for Tracking Beds and Patient Movement Within and Across VHA Facilities*, November 28, 2017.

[10] VHA Deputy Under Secretary for Health for Operations and Management (10N) memo, "Mental Health Residential Rehabilitation Treatment Programs (MH RRTP) CPRS Note Templates Implementation," July 30, 2018.

[11] John S. McCain III, Daniel K. Akaka, and Samuel R. Johnson VA Maintaining Internal Systems and Strengthening Integrated Outside Networks (MISSION) Act of 2018, Pub. L. No. 115-182, 132 Stat. 1393 (2018).

[12] VHA Office of Community Care, "Field Guidebook: Specialty Programs," updated November 3, 2021. The Office of Community Care determines a patient is eligible for community mental health care when the wait time is greater than 20 days or the drive time is greater than 30 minutes for a VHA outpatient mental health appointment.

[13] VHA Assistant Under Secretary for Health for Clinical Services memorandum, "Ensuring Access to Residential Treatment for Veterans with Mental Health and Substance Use Disorders during the Pandemic," February 11, 2021.

The OIG Found VA North Texas DOM SUD Wait Times Exceeded Requirements and Staff Failed to Refer Patients to Community Residential Care as Required

The OIG team reviewed 15 VA North Texas DOM SUD consults to determine admission wait times and evaluate whether staff offered community residential care. The team substantiated the allegation that VA North Texas staff placed patients on waitlists for two to three months and failed to offer community residential care referrals during most of fiscal years 2020 and 2021, inconsistent with VHA requirements. It is important to note that the OIG did not identify any adverse clinical outcomes due to the patients' delayed access to residential care.

In March 2020, due to the pandemic, facility leaders restricted access to the Dallas DOM SUD to local veterans, in accordance with VHA guidance. The Dallas DOM SUD subsequently reopened to a broader group of patients but still with reduced capacity in September 2020. The Bonham DOM SUD remained open during the pandemic at reduced capacity until January 2022, when admissions were halted until June 2022 due to COVID-19 concerns. VHA data indicated that the Dallas and Bonham DOM SUDs' average wait times were 30 days or greater from the third quarter of fiscal year 2020 through the second quarter of fiscal year 2021, likely due to pandemic-related restrictions.

Of the 10 North Texas patients' records the OIG reviewed, five had one DOM SUD consult placed and the other five had two consults placed, resulting in a total of 15 consults examined. Of the 15 consults, 13 were referrals to the Bonham DOM SUD and two were referrals to the Dallas DOM SUD. Seven consults were closed when the patients were admitted within 30 days, declined screening, or were not approved for admission. Among the eight remaining consults, two were closed when the patients declined admission and six resulted in patients waiting an average of 79 days before VA North Texas staff offered DOM SUD admission or removed the patient from the pending bed placement list. For seven of the eight consults, staff documented that the "anticipated admission date exceeds 30 days; however, there is no available alternative to consider at this time."

The OIG determined that the VA North Texas chief for Patient Administration Services, who oversees community care, misinterpreted community care guidance and provided inaccurate information to VA North Texas leaders and staff. Specifically, the Office of Community Care's guidance states that community care wait time standards were not applicable to MH RRTP. Facility staff should have instead followed VHA policy requiring a patient with a wait time of greater than 30 days be offered alternative residential treatment or another level of care. Alternative residential treatment could include a referral to a community program, another program in the VISN, or another program in another VISN.[14]

However, the Patient Administration Services chief told the OIG team during the review that MH RRTPs are "excluded from the MISSION Act" and not eligible for community care based on access standards—reflecting an inaccurate understanding of the Act. In contrast, the national director of the MH RRTP reported that although drive time and wait time standards do not apply to DOM SUDs, community care referrals are expected when a patient is determined to require a residential level of care and VHA is unable to provide treatment within the required timeframe.

In September 2020, the MH RRTP national program office released guidance that included instructions for community care referrals. In February 2021, VHA provided guidance that

[14] VHA Directive 1162.02.

VISN chief mental health officers and facility leaders must ensure that patients who require a residential level of care are offered a VA MH RRTP bed or community residential care. VHA further required that each facility provide the operational status of MH RRTP beds and "information on the availability of community based residential treatment options."[15] VISN 17's response to the February 2021 guidance indicated that the Dallas and Bonham DOM SUDs were not making community residential care referrals.

In December 2021, the OIG informed VISN 17 and VA North Texas leaders of staff's failure to comply with community residential care referral expectations and requested corrective action be taken to address staff education and potential patient treatment needs. VA North Texas leaders communicated referral requirements to Office of Community Care and Mental Health Services staff and reviewed all community residential care consults placed from October 1, 2019, through November 30, 2021.

Additionally, in response to the OIG's request, VA North Texas staff completed a clinical review to ensure appropriate follow-up for patients referred from October 1, 2019, through December 31, 2021, to the Dallas and Bonham DOM SUDs whose wait times were greater than 30 days.

Recommendations for Corrective Action

In contrast to VA North Texas's failures, the OIG's review of two patients referred to the Temple DOM SUD by VA North Texas staff indicated the VA Central Texas staff placed consults and scheduled patients in accordance with VHA policy. Further, VA Central Texas developed procedures for community residential care referrals when MH RRTP wait times were greater than 30 days.

The OIG made five recommendations in this report related to VA North Texas deficiencies and associated lack of oversight.[16] The first recommendation was for the VA North Texas director to ensure that staff provide alternative treatment options, including community care when MH RRTP admission wait times exceed 30 days. VA concurred with this recommendation. The second recommendation called on the director to conduct a comprehensive review of the management of community residential care referrals. VA concurred in principle with this recommendation. VA concurred with the remaining three recommendations described below.

There Was Inadequate VISN Oversight

The OIG determined that VISN 17 leaders did not ensure local facilities were adhering to the national MH RRTP policy. According to the MH RRTP directive, each VISN mental health

[15] VHA assistant under Secretary for health for clinical services, "Ensuring Access to Residential Treatment for Veterans with Mental Health and Substance Use Disorders during the Pandemic," memorandum.

[16] The OIG considers all five recommendations currently open pending the submission of sufficient documentation that would support that adequate progress has been made on implementing them. The OIG requests updates on the status of all open recommendations every 90 days, which are then reflected on the recommendation dashboard found on the OIG website. VA may, however, submit evidence of implementation sufficient to close a recommendation at any time. For this report, VA's first recommendation status update is due in mid-June.

lead is responsible for ensuring that all MH RRTPs in their region collect data sufficient for oversight related to VHA policy implementation.[17] Additionally, the national director of the MH RRTP confirmed the VISN has oversight responsibility to ensure eligible patients have access to a residential level of care, although there are not defined expectations related to community care utilization monitoring. The VISN 17 chief mental health officer provided guidance to VA North Texas leaders on three occasions in 2021 regarding the use of community residential care. However, she reported that the VISN role did not carry the authority to ensure policy adherence or "direct oversight" because "oversight is at the local facility management level." The third report recommendation was for the under secretary for health to make certain that VISN leaders provide adequate oversight to ensure that access to care for MH RRTPs is provided consistent with VHA policy.

Bonham MH RRTP Nonadherence with VHA Scheduling Requirements

During the inspection, the OIG team also identified that the Bonham MH RRTP standard operating procedure was inconsistent with VHA's minimum scheduling effort requirements, as it instructed schedulers to close a consult after three failed scheduling contact attempts with patients rather than the four required. Since 2016, VHA has required healthcare providers to document a request for other services in the referred patient's electronic health record. The second attempt must use a different method of contact and can be completed the same day as the first attempt, while the third and fourth attempts must be on different days. To allow the patient time to respond, providers' staff must wait a minimum of 14 calendar days from the second contact attempt before determining how to act on the consult request, such as closing the consult. Additionally, the Bonham MH RRTP staff were attempting to contact patients by phone and not using other modes of contact. Failure to adhere to VHA minimum scheduling requirements may hinder efficient patient scheduling and contribute to the barriers patients experience in accessing DOM SUD services. The fourth recommendation was for the VA North Texas director to ensure that Bonham MH RRTP scheduling procedures are consistent with VHA minimum scheduling effort requirements.

National Program Process Needed on Mental Health Treatment Coordinator Assignment

Finally, the OIG found that VA North Texas policy did not include information about the requirement for MH RRTP staff to assign a mental health treatment coordinator for patients awaiting admission to a residential program. Since 2012, VHA has required facility staff to assign a mental health treatment coordinator to patients who are receiving treatment in an outpatient mental health setting, have been admitted to an inpatient mental health setting, or are "waiting to engage in a different level of care," including an MH RRTP bed.[18] However, in an interview, the national director for the MH RRTP acknowledged not having an assignment

---

[17] VHA Directive 1162.02, Mental Health Residential Rehabilitation Treatment Program, July 15, 2019.

[18] VHA Deputy Under Secretary for Health for Operations and Management memorandum, *Assignment of the Mental Health Treatment Coordinator*, March 26, 2012.

process for patients waiting for MH RRTP admission. This failure to develop a national-level process likely contributed to the VA North Texas MH RRTP leaders' lack of knowledge that the VA North Texas policy should address the identification and assignment of a mental health treatment coordinator for accepted patients awaiting admission. Not only can this lack of policy awareness contribute to a coordinator not being assigned, it can also diminish the likelihood of patients' engagement in outpatient care while waiting for placement. The fifth report recommendation is related to strengthening coordinator assignment procedures for patients waiting for an MH RRTP bed.

Mismanagement of a Patient with Alcohol Withdrawal at the Tomah VA Medical Center

In 2021, the OIG issued a report reviewing allegations related to the care at the Tomah VA Medical Center of a patient suffering from alcohol withdrawal who subsequently died at another VA medical center from a presumed anoxic (lack of oxygen) brain injury.[19] The inspection team found that facility physicians' failure to prescribe an adequate medication regimen to address the patient's delirium tremens (withdrawal symptoms) effectively, review the patient's abnormal electrocardiogram prior to haloperidol administration, and transfer the patient earlier likely contributed to the patient's deterioration and ultimate death. The team substantiated that a non-VA paramedic documented that a supplemental oxygen flow was not active.[20] Tomah VA Medical Center leaders and staff reported they did not know about the failed oxygen delivery. The inspection team also found that the nursing staff did not complete all required alcohol withdrawal assessments; a physician improperly ordered restraints; nurses failed to obtain full vital signs while the patient was in restraints; and nurses did not receive restraint training as expected. Finally, leaders did not conduct an institutional disclosure with the patient's family in a timely manner, as required.

The OIG made 10 recommendations to the facility director related to educating personnel on alcohol withdrawal and cardiac risks, the need for a review to determine the causes of the failed oxygen delivery, identification of root causes and performance deficiencies, workgroup outcomes, alcohol withdrawal assessment protocol adherence, restraint management and training, compliance with admission criteria, emergency detention, and institutional disclosures. The Tomah VA Medical Center has provided documentation on sufficient corrective actions and the recommendations are closed.

Assessing and stabilizing patients who are at risk for life-threatening complications from alcohol withdrawal is critical. Failure to ensure appropriate staff training on such care puts patients at risk for severe consequences, including death. Because hospitals in rural settings often have limited specialty and intensive care services on-site that do not meet the need for

---

[19] VA OIG, *Mismanagement of a Patient at the Tomah VA Medical Center in Wisconsin*, August 21, 2021.

[20] Tomah VAMC Policy MS-03, *Emergency Services*, March 7, 2017, requires staff to respond to medical emergencies by calling "911," as necessary for non-VHA emergency assistance. The emergency medical services personnel who responded to the patient included a lead paramedic, a second paramedic, and an emergency medical technician. The paramedics performed an endotracheal intubation on the patient and the patient was transported to a non-VHA facility by helicopter. The lead paramedic completed the documentation that noted failed oxygen delivery. Three days later, the patient was transferred from the non-VHA hospital to another VA medical center.

higher-level care, clinical interventions related to assessment and stabilization are even more critical while patient transfer arrangements are made.

Other OIG Reports Citing Concerns with Community Care Coordination of Veterans with Complex Mental Health Needs

Coordinating medical care between VHA and community providers remains a challenge, particularly for addressing the needs of patients with complex mental health conditions. The OIG has identified persistent administrative and communication errors or failures among VHA, its third-party administrators, and community care providers, as well as between care providers and their patients.

These deficiencies challenge the considerable efforts of VHA personnel to ensure a seamless experience for veterans. Many OIG reports have described the frustrations and, most importantly, the risks to patients associated with referrals to the community when coordination and communication are inadequate. The following reports exemplify how poor care coordination contributes to sometimes tragic consequences for high-risk patients.

In a report on the deficiencies found in the care and administrative processes for a patient who died by suicide, the OIG review team found that administrative errors and confusion in the Phoenix VA healthcare facility's community referral process delayed specialized psychological testing for a veteran. The veteran died by suicide never having received the appropriate testing and resulting targeted treatment.[21]

Another oversight report focused on a patient who ultimately died by suicide after not receiving several authorized community care counseling sessions. This was due to deficiencies in the coordination of the patient's care between the Memphis VA facility's community care staff, providers in the community, and the third-party administrator.[22] In addition, the patient suffered from hyperthyroidism, a condition that can aggravate anxiety. The patient declined a referral to endocrinology at the facility, due to the distance from home, but was never offered a referral to the community.

An Ongoing Focus on Rural Veterans, Community Care Coordination, and Mental Health and Substance Use Disorders

Considering VA's persistent challenges caring for high-risk and complex patients identified in prior reviews, the OIG continues to initiate proactive projects to highlight threats to patient safety and quality of care as well as detail specific facilities' innovative solutions to these issues. The following work demonstrates the OIG's broad oversight footprint across VA and our continued focus on veterans who require mental health and substance use disorder treatment, with special consideration for those living in rural locations.

---

[21] VA OIG, *Deficiencies in Care and Administrative Processes for a Patient Who Died by Suicide, Phoenix VA Health Care System, Arizona*, March 31, 2021.

[22] VA OIG, *Deficiencies in Care, Care Coordination, and Facility Response to a Patient Who Died by Suicide, Memphis VA Medical Center in Tennessee*, September 3, 2020.

In the past two fiscal years, OIG's healthcare inspection teams conducting cyclical reviews visited nine medical centers designated by VA as rural.[23] OIG teams also performed inspections of 12 VISNs that are responsible for the management of 265 rural and highly rural facilities and community based outpatient clinics. During FY 2024, the OIG will be rolling out an updated healthcare facility inspection program that will use a more customized and data-driven approach to better highlight distinct challenges that affect the quality of healthcare delivery, such as those specific to rural settings.

The OIG's cyclical reviews of vet centers have focused on 36 locations, with three in rural and highly rural settings. Vet centers are community-based counseling centers that offer myriad services to eligible veterans, service members, and their families.[24] These centers are critical to VHA's efforts to expand outreach and support more veterans in getting the care they need, particularly mental health care.

Moreover, VA's 80 mobile vet centers are meant to be used for outreach and services to underserved populations—often in highly rural areas. The OIG's vet center review teams are including mobile vet centers in their current inspection cycle.

The OIG's newest planned cyclical review will inspect mental health inpatient units of all sizes across the system. Currently in the pilot phase, the planned launch is for FY 2024. In July 2023, a new VISN community care cyclical review is also being undertaken to evaluate the administrative and care coordination processes to veterans receiving care through VHA's Community Care Network (CCN).

A review will also soon be released that assessed care coordination for patients of the VA Eastern Kansas Health Care System who have been receiving care and dually prescribed opioids and benzodiazepines from CCN providers.[25] Veterans are at a higher risk of harm associated with concurrent use of opioid and benzodiazepine medication due to the prevalence and severity of chronic pain that is often accompanied by mental health comorbidities when compared to nonveterans. The OIG team assessed VHA and CCN providers' care coordination, documentation processes, and use of risk- mitigation strategies for patients, as well as VHA's oversight of CCN providers' opioid prescribing practices.

After Congress passed the SUPPORT for Patients and Communities Act in 2018, requiring the expansion of substance use disorder treatment, the Office of Mental Health and Suicide Prevention developed a large-scale national hiring initiative to expand the availability of such treatment to veterans at VA medical centers during FY 2022. This initiative included a requirement to hire 90 percent of the 1,180 approved positions before the end of September 2022. The OIG is currently assessing how well medical centers have met the FY 2022 substance use disorder hiring initiative goal. The review team has already analyzed national hiring data at 139 medical centers to determine if the facilities achieved the initiative goal. The team selected a statistical sample of four medical centers (two of which are located in rural areas) for a deeper review to understand how different VISNs and medical centers managed the initiative and to identify any internal obstacles to facilities' meeting the hiring goal.

Collectively, these OIG reviews and other oversight reports provide veterans and their families, VA staff and leaders, the public, and Congress with a comprehensive understanding of VA health care and mental health services delivered in a variety of settings.

---

[23] VHA has a total of 16 medical centers, hospitals, or healthcare systems in rural locations.

[24] For more information, visit the vet center website at www.vetcenter.va.gov/.

[25] VHA has been sent a copy of the report and it is under review for their comments.

Conclusion

Every veteran deserves high-quality, timely, and well-coordinated care. This is particularly critical for veterans in rural areas with limited resources who are at high risk due to their mental health and substance use conditions. The pandemic disrupted healthcare delivery in all practice areas, including addiction treatment, while escalating the demand for interventions. VHA will need to continue to rely on community providers to deliver care when veterans' needs cannot be met within VA's own facilities. As the reports highlighted in this testimony demonstrate, VHA faces numerous challenges in providing needed substance use and mental health treatments—exacerbated by the limited availability of appropriate treatment services for veterans living in rural and highly rural locations. The OIG will continue to focus on these matters to assist VA in mitigating the risks inherent in providing and coordinating behavioral health care both within VHA and with community partners.

Chairman Tester, Ranking Member Moran, and members of the committee, this concludes my statement. I would be happy to answer any questions you may have.

Geographic Availability of Substance Use Disorder Treatment for Veterans The Need for Data-Driven Solutions

Jonathan H. Cantor

For more information on this publication, visit www.rand.org/t/CTA2808-1.

Testimonies

RAND testimonies record testimony presented or submitted by RAND associates to federal, state, or local legislative committees; government-appointed commissions and panels; and private review and oversight bodies.

Limited Print and Electronic Distribution Rights

Geographic Availability of Substance Use Disorder Treatment for Veterans: The Need for Data-Driven Solutions

Testimony of Jonathan H. Cantor[26]

The RAND Corporation[27]
Before the Committee on Veterans' Affairs United States Senate
June 14, 2023

Chairman Tester, Ranking Member Moran, and members of the committee, I want to thank you for your invitation to testify today on what is a pressing and urgent public health problem. My name is Dr. Jonathan Cantor. I am a policy researcher at the RAND orporation. My training is in health policy research, and I have conducted extensive research on the geographic availability and accessibility of substance use disorder (SUD) treatment for veterans, military service members, and the civilian population.[28]

During my almost seven-year career as a RAND researcher, I have sought to develop and improve the quality of metrics to measure and track the geographic availability of SUD treatment—both where treatment is located and whether those in need can actually access this care. I have examined the marketplace of SUD care provided by the U.S. Department of Veterans Affairs (VA) and non-VA providers. In 2018, I was a task lead for a study that calculated novel measures of geographic accessibility of SUD treatment for a national sample ofU.S. veterans.[29] We found that, while many veterans lived within a 15-minute drive of an SUD treatment facility, most lived around an hour from a VA facility that provided specialized SUD treatment. While these data are useful, our research highlights significant challenges to accurately measuring the geographic availability and accessibility of SUD treatment. These challenges include an inability to access data on the total capacity of a facility, the services the facility offers for veterans particularly, the approximate wait time to the next appointment, and the quality of care received. Today, I will discuss how existing data limit our ability to comprehensively measure geographic availability of SUD treatment for veterans. I will also

---

[26] The opinions and conclusions expressed in this testimony are the author's alone and should not be interpreted as representing those of the RAND Corporation or any of the sponsors of its research.

[27] The RAND Corporation is a research organization that develops solutions to public policy challenges to help make communities throughout the world safer and more secure, healthier and more prosperous. RAND is nonprofit, nonpartisan, and committed to the public interest. RAND's mission is enabled through its core values of quality and objectivity and its commitment to integrity and ethical behavior. RAND subjects its research publications to a robust and exacting quality-assurance process; avoids financial and other conflicts of interest through staff training, project screening, and a policy of mandatory disclosure; and pursues transparency through the open publication of research findings and recommendations, disclosure of the source of funding of published research, and policies to ensure intellectual independence. This testimony is not a research publication, but witnesses affiliated with RAND routinely draw on relevant research conducted in the organization.

[28] According to Catherine McLaughlin and Leon Wyszewianski, "*Availability* measures the extent to which the provider has the requisite resources, such as personnel and technology, to meet the needs of the client. *Accessibility* refers to geographic accessibility, which is determined by how easily the client can physically reach the provider's location" (Catherine G. McLaughlin and Leon Wyszewianski, "Access to Care: Remembering Old Lessons," *Health Services Research*, Vol. 37, No. 6, December 2002, p. 1441. Emphasis in original).

[29] Eric R. Pedersen, Kathryn E. Bouskill, Stephanie Brooks Holliday, Jonathan Cantor, Sierra Smucker, Matthew L. Mizel, Lauren Skrabala, Aaron Kofner, and Terri Tanielian, *Improving Substance Use Care: Addressing Barriers to Expanding Integrated Treatment Options for Post-9/11 Veterans*, RAND Corporation, RR-4354-WWP, 2020, www.rand.org/pubs/research_reports/RR4354.html.

discuss how existing data inhibit our ability to calculate disparities in access based on where veterans live, as well as their personal attributes, such as sex, race, and ethnicity.

In this testimony, I will first discuss the complexity of SUD treatment for veterans given the frequent existence of co-occurring mental health problems. Second, I will provide a brief overview of the geographic accessibility of SUD treatment for veterans based on our research. Third, I will describe why it is difficult to assess disparities in the geographic accessibility of SUD treatment for veterans. Finally, I will recommend a few ways to improve data collection and reporting on providers to better understand the geographic availability and accessibility of treatment for SUD for veterans and ways it can be measured over time.

SUD Treatment for Veterans Is Complex Because of Co-Occurring Mental Health Problems

In 2020, around 12 percent of veterans 18 years of age or older had an SUD, according to the National Survey on Drug Use and Health.[30] Approximately 1.1 million veterans suffered from *both* an SUD and a mental illness.[31] Most individuals who present with a co-occurring mental health problem and an SUD do not receive treatment for either condition.[32] There are many possible contributors to this treatment gap. For example, addiction counselors lack awareness of mental health conditions and lack training on how to treat co-occurring disorders.[33] Other possible reasons for this treatment gap include personnel shortages and workforce burnout.[34] Burnout among mental health staff compromises the quality of the patient-provider relationship and has led many to leave the workforce.[35] In short, veterans may have more-complex requirements than nonveterans when seeking treatment for SUD, and they may seek treatment in the context of a more constrained workforce with limited expertise or capacity to provide them with effective care for their specific needs.

There are a multitude of other reasons why a veteran with an SUD would not receive the necessary care. First, some veterans who use substances do so to self-medicate their posttraumatic stress disorder (PTSD) symptoms.[36] These veterans may be hesitant to seek treatment because of their treatment providers' policies. For example, some behavioral health treatment programs will not accept a patient unless the patient is abstinent from substances for

[30] Substance Abuse and Mental Health Services Administration, "2020 National Survey on Drug Use and Health: Veteran Adults," presentation slides, July 2022, www.samhsa.gov/data/sites/default/files/reports/rpt37926/2020NSDUHVeteransSlides072222.pdf.

[31] Substance Abuse and Mental Health Services Administration, 2022.

[32] Katherine E. Watkins, Audrey Burnam, Fuan-Yue Kung, and Susan Paddock, "A National Survey of Care for Persons with Co-Occurring Mental and Substance Use Disorders," *Psychiatric Services*, Vol. 52, No. 8, August 2001.

[33] Substance Abuse and Mental Health Services Administration, *Substance Use Disorder Treatment for People with Co-Occurring Disorders*, Treatment Improvement Protocol (TIP) 42, SAMHSA Publication PEP20-02-01-004, March 2020.

[34] Claire Snell-Rood, Robin A. Pollini, and Cathleen Willging, "Barriers to Integrated Medication-Assisted Treatment for Rural Patients with Co-Occurring Disorders: The Gap in Managing Addiction," *Psychiatric Services*, Vol. 72, No. 8, August 2021.

[35] Committee to Evaluate the Department of Veterans Affairs Mental Health Services, National Academies of Sciences, Engineering, and Medicine, "Mental Health Workforce and Facilities Infrastructure," in *Evaluation of the Department of Veterans Affairs Mental Health Services*, National Academies Press, 2018.

[36] Howard D. Chilcoat and Naomi Breslau, "posttraumatic stress disorder and Drug Disorders: Testing Causal Pathways," *Archives of General Psychiatry*, Vol. 55, No. 10, October 1998.

a certain period of time.[37] Second, many veterans fear seeking mental health or SUD treatment because it could negatively affect their career advancement.[38] In qualitative interviews, a sample of veterans told researchers that they find it difficult to balance their recovery, which would benefit from treatment, with vocational goals that may require that they disclose that they are receiving such care.[39] Third, co-occurring disorders often go unidentified. A practitioner may identify an SUD or a mental health disorder but not necessarily both.[40] Finally, the appropriate treatment for an individual with an SUD and a co-occurring mental health disorder is more complex than treating one or the other alone. Many treatment facilities that specialize in either mental health or SUDs are not equipped to address the needs of veterans with co-occurring disorders. There are not enough opportunities for formal training in the treatment of co-occurring disorders;[41] thus, there are a limited number of providers able to provide evidence-based care for co-occurring disorders. This could be particularly pronounced in areas of the country with a dearth of behavioral health care providers—called Mental Health Professional Shortage Areas.

Fortunately, the Veterans Health Administration (VHA) appears to be addressing this problem. According to the 2018 National Mental Health Services Survey, more than half—around 56 percent—of VA medical centers (VAMCs) had a specialized treatment program for co-occurring disorders.[42] More-recent data indicate that this percentage has been increasing.

Geographic Access to SUD Treatment Is Difficult to Measure with Existing Data Resources

Recent national research found that less than 10 percent of veterans with an SUD in 2020 received any treatment.[43] A key determinant for whether an individual receives SUD treatment is how far they have to travel for care.[44] To date, there have been few studies that have examined distance to SUD treatment (geographic accessibility) as a barrier to care for a national sample

---

[37] Alan Bernhardt, "Rising to the Challenge of Treating OEF/OIF Veterans with Co-Occurring PTSD and Substance Abuse," *Smith College Studies in Social Work*, Vol. 79, No. 3–4, July–December 2009; Karen H. Seal, Greg Cohen, Angela Waldrop, Beth E. Cohen, Shira Maguen, and Li Ren, "Substance Use Disorders in Iraq and Afghanistan Veterans in VA Healthcare, 2001–2010: Implications for Screening, Diagnosis and Treatment," *Drug and Alcohol Dependence*, Vol. 116, No. 1–3, July 1, 2011.

[38] Ann M. Cheney, Christopher J. Koenig, Christopher J. Miller, Kara Zamora, Patricia Wright, Regina Stanley, John Fortney, James F. Burgess, and Jeffrey M. Pyne, "Veteran-Centered Barriers to VA Mental Healthcare Services Use," *BMC Health Services Research*, Vol. 18, No. 591, 2018.

[39] Brian J. Stevenson, Ummul Kathawalla, Camille Smith, and Lisa Mueller, "Career Development in Transitional Work Settings: A Qualitative Investigation Among Veterans and Vocational Counselors," *Journal of Career Development*, October 28, 2022.

[40] Mary Ann Priester, Teri Browne, Aidyn Iachini, Stephanie Clone, Dana DeHart, and Kristen D. Seay, "Treatment Access Barriers and Disparities Among Individuals with Co-Occurring Mental Health and Substance Use Disorders: An Integrative Literature Review," *Journal of Substance Abuse Treatment*, Vol. 61, February 2016.

[41] Howard Padwa, Erick G. Guerrero, Joel T. Braslow, and Karissa M. Fenwick, "Barriers to Serving Clients with Co-Occurring Disorders in a Transformed Mental Health System," *Psychiatric Services*, Vol. 66, No. 5, May 2015.

[42] Substance Abuse and Mental Health Services Administration, *National Mental Health Services Survey (N- MHSS): 2018: Data on Mental Health Treatment Facilities*, 2019.

[43] Substance Abuse and Mental Health Services Administration, 2022.

[44] Kyle Beardsley, Eric D. Wish, Dawn Bonanno Fitzelle, Kevin O'Grady, and Amelia M. Arria, "Distance Traveled to Outpatient Drug Treatment and Client Retention," *Journal of Substance Abuse Treatment*, Vol. 25, No. 4, December 2003.

of veterans. A study of 266,301 female veterans who received any care from VHA in 2009 found that the longer the drive time to a provider, the less likely the veteran received outpatient care in the following two years.[45] Distance also predicts whether veterans obtain step-down aftercare, which is incredibly important for achieving long-term treatment success, after discharge from inpatient SUD treatment. Less than half of patients who received inpatient SUD treatment and lived more than 25 miles from their nearest outpatient mental health care facility received any follow-up care.[46]

Under the Maintaining Internal Systems and Strengthening Integrated Outside Networks Act (MISSION Act) of 2018, VA established an access standard of a 60-minute drive time for specialty care, including SUD treatment.[47] In 2019, the Wounded Warrior Project (WWP) partnered with RAND researchers to understand geographic accessibility of co-occurring mental health and SUD treatment.[48] We used two national databases to assess geographic accessibility of mental health and SUD treatment facilities nationwide. We linked these data with two different sets of data from the WWP, which included information on WWP alumni veterans' zip codes of residence. Our calculations indicated that, on average, WWP alumni lived 12 minutes from a mental health facility that had a co-occurring SUD program and 11 minutes from the nearest SUD treatment facility that had a co-occurring mental health program. For these veterans, the closest VAMCs or VA-affiliated facilities that provided treatment for co-occurring mental health disorders and SUDs were, on average, 57.0 and 66.3 minutes from where the veterans lived, "for mental health and substance use treatment facilities, respectively."[49] Our results were encouraging: Most WWP alumni veterans were able to access treatment programs for co-occurring mental health conditions and SUDs within the 60-minute drive time standard.

One major limitation of this line of research is that while a facility may be within a 60-minute drive time, it may not be able to accept the veteran as a patient. Our study did not incorporate measures of treatment capacity or wait times. Currently, there is no national database that includes these measures for all VA and non-VA facilities that provide SUD treatment. A second limitation of this work is that a veteran's zip code is a pretty broad indicator of where the veteran lives, and our estimates would be more accurate if we used veterans' specific addresses. Finally, our study was based on a sample of WWP alumni veterans, and whether these findings hold for all veterans is unknown.

Disparities Are Also Difficult to Measure Using Existing Data Resources

Figures 1 and 2 are heat maps that demonstrate the large variability in geographic accessibility of mental health and SUD treatment facilities with specialized treatment programs for co-

---

45 Sarah A. Friedman, Susan M. Frayne, Eric Berg, Alison B. Hamilton, Donna L. Washington, Fay Saechao, Natalya C. Maisel, Julia Y. Lin, Katherine J. Hoggatt, and Ciaran S. Phibbs, "Travel Time and Attrition from VHA Care Among Women Veterans: How Far Is Too Far?" *Medical Care*, Vol. 53, No. 4, Supp. 1, April 2015.

46 Susan K. Schmitt, Ciaran S. Phibbs, and John D. Piette, "The Influence of Distance on Utilization of Outpatient Mental Health Aftercare Following Inpatient Substance Abuse Treatment," *Addictive Behaviors*, Vol. 28, No. 6, August 2003.

47 U.S. Department of Veterans Affairs, "VA Launches New Health Care Options Under MISSION Act," news release, June 6, 2019.

48 Pedersen et al., 2020.

49 Pedersen et al., 2020, p. 74.

occurring disorders and WWP alumni. Areas in white are zip codes that lack one of these facilities within a 60-minute drive time from the veteran's zip code. The maps show that VAMCs and VA-affiliated facilities tend to be located in areas of the country with the largest number of non-VA facilities that serve veterans (as shown by the darker blue shading). In other words, facilities that serve veterans, be they VA or non-VA, cluster together. However, additional analyses by our research team indicated that, if we were to remove the VAMCs and VA- affiliated facilities from the maps, there would be less geographic accessibility for veterans to receive treatment, highlighting the critical role that VA plays in substance use treatment for veterans.

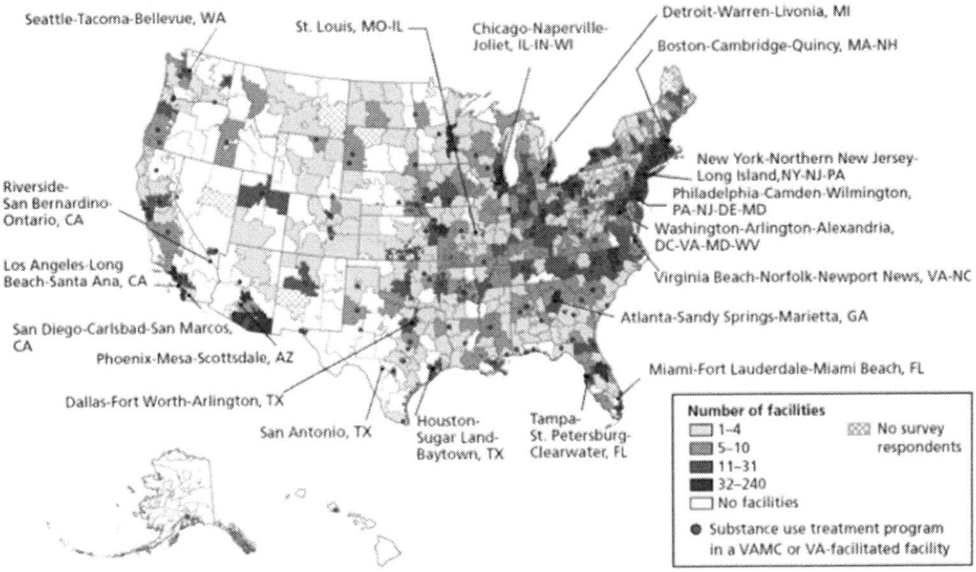

NOTES: Darker blue shading indicates increasing availability of facilities within a 60-minute drive time from the centroid of 2019 WWP Alumni Survey respondents' three-digit zip codes. White areas had no facilities within a 60-minute drive time. Areas with a hatch pattern had no survey respondents residing in them. Core-based statistical areas (CBSAs) with 200,000 or more veteran residents, according to the VetPop data, are labeled on the map, with the lines pointing to the CBSAs' centroids.

Source: Reproduced from Pedersen et al., 2020.

Figure 1. SUD Treatment Facilities with a Specialized Co-Occurring Disorders Program and a Specialized Treatment Program for Veterans.

Almost one-quarter of U.S. veterans reside in rural communities.[50] There is a concern that it is more difficult for rural veterans to receive care given that they must travel farther than veterans who live in urban areas. Treatment services in rural areas have challenges that include a shortage of specialized providers and a lack of accessible public transportation. In one study of 15 VHA primary care clinics in eight Midwestern states, distance was listed as a significant barrier for rural veterans seeking health care. And the effect of distance can be compounded by other factors, such as a veteran's health status, functional impairment, travel cost, and work or

[50] Office of Rural Health, U.S. Department of Veterans Affairs, "Rural Veterans: Rural Veteran Health Care Challenges," webpage, undated, www.ruralhealth.va.gov/aboutus/ruralvets.asp.

family obligations.[51] In 2019, the U.S. Government Accountability Office examined whether there was a disparity in SUD treatment utilization based on whether the veteran resided in an urban or a rural locality. The study found that veterans in urban and rural localities used VA SUD treatment services at a similar rate.[52] Thus, while there is a concern that there is a geographic disparity in health care access between rural and urban veterans, this disparity does not appear to affect utilization rates for SUD treatment. But more work is needed to confirm this result.

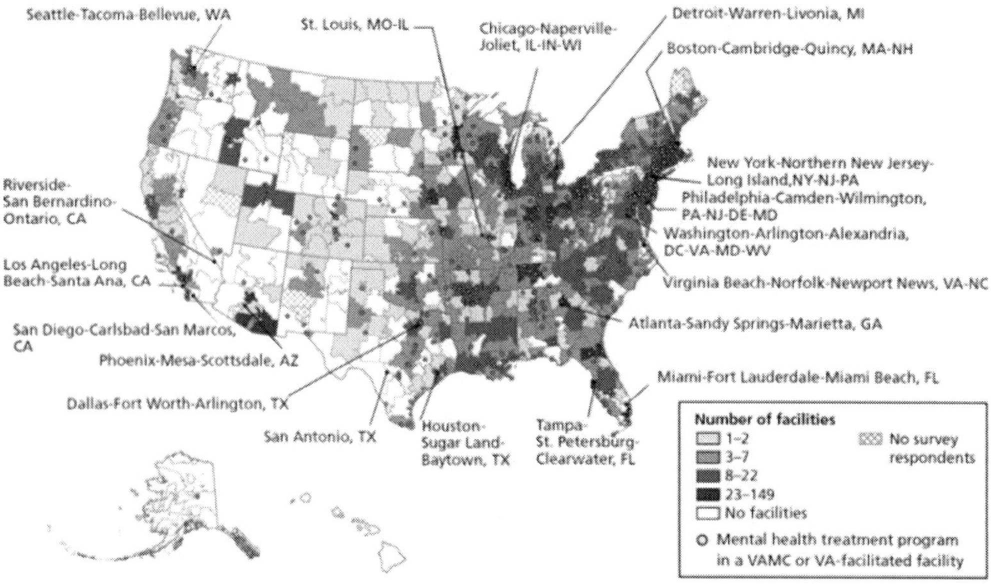

NOTES: Darker blue shading indicates increasing availability of facilities within a 60-minute drive time from the centroid of 2019 WWP Alumni Survey respondents' three-digit zip codes. White areas had no facilities within a 60-minute drive time. Areas with a hatch pattern had no survey respondents residing in them. Core-based statistical areas (CBSAs) with 200,000 or more veteran residents, according to the VetPop data, are labeled on the map, with the lines pointing to the CBSAs' centroids.

Source: Reproduced from Pedersen et al., 2020.

Figure 2. Mental Health Treatment Facilities with a Specialized Co-Occurring Disorders Program and a Specialized Treatment Program for Veterans.

The geographic accessibility of SUD care could also vary based on the sociodemographic characteristics of veterans. For example, women veterans, racial or ethnic minority veterans, or older veterans may disproportionately live in areas with fewer SUD facilities. Our study did not focus on these potential disparities. There are extensive data challenges in quantifying these differences. Such analyses would require detailed data on the addresses, or at least zip codes, of veterans, as well as data on their race/ethnicity, age, and gender. Finally, and perhaps most challenging, the data would need to include whether the veterans suffered from SUDs only or SUDs and mental health problems.

---

[51] Colin Buzza, Sarah S. Ono, Carolyn Turvey, Stacy Wittrock, Matt Noble, Gautam Reddy, Peter J. Kaboli, and Heather Schacht Reisinger, "Distance Is Relative: Unpacking a Principal Barrier in Rural Healthcare," *Journal of General Internal Medicine*, Vol. 26, No. 2, Supp. 2, November 2011.

[52] U.S. Government Accountability Office, *Veterans Health Care: Services for Substance Use Disorders, and Efforts to Address Access Issues in Rural Areas*, GAO-20-35, December 2019.

Recommendations

Drawing on my research and existing work, I have several recommendations. Each recommendation pertains to the relative dearth of detailed data that we have on providers or patients. For providers, it would be important for VA to consider updating its SUD programs website to include additional details on the specific types of SUD treatment that a particular facility provides.[53] The existing information includes locations, names, addresses, and phone numbers of existing services, but it may be difficult for a veteran to identify the provider that best serves their unique needs. Veterans would benefit from knowing the types of services provided or the specific substances that the facility offers treatment for. Similarly, there is no listing of wait times or capacity for treatment that VA keeps detailed information for.[54] Pieces of this information are included on other portions of the VA website,[55] but it would be useful to have all the data integrated into one location.

VA's SUD programs website refers individuals to the Substance Abuse and Mental Health Services Administration's (SAMHSA's) Behavioral Health Treatment Services Locator for treatment outside VA.[56] This locator has historically been based on annual surveys of both mental health and SUD treatment facilities to understand the availability of treatment resources and to help patients identify a provider. (The surveys have since been combined into one.) SAMHSA could consider asking treatment facilities additional specific questions in its annual survey of providers that informs the locator. One approach would be to ask whether specific treatment approaches are available for veterans. Currently, the survey asks about the types of specialized treatment programs that are present at the responding facility. However, the questionnaire does not ask what treatment approaches are used within those programs. Using 2019 SAMHSA data, we identified 3,782 mental health treatment facilities that contained both a specialized treatment program for veterans and specialized treatment for PTSD and co-occurring disorders. Similarly, we found that there were 5,484 SUD treatment facilities that offered a specialized treatment program for veterans and specialized treatment for trauma and co- occurring disorders.[57] However, SAMHSA's data do not describe what the specialized treatment programs for each of these facilities entail. The most recent iteration of the National Substance Use and Mental Health Services Survey, the survey that the locator is based on, has supplementary questionnaires for substance use VA facilities and mental health VA facilities on specific treatment approaches related to suicide.[58] This could be one model to use for asking more-detailed questions on treatments for co-occurring disorders. Separately, one recent audit study of the Behavioral Health Treatment Services Locator data asked targeted questions about

---

53 U.S. Department of Veterans Affairs, "Locations: Substance Use Disorder (SUD) Program," webpage, last updated November 3, 2021, www.va.gov/directory/guide/SUD.asp.

54 U.S. Department of Veterans Affairs, "Average Wait Times at Individual Facilities Search," web tool, undated, www.accesstocare.va.gov/PWT/SearchWaitTimes.

55 U.S. Department of Veterans Affairs, "Find VA Locations," web tool, undated, www.va.gov/find-locations/.

56 Substance Abuse and Mental Health Services Administration, Behavioral Health Services Locator, web resource, undated, www.samhsa.gov/resource/dbhis/behavioral-health-treatment-services-locator?gclid=CjwKCAjw-IwkBhBTEiwA2exyO_ry7dxpmu35RCm5ybl9kx7RxOgUTWcn7C9od3MGCif0XLOMdIdQ_xoC3-EQAvD_BwE. See also Substance Abuse and Mental Health Services Administration, FindTreatment.gov, homepage, undated, findtreatment.gov.

57 Pedersen et al., 2020.

58 Substance Abuse and Mental Health Services Administration, "Supplement for Mental Health Veterans Affairs Facilities," supplementary questionnaire for National Substance Use and Mental Health Services Survey, March 31, 2023.

residential treatment programs, including questions concerning the costs of services, average wait times, and travel-based inducements to receive treatment at the facility, such as car transportation.[59] Many of these measures could be collected by SAMHSA in its annual survey or in audits of the responses of specific facilities in a given year. An eventual long-term goal should be to incorporate quality-of-care measures for these facilities.

A separate limitation of the SAMHSA Behavioral Health Treatment Services Locator data is that the information on the treatment services that the facility provides is outdated and not easily understandable by the user.[60] Previous studies have found that contacting these providers and posing as a patient provides a more accurate measure of the payments accepted, treatments provided, and time to the next available appointment. Either SAMHSA or VA should consider conducting regular audit studies among non-VA facilities to get a more accurate understanding of the forms of treatment offered, approximate wait times to the next appointment, and total capacity of the facilities for SUD treatment.

Similarly, we lack information on disparities in geographic access to facilities based on sociodemographic characteristics of patients. Given that there may be differences in treatment approaches based on these characteristics, the audits should include calls to treatment facilities by individuals with different genders, races, and ethnicities.

Finally, it would be important for VA to consider alternative ways to expand treatment availability and accessibility of resources. Since the onset of the coronavirus disease 2019 (COVID-19) pandemic, there has been a rapid rise in the use of telehealth services. Preliminary work has shown that telehealth has increased treatment initiation for SUD in at least one VA hospital outpatient alcohol and drug treatment clinic.[61] While telehealth may increase retention for new and continuing opioid use disorder patients, it may do so differently based on characteristics of veterans.[62] Research should continue to be conducted on the effectiveness of telehealth in the population of veterans with SUDs and co-occurring mental health problems to reduce geographic disparities.

Conclusion

Far too many Americans, and especially veterans, fail to receive treatment for SUD each year. I am confident that we can increase the number of veterans who receive treatment and prevent unnecessary drug overdose deaths, but that will require an infusion of funding to improve current data collection systems and ensure that veterans can access the information necessary to make treatment decisions. It will also require research on best practices for identifying high-quality providers that meet the needs of veterans. In my testimony today, I outlined several data

---

[59] Tamara Beetham, Brendan Saloner, Marema Gaye, Sarah E. Wakeman, Richard G. Frank, and Michael Lawrence Barnett, "Admission Practices and Cost of Care for Opioid Use Disorder at Residential Addiction Treatment Programs in the US," *Health Affairs*, Vol. 40, No. 2, February 2021.

[60] Aneri Pattani, "National Addiction Treatment Locator Has Outdated Data and Other Critical Flaws," KFF Health News, May 9, 2022.

[61] Rebecca E. Sistad, Justin Enggasser, Nicholas A. Livingston, and Deborah Brief, "Comparing Substance Use Treatment Initiation and Retention Between Telehealth Delivered During COVID-19 and In-Person Treatment Pre- COVID-19," *American Journal on Addictions*, Vol. 32, No. 3, May 2023.

[62] Madeline C. Frost, Lan Zhang, H. Myra Kim, and Lewei (Allison) Lin, "Use of and Retention on Video, Telephone, and In-Person Buprenorphine Treatment for Opioid Use Disorder During the COVID-19 Pandemic," *JAMA Network Open*, Vol. 5, No. 10, October 2022.

limitations and how we might be able to address data gaps to understand the availability of SUD treatment resources for veterans. The lack of real-time measures on the capacity and wait times for both VA and non-VA providers for SUD treatment is a significant barrier that hinders our ability to monitor the availability of SUD treatment for veterans. Thank you for giving me the opportunity to speak on such an important issue, and I look forward to your questions.

Statement of Naomi Mathis
Associate National Legislative Director of the Disabled American Veterans for the Senate Committee on Veterans' Affairs
June 14, 2023

Chairman Tester, Ranking Member Moran and Members of the Committee:

On behalf of DAV's (Disabled American Veterans) more than 1 million members, thank you for inviting us to provide testimony for the Senate Veterans' Affairs Committee hearing titled, "Connections to Care: Improving Substance Use Disorder Care for Veterans in Rural America and Beyond."

DAV members are wartime service-disabled veterans who were wounded, injured, or made ill during their service. They utilize Department of Veterans Affairs (VA) benefits and Veterans Health Administration (VHA) services at extremely high rates, which many depend on as their sole source of health care. Our members live in locales across the country and beyond, which provides us with an insight into the plight of rural veterans and their unique struggles with access to care.

Today's hearing on rural veterans and access to health care for substance use disorders (SUD) is very important to DAV and our membership. Many of our members have benefited from these specialized programs and services. Our testimony will address VA's existing SUD programs and the unique challenges and barriers to care that exist for rural veterans and women veterans and a few recommendations.

Existing Va Substance Use Disorder Programs

VA offers a range of services to treat veterans with SUD. This includes short- term inpatient medication management for withdrawal, long-term medication management, individual and group behavioral health interventions, and residential rehabilitation treatment programs (RRTP) to manage addiction and develop new life skills simultaneously.

VA's residential rehabilitation units provide a comprehensive and intensive level of care. The Mental Health RRTP mission is to provide state-of-the-art, high-quality residential treatment services for veterans with co-occurring mental health and substance use disorders, medical concerns, and/or psychosocial needs such as homelessness and unemployment. This includes 24/7 nursing coverage and support for medication compliance and administration. In addition, VA's SUD treatment programs focus on a whole health model of care and provide alternatives to traditional medicine such as meditation, yoga, acupuncture, and tai chi.

VA is currently working on using innovative ways to reach veterans dealing with SUD such as peer specialists and mobile apps. Peer support specialists are often helpful in personalizing a veteran's health care experience, especially if specialists have had similar lived experiences as those they are working with and are in recovery from issues such as SUD, post-traumatic stress disorder (PTSD), eating disorders, or the effects of military sexual trauma (MST). For women veterans, who are more likely to indicate they have poor social networks than male peers, connections to other women veterans may be critical to their recovery and long-term abstinence. VA has stated it plans to use more peer support in mental health settings, including SUD programming, to improve veterans' retention and engagement in evidence-based treatment.

In May 2018, VHA launched the Stepped Care for Opioid Use Disorder – Train the Trainer (SCOUTT) initiative. The SCOUTT program has demonstrated that medication-assisted opioid use disorder treatment can be successfully provided outside of specialty care and that a stepped-care approach to treatment provides opportunities to address the broader spectrum of SUD treatment needs.

The Office of Rural Health (ORH) has approved two notable enterprise-wide initiatives to increase access for rural veterans by leveraging Clinical Pharmacist Practitioner (CPP) providers in SUD care.

At least 15 VA Medical Centers (VAMCs) currently operate Syringe Service Programs, which provide veterans who are IV drug users with clean and safe syringes. When combined with medications that treat opioid dependence (also known as medication-assisted treatment), there is a demonstrated reduction in HIV transmission.

Coaching into Care is a free service for families and friends of veterans where responders briefly assess a caller's concerns and provide appropriate resources and referrals. Through 10 to 30-minute calls, licensed psychologists and social workers offer guidance and help for starting conversations with a veteran who might be dealing with substance use and motivating them to seek treatment if it is needed.

According to VA, in 2022, more than 550,000 unique veterans were seen in VHA with a substance use disorder diagnosis. VA acknowledges fewer than 15% of veterans with a SUD diagnosis in 2022 received treatment. Of those who do receive VHA care, fewer than half receive such care in specialized settings and only about 46% of veterans diagnosed with opioid use disorder and 14% of those with alcohol use disorder received medications recommended under VA and DOD's clinical practice guideline.

VA has one of the country's premier SUD programs, providing high-quality evidence-based therapies and treatments. However, there are many challenges to adequately fund and staff this specialized programming, which is particularly concerning for the 4.7 million rural veterans in the United States, 58% of whom are enrolled in VHA.

It is clear that, due to these challenges and barriers, rural veterans are less likely to receive the standard of care for SUD.

Challenges and Barriers to Rural Health Care

In general, rural veterans have lower average household incomes than other veterans (52% have annual incomes of less than $35,000); 27% do not access the internet at home; they often face long driving distances to access quality health care; and there are fewer health care providers and nurses per capita in rural areas. This coupled with VHA inconsistencies in staffing and a lack of transportation, creates disparity for rural veterans trying to access primary health care and specialty treatment for SUD.

Inconsistent Policy

Consistency in implementing standards across VHA continues to be a challenge due to each facility's interpretation of VA policy as noted in a recent January 2023 Office of Inspector General (OIG) report. The report showed VA staff at a facility in North Texas misinterpreted policy when referring patients to residential care, which included a rural facility.

The U.S. Government Accountability Office (GAO) also noted similar findings as indicated in its Watch Blog from May 16, 2023, "...about one-third of veterans enrolled in the Veterans Health Administration (VHA) live in rural areas. However, in our review of VHA data, we found that rural veterans use intensive mental health care services, such as residential care or intensive case management, less than urban veterans, raising questions about access."

During a recent House Veterans' Affairs Committee hearing on SUD, witnesses stated there is a very short window from the moment a veteran with substance use disorder indicates they are willing to go to inpatient treatment, to successfully get them into care. When asked what would be a reasonable timeline, a witness indicated 72 hours would be the maximum amount of time. We understand the challenges VA faces when getting this cohort into care, but having a veteran wait 30 days for treatment (the current access standard for routine admission) is a far cry from 72 hours. SUD is also associated with an increased risk of suicidal ideation, suicide attempts, and death by suicide, making it imperative that veterans ready to start treatment have expedited access to care.

Transportation Concerns

Rural veterans face issues accessing health care similar to those faced by the general population, including a lack of transportation. In rural communities, distance to a health care facility, time, cost of fuel, and access to transportation are all exacerbated and known barriers to care. Veterans may lack access to public transportation or are no longer able to drive because of age, health status, or driving restrictions. Some rely on family, friends, or community service organizations.

DAV's Transportation Network

DAV operates a fleet of vehicles around the country to provide free transportation to VA medical facilities for injured and ill veterans. DAV stepped in to help veterans get the care they need at the time when the federal government terminated its program in the 1980s, which helped many of them pay for transportation to and from medical facilities. The vans are driven by volunteers, who are recruited and organized by DAV, and the rides are coordinated by more than 156 DAV Hospital Service Coordinators around the country.

Since the program's inception in 1987, DAV departments and chapters have donated 3,665 vehicles to VA, along with Ford Motor Co., which has donated 256 vehicles at a cost of more than $92 million. Volunteer drivers have logged over 700 million miles. Last year alone, they drove over 9 million miles. While this program is highly successful and beneficial for the veterans we serve, we continue to face administrative challenges with expediting volunteer driver examinations. Specifically, there is a breakdown in the onboarding process for our volunteer drivers nationally. For example, our transportation coordinator in Montana tells us they had 30 applications for volunteer drivers, and by the time VA completed onboarding a year and a half later, they were left with only two applicants. Montana is not unique in this extraordinary delay.

Unfortunately, there is no standard onboarding process for volunteers and local cooperation can vary highly. Some VA facilities do not make volunteer physicals a priority and do not realize delays create a barrier to access for veterans who need our services. DAV proudly serves and will continue to serve rural states to include Montana, Kansas, North Dakota, South Dakota, Ohio and Nebraska among others.

Recommendation

- Standardize and expedite the volunteer driver onboarding process VHA-wide, as soon as possible.

Telehealth

The ability to offer telehealth services provides options for patients and provides a potential path to address a health issue timely and conveniently but is impacted by barriers in rural communities regarding the availability of equipment and adequate bandwidth. Too many of our rural and tribal veterans are unable to participate in the programs established by VA such as Telehealth, TelePain, and eConsults. A July 2020 OIG report found that these programs are underutilized in highly rural Community- Based Outpatient Clinics (CBOC). While funds exist to expand the capacity of the programs, it may not be feasible due to a lack of broadband access in rural areas.

Recommendations

Continue to expand telehealth options when and where appropriate to supplement in- person SUD treatment

- *Expand Rural Veteran Tablet Program.* This VA program distributes video- enabled tablets to veterans, allowing them access to their primary and specialty care providers. Research indicates high satisfaction with the program and increasing it would provide greater access to SUD treatment and continuity of care.

- *Increase number of Clinical Resource Hubs (CRHs).* To aid veterans who live in areas that experience bandwidth problems, but are still too rural for easy access to care at a VAMC; paired with telehealth technology, CRHs allow veterans to connect with distant primary care, mental health, and specialty care teams to improve access to health care.
- *Expand and fund Virtual Living Rooms.* In partnership with the Rural Broadband Association, this program leverages locations where there is broadband access in a comfortable, private area such as a library, church, community center, or a local fraternal building.

Staffing for primary care is a major challenge in rural America, but specialty care is even scarcer. Compounded with the often complex needs of a veteran—the medical care and services they need are just not there. Even in terms of using community care, these specialty care providers are often not available. Particularly in areas outside of the continental United States (CONUS).

Veterans Outside the Continental United States (CONUS)

The Philippines is the only foreign country in which there is a VA Outpatient Clinic to serve eligible veterans. Recently, we began receiving complaints from our members who indicated VA had completely stopped dispensing Schedule 1 medication. This was not without advance notice to the veterans affected; however, the options faced by this population of veterans were to either travel to Guam, go into the community, stop the medication, or travel to the United States whenever a refill was needed. Further, the community-dispensed medication is not FDA-approved; therefore, the quality of these medications is not regulated or guaranteed. VA's own website under the Foreign Medical Program states, "physicians should only prescribe medications that are legally available within the veteran's country of residence and are accepted by VA and the U.S. Food and Drug Administration (FDA)." Service-disabled veterans deserve access to high-quality care and should not have to travel to great lengths to receive needed medications.

Guam, American Samoa, Puerto Rico, U.S. Virgin Islands, and the Northern Mariana Islands face even greater challenges due to limited or poor infrastructure.

Veterans living in these areas sometimes have to take commercial aircraft, which are frequently not disability friendly, to get to appointments or fill prescriptions. Severe weather events affect these areas differently than rural areas within CONUS. According to VA's website, not one of the outside CONUS sites has a specialty SUD program.

A new Mental Health RRTP is scheduled to open in San Juan, Puerto Rico in 2024 to treat veterans on the island who are in desperate need of these services.

Puerto Ricans serve in the Armed Forces at higher numbers per capita, than many states within the union. We hope there will be a concerted effort to treat veterans with SUD and particularly gender-specific programming, to include a separate section for women veterans.

An additional barrier facing veterans residing outside of the United States is the Beneficiary Travel Self-Service System, which was designed to automate the travel reimbursement claims process. A May 2023 OIG report found significant problems with this system. While DAV supports this modernization effort, there continue to be complaints regarding the slow processing of payments, and improper payments made to beneficiaries.

Consider a service-disabled veteran who is wheelchair-bound and lives in Guam. That veteran experiences severe back pain that requires a medical procedure, but due to the lack of specialty care on the island, they are forced to travel to Hawaii, over 3,000 miles away, for their care. The veteran is eligible to take a military plane, but there are none available, so they must take a commercial flight, which the veteran must pay for up-front, and could cost $1,200. The veteran then needs transportation to the VHA facility, as well as a hotel—again, an up-front expense to the veteran. After spending thousands of dollars and flying 16 hours roundtrip for their medical care, the veteran finally returns home and files a claim using VA's travel reimbursement portal if they are technologically informed and/or have access.

They now have to wait weeks and very often, months, to get reimbursed, and not always the full amount that they originally paid out. This scenario is not just true for our veterans living outside of the continental United States, but also occurs in rural America.

Recommendation

- VA should conduct a needs assessment to determine if adding SUD programming for outside CONUS communities is warranted. As noted above, there are no SUD programs in any of the outside CONUS territories. In fact, many of these areas do not have VA facilities at all, making it difficult for veterans to access even basic health care.

Women Veterans and SUD

Unfortunately, not only rural veterans face challenges with SUD treatment.

Women veterans have a different and unique set of roadblocks to these specialized services and care. Like their male counterparts, rural women veterans also deal with health care access disparities due to long distances to medical facilities and lack of transportation. But for women veterans, there is also limited gender-specific programming for SUD services. Currently, there are only two gender-specific residential treatment programs with two pending. While VA has 13 gender-specific programs across nine locations, it is limited in what it can provide to women veterans in locations without more comprehensive residential treatment programs.

VA will provide beneficiary travel to the closest available facility offering the care, but it must work within current authorities, or coordinate other arrangements if the veteran is ineligible for beneficiary travel. Child care or concern over losing custody of children because of care-seeking for significant mental health conditions and/or SUD may be another barrier for women who need more intensive specialized care. Average and median wait times for women's care in domiciliaries were found to be slightly higher for women than men. VA reports that wait times are, on average, 24 days for women compared to 22 days for men. While 72 hours is VA's goal from screening to admission, fewer than 16% of women and 20% of men are admitted within this timeframe.

Some of the additional waiting time for women may be due to VA's lower capacity to address women's needs. VA reports fewer than half of all residential facilities have separate dorm space for women veterans and only 13 programs have gender-specific services for women veterans compared to 27 programs exclusive to men.

SUDs are associated with family instability, decreased worker productivity and declining health, and increased risk for suicidal behavior in veterans, especially in women. Women's bodies also respond differently to substance use and withdrawal, and their reasons for both using substances and stopping or reducing their substance use may be different from those of men. Understanding these differences is important to providing effective care. Additionally, while access to more tailored care is necessary for improving screening and SUD services for women veterans, it is critical that VA ensures safe and private therapeutic settings conducive to their recovery. Women are shown to be more likely than male veterans or non-veteran women to have co-occurring psychiatric and medical impairments, in many instances linked to a history of sexual trauma or domestic violence.

A 2020 study noted that women veterans of Operation Iraqi Freedom/Operation Enduring Freedom in Puerto Rico, utilized VA health care services at higher rates and had greater barriers to care than their U.S. counterparts.

Recommendation

- Conduct a nationwide analysis of the need and efficacy of women-specific programs that treat and rehabilitate women veterans with drug and alcohol dependency to determine if expanding gender-specific SUD inpatient care is warranted.

In closing, DAV is grateful for VA's whole-health integrated model of care along with top-tier evidence-based treatment and supportive services for veterans struggling with substance use disorders; however, only a small percentage of veterans diagnosed with SUD seek specialized treatment for their condition. This, coupled with the access challenges for rural and women veterans, make it clear that we need to address existing barriers to treat all veterans who need this life-saving specialized care. We appreciate the Committee's consideration of our recommendations to improve and expand these important services throughout this testimony.

We thank the Committee for the opportunity to testify on this important issue and are pleased to answer any questions you may have.

Statement of Chelsey Simoni, APRN, MSN, Ph.D.(c), Clinical Nurse Researcher & Executive Director of the HunterSeven Foundation

Chairman Tester, Ranking Member Moran, and members of the Senate Veterans Affairs Committee, I appreciate the opportunity to come and speak this evening on substance use in the veteran community.

Today, I speak before the committee as a licensed healthcare provider with advanced medical degrees, including public health and epidemiology specialty certifications. I've spent over fifteen-thousand hours working in emergency medicine, long- and short-term substance use settings, and military veteran-specific mental health clinics. I've published in numerous academic journals and presented at conferences nationwide. However, I speak to the committee today as the sister of a combat-wounded Marine losing his battle with addiction… as the child of an alcoholic and heroin-addicted father. I speak today as a disabled Army veteran dealing with constant, debilitating pain and the uninterrupted emotional burden I face daily. The testimony I share today is, unfortunately, entirely true.

I am the youngest of five. My sister and I share a mother, while my three brothers and I share a father. My three brothers lived with our aunt, as my father was preoccupied with shooting heroin and rotating between a "halfway house" and jail. Growing up, I thought drug use was regular for most adults. Everywhere I turned, I'd find a hypodermic needle or a spoon with a rubber band nearby. Sometimes I'd see the ambulance come to our apartment complex, and shortly after, a stretcher with a black body bag would roll by where I was playing. Some nights I'd stay awake crying, wondering if my parent would come home that night and if they did, I'd pray they wouldn't be so intoxicated that they would fall. I was always afraid when they drank because they would get hurt. While most ten-year-old kids enjoy sleepovers with their friends on the weekends, I was busy caring for my parent, confirming they got into bed, and checking on them throughout the night to ensure they were still breathing.

By fourteen, I needed to get a job; I skipped school and had never done my homework. I got into fights and did everything I wasn't supposed to, so I failed my freshman year of high school. At fifteen years old, I lost my oldest brother to an overdose. My mother told me my 24-year-old brother planned to enter substance use treatment the following Monday. He didn't make it. He had shot up the night before with friends of my fathers; he had fallen asleep and began to throw up… instead of calling 9-1-1 and keeping him awake, those he was with had moved his body into the hallway, where he choked on his vomit and died.

Shortly after his death, I was expelled from school. My behavior was self-destructive and lacked structure and discipline. It was difficult to talk about my situation at home with those who didn't understand, especially with those who just thought I was a "bad kid" but never figured to ask why. By sixteen, in 2007, my youngest brother had signed up to serve as an infantryman in the United States Marine Corps; we wrote to each other often while he was in boot camp at Parris Island. He loved it, every single minute of it. I had just graduated high school when my brother told me he would be deployed as one of the first waves into Marjah, Afghanistan, under President Obamas' "Surge," to disrupt Taliban forces. He spent seven months in southern Afghanistan.

While he was deployed, I'd sit at night and watch the evening world news to keep myself in the loop of what was happening in the war. Every time I heard about unnamed Marine casualties, my heart sank. It was almost daily. In total, 68 Marines were killed in action during that seven-month deployment, and 697 Marines were wounded in action.[63] In turn, I enlisted in the United States Army.

In August 2011, he redeployed to Sangin, Afghanistan, for eight months. Thirty Marines had been killed in action, while 582 Marines were wounded in action. One of those wounded Marines was my brother. While he had lost men he considered brothers, and witnessed his closest friends suffer near-death amputations from hidden improvised explosive devices and others who had been physically ripped apart from RPK machine gun rounds, my brother felt

[63] Defense Casualty Analysis System (June 9, 2023). U.S. Military Casualties - Operation Enduring Freedom (OEF) Casualty Summary by Month and Service. Retrieved from: https://dcas.dmdc.osd.mil/.

lucky. He had sustained outrageous blast injuries from explosions and rocket-propelled grenades. One blast so severe his MRAP vehicle had flipped over, throwing him from the turret, causing him to break four ribs, fracture his skull and sections of his lower back. He came home, but the physical pain was moot compared to the emotional guilt and moral injury he tried so hard to hide.

Over the next year, he struggled with physical pain and depression; the guilt overwhelmed his life. What began as a short- term Vicodin prescription for pain management became a full-blown addiction where he would steal Fentanyl patches from the regiments Navy corpsmen. He had kept his habit under the radar until a random drug test found opiates in his system.

Sixteen days later, he was discharged under "Other than Honorable" conditions for illicit drug use. He was homeless, jobless, emotionally and physically unstable, and addicted. He was too embarrassed to seek help; he suffered in silence and ended up sleeping on our aunts' couch.

Around the same time, I suffered a severe spinal injury while serving in the Army. I remember the electrifying pain, it wasn't like any pain I had experienced before, but my adrenaline was high, and the mission made the pain seem nonexistent. It wasn't until later that evening that I lost control of my bladder, and pins and needles drove up my leg, causing a debilitating painful paralysis. At 21 years old, I was told my injury led the discs in my lower back to partially paralyze my spinal cord, and I needed surgery. My military career was placed on hold, but that wasn't the case for the rest of my team. In the months leading up to the major surgery I was scheduled for, I was given more than 300 pills of the mild opiate hydrocodone-acetaminophen, better known as "Vicodin." I was told to take them every 6 hours for pain. In case the Vicodin wasn't working, I was given 100 pills of Tramadol, a synthetic opioid that reduces the pain felt through the central nervous system. To lessen the right-sided leg numbness, severe neuropathy, and muscle spasms, I was given 100 pills of Flexeril.

My anxiety was front-and-center at all of this, so I was given 30 pills of Lorazepam, an anti-anxiety benzodiazepine, to take "as needed" for anxiety.

Two weeks later, I received a call that one of my closest friends I had known since I was 14, was killed in Dawlat Shah, Afghanistan. I felt helpless, motionless, stuck in time; I couldn't move. The "pain" had gotten worse. The more of these pills I took, the less "pain" I had. And as time went on, everything became easier to deal with; or at least that is what I had thought.

I went through a three-hour surgery and was on the road to recovery. The first few nights were hell. I had severe nightmares; dreams I'd never wish anyone would experience; I'd wake up covered in sweat and unable to move. The pain worsened; I was given 60 pills of oxycodone-acetaminophen (Percocet) and told to stop taking the Vicodin as it may have been an adverse reaction. I couldn't swallow the pills without vomiting, worsening the post-operative pain. I was sent home with an 8oz. bottle of "Oxydose" - liquid oxycodone.

It helped with the pain; eventually, it subsided as I healed. I felt great. Looking back, I cannot remember a time in my life when I felt that relaxed or carefree. I could sleep. My mind stopped overthinking, and my heart stopped racing. I wasn't sad. I wasn't worried about the future; I was enjoying the present. And when I started to feel myself come back to reality, I'd grab the medicine bottle and take another sip. Like most 21-year-olds, I didn't have a way to measure the amount I was taking. Instead, I'd rely on my balance to let me know if I had taken enough. I don't remember much besides laying in my bed thinking, isn't life great.

I loved how I felt in those moments; it was an unmatched feeling. I took medication not for the physical pain but to cover my emotional pain, which worked very well – until it almost killed me. Late one night, I was lying in bed and had drunk too much. I laid back and felt a sudden sickness; I went to get up and felt my legs get weak. Using the side of my bed, I slowly slid to the ground… I don't remember much afterward until I woke up minutes later, covering my floor with vomit. I cried; I knew what happened. The next day I knew I had to get rid of it, which wasn't easy. But what kept me motivated was returning to uniform and being with my team again. There is a reasonable probability that is what kept me alive. To this day, I know I cannot take Percocet – I enjoy it too much.

While dealing with my situation, my brother battled something similar. He was figuring out his next steps, but none knew he was battling addiction. While staying with our aunt, he had been taking prescription opiates… when those ran out, and he couldn't get more, he turned to heroin.

He was alone one night and had shot up heroin that we later discovered had traces of fentanyl. He passed out on the couch, and when our aunt found him, he was covered in vomit and not breathing. She called 9-1-1 and began CPR; his lips were dusky and cold. He was given Narcan, intubated, and rushed to the emergency department, where the medical team worked to save his life. The doctor said it was a miracle he survived because he shouldn't have. They were cautiously optimistic as his brain was oxygen-deprived for some time, and we wouldn't know the severity until he was out of a coma.

He was transferred to the intensive care unit at the Department of Veterans Affairs in Boston, where he would spend the next few weeks hooked up to a breathing machine. Every night after dinner, I would sit with him; I'd play his favorite band, Stone Temple Pilots, while he lay there on life support. I'd wash his face and brush his hair. Weeks later, he was brought out of the coma, his neurological function was intact, but his attitude was almost careless – which surprised me the most. He had told me everything that had happened, from his other-than-honorable discharge to his lack of ability to receive services within the VA Healthcare System, as he had difficulty enrolling in care. He didn't have a backup plan and felt trapped as if he had returned to the bottom where he started. It took more than seven years to enroll him in substance use treatment and nearly ten years to have his military service discharge overturned.

While my brother faced his battles, I received medical clearance to remain in the Army despite having just had a life- changing surgery. My provider had told me that the chances of another injury occurring are inevitable and that I may not be so lucky this time around. Against his medical advice and warning of imminent pain and suffering, I knew it was where I belonged. It was my comfort zone; it was the family I never had. But as predicted, years later, I suffered a re-injury. This time was equally painful, but I could still move and manage. For me, long story short, my career was over. Discharged.

It will always be the most dangerous time in any service member-turned-veterans' life. You are leaving a tight-knit group, leaving a feeling of "belonging," and reintegrating into a society that couldn't give a shit about you, your service, your situation, or your struggles. There is no "team" or "tribe" that you can turn to or fall back on; there is no safety net or mirroring experience in a fellow veteran for you to voice your thoughts and feelings with.

I went to bed as a service member and woke up the following day as a civilian. My pain had become increasingly worse. My temper became short, my anger and frustration grew, and my anxiety worsened. I was alone with myself and my thoughts.

My grandparents had invited me to stay with them while I figured out my situation; with their help, I enrolled in school in hopes of receiving my undergraduate degree in nursing. Opposite to my time in high school, college became much easier for me. I was structured, disciplined, motivated, and mission-focused, but it felt like I was passing the time. I didn't feel like I was where I belonged.

I woke up one morning during my senior year of college, and it was like a trap door had fallen from underneath me. The best way to describe it is that I felt like I was running full speed on a treadmill. What that something was, I do not know. But I hit the lowest point in my life. I was running on empty. I couldn't stop crying – and I didn't know why. I couldn't eat or keep any food down. Instead, I drank whiskey to keep the anxiety and emotions at bay, leading to an ulcer eating my stomach lining. I hid my sadness from my family and friends. I was alone as if I was on the outside looking in. I had lost any meaningful purpose in my life, and I knew I didn't belong.

You can only run so much before you are on empty. And I was on empty.

I had a commemorative military pistol from the unit, a Sig Sauer P250, .45 ACP, underneath my bed, and I laid down on my bedroom floor looking up at the ceiling with the pistol in my right hand. I pointed the gun toward myself and placed the barrel in my mouth. I can remember the cold feeling and taste of steel. The only reason why I am still here today is two-fold.

I couldn't kill myself in my grandparents' house. I couldn't do that to them or have them wondering why for the rest of their lives. I got in my car and drove; I pulled over and texted, "I'm not okay," to the only person I knew would understand. My nursing professor a 29-year Air Force veteran and flight nurse. She understood. Thirty minutes later I was at the VA Hospitals' mental health urgent care getting the support I needed.

I didn't tell you all my life story for sympathy but to emphasize the importance of understanding the "bigger picture" concerning substance use, pain management, mental health, and recovery in military veterans. As difficult as it is to share at times, it is a lived experience that will provide some context for what I am about to say and hopefully guide your decision-making process regarding how post-9/11 military veterans receive potentially life-saving care.

Adverse Childhood Experiences

Adverse childhood events (ACE) are a list of eight negative experiences that occurred during one's childhood before age 18. These include living with a person who is mentally ill, depressed, or suicidal, living with an alcoholic, living with a person who used or abused illegal or prescription drugs, living with someone who had been incarcerated, parental divorce or separation, witnessing intimate partner violence, and being physically, emotionally, or sexually abused. Notably, a shift toward an all-volunteer military force has provided insight that children who experience adverse childhood events (ACE) are more than twice as likely to enlist in the Armed Forces.[64] For those who experienced situations similar to my brother and I, enlisting in the military served as an instrumental, live-changing choice to escape a dangerously destructive environment. Like myself, many of those who experienced adverse childhood events… crave regularity, routineness, safety, reliability, and structure—everything the military gives us.

[64] Bloshnich, J., Dichter, M., Cerulli, C., Batten, S. & Bossarte, R. (2014). Disparities in adverse childhood experiences among individuals with a history of military service. *Journal of the American Medical Association Psychiatry*, 71(9): 1041-1048. https://doi.org/10,1001/jamapsychiatry.2014.724.

In contrast, comparing those veterans who experienced no adverse childhood events, veterans who had experienced at least one were more than twice as likely to attempt suicide, while those with four or more adverse events during childhood were nearly four times more likely to attempt suicide.[65] Additionally, those who experienced adverse childhood events were upwards of ten times as likely to report substance use and addiction, and for those who had overlapping adverse childhood events and a substance use history, their risk of attempted suicide increased by 60%.[66]

Physical Health

Since 2001, more than three million veterans have served in the Global War on Terror / Post-9/11 era. Notably, various studies across different spectrums have determined that the following service, post-9/11 era veterans have poor physical health and higher levels of disability within specific body systems.[67] Post-9/11 veterans, when compared to non-veterans, experience significant elevations in prevalence with back and neck pain (49.3%), fractures and bone-joint injuries (47.6%), and arthritis (26.2%), leading to a relative risk of roughly three-and-a-half-times more likely to experience these issues following military service.

Furthermore, musculoskeletal conditions in veterans have also been associated with poor mental health status. In a study of Iraq War veterans, physical pain was twice as high in Iraq veterans diagnosed with post-traumatic stress (50%) than those without (26%).[68] Not only can post-traumatic stress and related depression limit any desire for physical activity, but post-traumatic stress and constant elevated "fight or flight" can also exacerbate injury through inflammatory pathways.[69] For some, such as myself, when we experience pain, we can be particularly susceptible to experiencing elevated anxiety due to pain but also injurious limitations and feeling "stuck." Utilizing medicinal or prescription opiates to treat chronic pain in post-9/11 military veterans is a dangerous downward slope, as it can be used as a temporary Band-Aid for a much larger problem.

Emotional Health & Suicidal Ideation

If you ask any veteran if they miss serving in uniform, they will say yes, through good and bad times, even while at war. It is a complex, paradoxical relationship – but it is critical to understand the deeper meaning behind the "why." When my brother came home and told me what had happened while deployed during the height of the war, I figured his response and

---

[65] *Ibid.*

[66] Douglas, K. et al. (2010). Adverse childhood events as risk factors for substance dependence: Partial mediation by mood and anxiety disorders. *Addictive Behaviors*, 35(1): 7-13. https://doi.org/10.1016/j.addbeh.2009.07.004.

[67] Cypel, Y. et al. (2023). Physical health of Post-9/11 U.S. Military veterans in the context of Healthy People 2020 targeted topic areas: Results from the Comparative Health Assessment Interview Research Study. *Preventive Medicine Reports*, 32. https://doi.org/10.1016/j.pmedr.2023.102122.

[68] Nazarian, D., Kimerling, R. & Frayne, S. (2012). Posttraumatic stress disorder, substance use disorders, and medical comorbidity among returning U.S. veterans. *Journal of Traumatic Stress*, 25(2): 220-225. https://doi.org/10.1002/jts.21690.

[69] Banihashemi, L., Wallace, M., Peng, C., Stinley, M., Germain, A. & Herringa, R. (2020). Interactions between childhood maltreatment and combat exposure trauma on stress-related activity within the cingulate cortex: A pilot study. *Military Psychology*, 32(2): 176-185. https://doi.org/10.1080/08995605.2019.1702831.

reaction would be more traumatic. He visually described his teammate that rescued two wounded Marines while running under a hail of gunfire and eventually stepping on a pressure-plate bomb that tore his legs cleanly from the bone. He told me war is destructive and dangerous, and there is no shortage of suffering – he said it was no worse than being at home, but at least in Afghanistan, he had his brothers by his side. Emotional suffering is much less evident and damaging if surrounded by others who understand. Most importantly, it gave each marine a sense of purpose, meaning, and identity more significant than themselves.[70]

The first six months to a year are considered the "transition" period following separation from military service and reintegration into civilian life. Veteran suicide risk appears particularly elevated during this first year. Historically, during this period, veterans have a suicide rate 2.5 times higher than that of active-duty service members.[71] It can be similar to a culture shock when leaving service and losing the close-knit cohesion and interdependence obtained in service, mixed with modern-day civilian societies' level of isolation and disconnection can perceive the feeling of individual alienation and lack of belonging. Suppose you are one of those veterans who had a forced end to your military career from addiction or other maladaptive behaviors, physical injury, or mental health disorders. In that case, your risk for self-harm, substance use, and suicide increases dramatically, and if compounded with a history of adverse childhood events, your chances of survival are slim, and the worst part is that you are alone.

Substance Use & Addiction

The most effective way to explain why veterans become addicts at increasingly higher rates is best reflected by the "Rat Park Experiment" conducted by psychologist Bruce K. Alexander.[72] The experiment aimed to explore the role of social and environmental factors in drug addiction. Traditionally, addiction research had predominantly focused on individual drug exposure and chemical dependency. The Rat Park experiment sought to challenge this perspective by examining the influence of social and environmental factors on drug-seeking behavior. In the experiment, researchers created two distinct environments for laboratory rats.

The first environment was a traditional small cage with solitary housing, where rats had access to two water bottles: one containing plain water and the other laced with morphine. The second environment was a larger enclosure called "Rat Park," which provided an enriched social and physical environment with a variety of stimuli, such as toys, wheels, and the presence of other rats. Similarly, the rats in Rat Park had access to the same two water bottles. The study results showed that the rats in Rat Park consumed little-to-no morphine-laced water than solitary housing rats. The researchers concluded that the rats in Rat Park, with their enriched environment and social interactions, were less inclined to become addicted to morphine. They hypothesized that the rats in solitary housing were more susceptible to drug addiction due to

---

[70] Hedges, C. (2003). *War is a force that gives us meaning*. Anchor Books, Random House, Inc. 1st edition. ISBN: 978-1-61039-359-1.

[71] Ravindran, C., Morley, S., Stephens, B., Stanley, I. & Reger, M. (2020). Association of suicide risk with transition to civilian life among U.S. military service members. *Journal of American Medical Association*, 3(9): e201621. https://doi.org/10.1001/jamanetworkopen.2020.16261.

[72] Alexander, B., Coambs, R. & Hadaway, P. (1978). The effect of housing and gender on morphine self-administration in rats. *Psychopharmacology*, 58(2): 175-179. https://doi.org/10.1007/BF00426903.

their lack of social and environmental stimulation, challenging the idea that addiction is solely based on chemical dependency.[73] Healing veteran addiction is possible through community, not through a rural clinic hours away.

While various factors were touched upon, from musculoskeletal injuries to childhood experiences, mental health, suicidal ideation, and transition, everything mentioned in this testimony is critical in understanding how to treat best (and prevent) military veteran addiction. While the Department of Veterans Affairs does a fine job with non-emergent, chronic conditions, the same isn't to be said for veterans dealing with polytrauma and dual diagnoses. Instead of treating these conditions separately, they must be treated simultaneously and from a whole-body, head-to-toe approach.

After reviewing services within the Department of Veterans Affairs Healthcare System nationwide for care related to addiction, 365 VA facilities offered new patient substance use programs. Of those, an initial appointment's average wait time is nine days. While some locations had no wait time data, and others didn't offer substance use treatments (i.e., Guam), other locations had upwards of 40 to 99 waiting days for substance use treatment. As mentioned above, mental health and co-morbid post-traumatic stress often overlap with military veterans who suffer from substance use. The most effective way to approach and successfully treat addiction is to look at the big picture holistically. After gathering the wait days for substance use, the process was repeated for a new veteran patient(s) wait days for mental health and post-traumatic stress, respectfully. The average wait for mental health services was 32 days, while post-traumatic stress-specific services were widely unavailable in more than half of the locations treating veteran substance use. I invite the Committee to review this chart included in the appendix.

In Montana, for example: if a veteran lives in Glacier County, the closest VA facility offering substance use treatment is Great Falls which is only 1.5 hours away and has no wait time for new patients. However, it doesn't provide PTSD-specific care and has a 74-day wait list for mental health treatment. The next closest facility is in Kalispell; the wait is only 26 days for substance use and 13 days for mental health, PTSD-specific care isn't available, but the drive is more than 2.5 hours away. This isn't a feasible option for rural area veterans. Many of us who have faced substance use disorders and co- occurring post-traumatic stress, depression, or any type of mental health disorder do not have the time to wait. Most who suffer from dual-diagnosis disorders such as mental health and substance use do not have the means to travel 2.5 hours away for care, nor do many have the transportation resources. Successful treatment for addiction begins with, first, the individual determining they have a problem and, second, their willingness and readiness to seek treatment. Neither of which can wait 26 days.

To positively change and impact military veteran care, *the approach should be less about the Department of Veterans Affairs and more about the veterans themselves.* Meeting the veteran where they are and allowing them to be the Captain of their ship giving them the slightest bit of self-control and self-determination regarding their healthcare. I ask that the committee consider civilian and non-Veterans Affairs options, access, and coverage to substance use and mental health / post-traumatic stress-specific care in the community. Mr. Chairman, and members of the Senate Veterans Affairs Committee, I appreciate your listening to my story and many other military veterans nationwide. That concludes my statement, and I would be pleased to answer any questions you or the Committee members may have.

---

[73] *Ibid.*

VA NAME	CITY	STATE	ZIP	SUBSTANCE USE WAIT (DAYS)	MENTAL HEALTH WAIT (DAYS)	PTSD SPECIFIC WAIT (DAYS)
ALASKA VAHCS (JBER)	ANCHORAGE	AK	99504	0	28	NOT OFFERED
BIRMINGHAM EAST VA CLINIC	IRONDALE	AL	35210	0	52	0
TUSCALOOSA VA MEDICAL CENTER	TUSCALOOSA	AL	35404	3	43	18
HUNTSVILLE VA CLINIC	HUNTSVILLE	AL	35805	0	45	NOT OFFERED
CENTRAL ALABAMA VAMC	MONTGOMERY	AL	36109	15	46	0
CENTRAL ALABAMA VAMC	TUSKEEGEE	AL	36083	0	28	0
EUGENE TOWBIN HEALTHCARE CENTER	NORTH LITTLE ROCK	AR	72114	0	38	0
FAYETTEVILLE VAMC	FAYETTEVILLE	AR	72703	0	12	1
FORT SMITH VA CLINIC	FORT SMITH	AR	72903	71	25	NOT OFFERED
CONRAD VAHC CLINIC	GILBERT	AZ	85297	0	63	0
MESA VA CLINIC	MESA	AZ	85212	8	65	NOT OFFERED
HAYDEN VAMC	PHOENIX	AZ	85012	46	34	NOT OFFERED
TUCSON VAMC	TUCSON	AZ	85723	40	39	0
SOUTH TUCSON VA CLINIC	TUCSON	AZ	85747	0	40	NOT OFFERED
BOB STUMP VAMC	PRESCOTT	AZ	86313	6	25	50
REDDING VA CLINIC	REDDING	CA	96002	0	48	0
CHICO VA CLINIC	CHICO	CA	95923	1	36	NOT OFFERED
YUBA CITY VA CLINIC	YUBA CITY	CA	95991	0	3	NOT OFFERED
MCCLELLAN VA CLINIC	MCCLELLAN PARK	CA	95652	0	31	0
FAIRFIELD VA CLINIC (TRAVIS AFB)	TRAVIS AIR FORCE BASE	CA	94535	0	9	NOT OFFERED
MARE ISLAND VA CLINIC	MARE ISLAND	CA	94592	0	1	NOT OFFERED
SACRAMENTO VAMC	MATHER	CA	95655	1	15	0
MARTINEZ VAMC	MARTINEZ	CA	94553	0	64	0
SAN FRANCISCO VAMC	SAN FRANCISCO	CA	94121	40	33	0
21ST STREET VA CLINIC	OAKLAND	CA	94612	8	43	0
PALO ALTO VAMC	PALO ALTO	CA	94304	0	29	0
FREMONT VA CLINIC	FREMONT	CA	94538	0	48	NOT OFFERED
STOCKTON VA CLINIC	FRENCH CAMP	CA	95231	0	77	NOT OFFERED
ROSEMARY MARINER OUTPATIENT CLINIC	VENTURA	CA	93003	13	39	NOT OFFERED
SEPULVEDA VAMC	SEPULVEDA	CA	91343	78	59	0
WEST LOS ANGELES VAMC	LOS ANGELES	CA	90073	64	116	0
LOS ANGELES VA CLINIC	LOS ANGELES	CA	90012	3	58	0
CABRILLO VA CLINIC	LONG BEACH	CA	90806	0	NOT OFFERED	NOT OFFERED
TIBOR RUBIN VAMC	LONG BEACH	CA	90822	33	24	50
PLACENTIA VA CLINIC	PLACENTIA	CA	92870	0	75	NOT OFFERED
ESCONDIDO VA CLINIC	ESCONDIDO	CA	92025	5	82	NOT OFFERED
JENNIFER MORENO VAMC	SAN DIEGO	CA	92161	12	23	97
MURRIETA VA CLINIC	MURRIETA	CA	92562	0	148	NOT OFFERED
KEARNEY MESA VA CLINIC	SAN DIEGO	CA	92123	7	39	60
RIO VA CLINIC	SAN DIEGO	CA	92108	15	0	123
CHULA VISTA VA CLINIC	CHULA VISTA	CA	91910	6	37	0
SANTA ANA VA CLINIC	SANTA ANA	CA	92705	0	60	NOT OFFERED
JERRY PETTIS VETERANS HOSPITAL	LOMA LINDA	CA	92357	18	0	NOT OFFERED
LOMA LINDA VA CLINIC	LOMA LINDA	CA	92373	18	63	NOT OFFERED
GRAND JUNCTION VAMC	GRAND JUNCTION	CO	81501	0	12	5
SALIDA VA CLINIC	SALIDA	CO	81201	0	0	NOT OFFERED
ALAMOSA VA CLINIC	ALAMOSA	CO	81101	0	0	NOT OFFERED
GOLDEN VA CLINIC	GOLDEN	CO	80401	36	65	0
LINDSTROM VA CLINIC	COLORADO SPRINGS	CO	80907	0	32	0
ROCKY MOUNTAIN REGIONAL VAMC	AURORA	CO	80045	29	61	0
LOVELAND VA CLINIC	LOVELAND	CO	80538	0	0	0
NORTHERN COLORADO VA CLINIC	LOVELAND	CO	80538	6	65	0
JAMES DUNN VA CLINIC	PUEBLO	CO	81008	0	26	NOT OFFERED
WEST HAVEN VAMC	WEST HAVEN	CT	6516	15	39	0
ERRERA VA CLINIC	WEST HAVEN	CT	6516	0	0	NOT OFFERED
NEWINGTON VA CLINIC	NEWINGTON	CT	6111	16	11	NOT OFFERED
WASHINGTON VAMC	WASHINGTON	DC	20422	1	16	16
KENT COUNTY VA CLINIC	DOVER	DE	19901	0	8	NOT OFFERED
SUSSEX COUNTY VA CLINIC	GEORGETOWN	DE	19947	0	19	NOT OFFERED
WILMINGTON VAMC	WILMINGTON	DE	19805	10	7	NOT OFFERED
BRUCE CARTER VAMC	MIAMI	FL	33125	0	25	6
WILLIAM KLING VA OUTPATIENT CLINIC	SUNRISE	FL	33351	0	6	0
WEST PALM BEACH VAMC	WEST PALM BEACH	FL	33410	1	19	0
LEE COUNTY VA CLINIC	CAPE CORAL	FL	33909	34	18	NOT OFFERED

VIERA VA CLINIC	VIERA	FL	32940	25	25	16
WEST LAKELAND VA CLINIC	LAKELAND	FL	33811	0	0	NOT OFFERED
ORLANDO VAMC	ORLANDO	FL	32827	6	11	20
SOUTH HILLSBOROUGH VA CLINIC	RIVERVIEW	FL	33579	0	6	NOT OFFERED
LAKE BALDWIN VA CLINIC	ORLANDO	FL	32803	0	12	0
46TH STREET SOUTH VA CLINIC	TAMPA	FL	33617	0	3	0
JAMES HALEY VAMC	TAMPA	FL	33612	0	21	0
C.W. BILL YOUNG VAMC	BAY PINES	FL	33744	4	27	10
BROOKSVILLE VA CLINIC	BROOKSVILLE	FL	34613	0	22	NOT OFFERED
WESTSIDE PAVILION VA CLINIC	DAYTONA BEACH	FL	32114	0	53	0
THE VILLAGES VA CLINIC	THE VILLAGES	FL	32162	5	91	0
LEO CHASE JR VA CLINIC	SAINT AUGUSTINE	FL	32086	2	45	NOT OFFERED
OCALA VA CLINIC	OCALA	FL	34474	5	16	NOT OFFERED
JACKSONVILLE SOUTHPOINT VA CLINIC	JACKSONVILLE	FL	32216	58	27	0
GAINESVILLE 1 VA CLINIC	GAINESVILLE	FL	32608	27	25	16
LAKE CITY VAMC	LAKE CITY	FL	32025	28	29	0
ERNEST THOMAS VA CLINIC	TALLAHASSEE	FL	32311	43	93	0
MACON VA CLINIC	MACON	GA	31220	17	51	NOT OFFERED
CARL VINSON VAMC	DUBLIN	GA	31021	20	6	NOT OFFERED
ROBERT POYDASHEFF VA CLINIC	COLUMBUS	GA	31904	0	43	NOT OFFERED
FORT MCPHERSON VA CLINIC	ATLANTA	GA	30310	0	70	NOT OFFERED
JOSEPH MAXWELL CLELAND VAMC	DECATUR	GA	30033	44	22	NOT OFFERED
HENDERSON MILL VA CLINIC	ATLANTA	GA	30345	0	0	1
COBB COUNTY VA CLINIC	MARIETTA	GA	30062	0	38	NOT OFFERED
AUGUSTA VA MEDICAL CENTER (UPTOWN)	AUGUSTA	GA	30904	11	17	53
OAKWOOD VA CLINIC	FLOWERY BRANCH	GA	30542	0	0	0
WAYCROSS VA CLINIC	WAYCROSS	GA	31501	20	19	NOT OFFERED
VALDOSTA VA CLINIC	VALDOSTA	GA	31601	8	32	NOT OFFERED
SAVANNAH VA CLINIC	SAVANNAH	GA	31419	27	43	NOT OFFERED
GUAM VA CLINIC	AGANA HEIGHTS	GU	96910	NOT OFFERED	71	NOT OFFERED
MATSUNAGA VAMC	HONOLULU	HI	96819	0	12	29
CEDAR RAPIDS VA CLINIC	CEDAR RAPIDS	IA	52404	0	92	0
CORALVILLE VA CLINIC	COARLVILLE	IA	52241	22	63	68
DAVENPORT VA CLINIC	DAVENPORT	IA	52801	12	0	NOT OFFERED
DES MOINES VAMC	DES MOINES	IA	50310	40	24	0
DUBUQUE VA CLINIC	DUBUQUE	IA	52003	0	77	0
IOWA CITY VAMC	IOWA CITY	IA	52246	0	31	NOT OFFERED
LINN COUNTY VA CLINIC	CEDAR RAPIDS	IA	52402	0	NOT OFFERED	NOT OFFERED
OTTUMWA VA CLINIC	OTTUMWA	IA	52501	0	11	NOT OFFERED
WATERLOO VA CLINIC	WATERLOO	IA	50701	1	50	NOT OFFERED
BOISE VAMC	BOISE	ID	83702	20	36	0
AUBURN GRESHAM VA CLINIC	CHICAGO	IL	60620	0	31	NOT OFFERED
BOB MICHEL VA OUTPATIENT CLINIC	PEORIA	IL	61615	0	37	0
JAMES LOVELL FEDERAL HEALTH CENTER	NORTH CHICAGO	IL	60064	0	13	29
CHICAGO HEIGHTS VA CLINIC	CHICAGO HEIGHTS	IL	60411	0	0	NOT OFFERED
DANVILLE VAMC	DANVILLE	IL	61832	8	31	0
EDWARD HINES JR. HOSPITAL	HINES	IL	60141	0	11	0
JESSE BROWN VAMC	CHICAGO	IL	60612	32	13	3
MARION VAMC	MARION	IL	62959	3	8	0
ROCKFORD VA CLINIC	ROCKFORD	IL	61107	0	0	NOT OFFERED
STERLING VA CLINIC	STERLING	IL	61081	0	64	NOT OFFERED
ADAM BENJAMIN JR VA OUTPATIENT CLINIC	CROWN POINT	IN	46307	0	27	NOT OFFERED
BROWNSBURG VA CLINIC	BROWNSBURG	IN	46112	0	51	NOT OFFERED
EVANSVILLE VA CLINIC	EVANSVILLE	IN	47715	6	29	0
FORT WAYNE VA CLINIC	FORT WAYNE	IN	46805	12	52	45
JACKIE WALORSKI VA CLINIC	MISHAWAKA	IN	46545	99	51	116
LAFAYETTE VA CLINIC	LAFAYETTE	IN	47905	0	97	NOT OFFERED
MARION VAMC	MARION	IN	46953	37	38	72
MUNROE COUNTY VA CLINIC	BLOOMINGTON	IN	47403	0	11	NOT OFFERED
NEW ALBANY VA CLINIC	NEW ALBANY	IN	47150	0	52	0
RICHARD ROUDEBUSH VAMC	INDIANAPOLIS	IN	46202	0	8	0
RICHMOND VA CLINIC	RICHMOND	IN	47374	0	24	NOT OFFERED
TERRE HAUTE VA CLINIC	TERRE HAUTE	IN	47803	0	78	NOT OFFERED
WAKEMAN VA CLINIC	EDINBURGH	IN	46124	1	79	NOT OFFERED
COLMERY-ONEIL VAMC	TOPEKA	KS	66622	8	25	28
EISENHOWER VAMC	LEAVENWORTH	KS	66048	0	13	22
HUTCHINSON VA CLINIC	HUTCHINSON	KS	67502	0	22	0
ROBERT DOLE VAMC & REGIONAL OFFICE	WICHITA	KS	67218	0	21	56

BEREA VA CLINIC	BEREA	KY	40403	0	29	NOT OFFERED
FLORENCE VA CLINIC	FLORENCE	KY	41042	0	29	NOT OFFERED
FORT KNOX VA CLINIC	FORT KNOX	KY	40121	0	52	0
FRANKLIN SOUSLEY CAMPUS	LEXINGTON	KY	40511	19	21	1
GRAYSON COUNTY VA CLINIC	CLARKSON	KY	42726	0	0	0
GREENWOOD VA CLINIC	LOUISVILLE	KY	40258	0	40	0
NEWBURG VA CLINIC	LOUISVILLE	KY	40218	0	48	0
PADUCAH VA CLINIC	PADUCAH	KY	42001	12	23	NOT OFFERED
ROBLEY REX VAMC	LOUISVILLE	KY	40206	18	26	NOT OFFERED
SOMERSET VA CLINIC	SOMERSET	KY	42503	0	0	NOT OFFERED
STONYBROOK VA CLINIC	LOUISVILLE	KY	40299	0	38	0
ALEXANDRIA VAMC	PINEVILLE	LA	71360	0	26	19
LAFAYETTE CAMPUS B VA CLINIC	LAFAYETTE	LA	70506	0	98	NOT OFFERED
BATON ROUGE SOUTH VA CLINIC	BATON ROUGE	LA	70810	10	25	0
HAMMOND VA CILNIC	HAMMOND	LA	70403	0	37	NOT OFFERED
NEW ORLEANS VAMC	NEW ORLEANS	LA	70119	4	46	196
SLIDELL VA CLINIC	SLIDELL	LA	70460	0	15	NOT OFFERED
OVERTON BROOKS VAMC	SHREVEPORT	LA	71101	24	71	32
BROCKTON VAMC	BROCKTON	MA	2301	23	41	96
BEDFORD VAMC	BEDFORD	MA	1730	9	16	NOT OFFERED
EDWARD BOLAND VAMC	LEEDS	MA	1053	10	25	NOT OFFERED
JAMAICA PLAIN VAMC	BOSTON	MA	2130	13	15	36
SPRINGFIELD VA CLINIC	SPRINGFIELD	MA	1104	0	18	NOT OFFERED
WORCESTER VA CLINIC	WORCESTER	MA	1604	51	62	NOT OFFERED
BALTIMORE VAMC	BALTIMORE	MD	21201	1	57	42
CUMBERLAND VA CLINIC	CUMBERLAND	MD	21502	0	53	NOT OFFERED
BANGOR VA CLINIC	BANGOR	ME	4401	0	108	NOT OFFERED
TOGUS VAMC	AUGUSTA	ME	4330	16	109	0
BATTLE CREEK VAMC	BATTLE CREEK	MI	49037	44	22	0
GLADSTONE VA CLINIC	GLADSTONE	MI	49837	0	30	NOT OFFERED
HANCOCK VA CLINIC	HANCOCK	MI	49930	0	14	0
IRONWOOD VA CLINIC	IRONWOOD	MI	49938	0	0	0
JOHN DINGELL VAMC	DETROIT	MI	48201	7	18	0
LANSING VA CLINIC	LANSING	MI	48911	0	22	NOT OFFERED
CHARLES KETTLES VAMC	ANN ARBOR	MI	48105	19	57	32
MANISTIQUE VA CLINIC	MANISTIQUE	MI	49854	0	26	0
MARQUETTE VA CLINIC	MARQUETTE	MI	49855	0	63	0
MENOMINEE VA CLINIC	MENOMINEE	MI	49858	0	17	NOT OFFERED
SAGINAW VA CLINIC	SAGINAW	MI	48603	21	24	42
WYOMING VA CLINIC	WYOMING	MI	49519	7	28	NOT OFFERED
BEMIDJI VA CLINIC	BEMIDJI	MN	56601	0	95	NOT OFFERED
FERGUS FALLS VA CLINIC	FERGUS FALLS	MN	56537	0	0	NOT OFFERED
MINNEAPOLIS VAMC	MINNEAPOLIS	MN	55417	0	29	0
ST CLOUD VAMC	ST CLOUD	MN	56303	0	7	NOT OFFERED
BRANSON VA CLINIC	BRANSON	MO	65616	0	18	NOT OFFERED
FARMINGTON VA CLINIC	FARMINGTON	MO	63640	16	14	NOT OFFERED
GENE TAYLOR VETERANS OUTPATIENT CLINIC	SPRINGFIELD	MO	65807	1	4	NOT OFFERED
HARRY TRUMAN VETERANS HOSPITAL	COLUMBIA	MO	65201	0	38	0
JOHN PERSHING VAMC	POPLAR BLUFF	MO	63901	0	18	0
JOPLIN VA CLINIC	JOPLIN	MO	64804	0	20	NOT OFFERED
KANSAS CITY VAMC	KANSAS CITY	MO	64128	18	12	NOT OFFERED
WEST PLAINS VA CLINIC	WEST PLAINS	MO	65775	20	40	NOT OFFERED
BILOXI VAMC	BILOXI	MS	39531	1	73	NOT OFFERED
GV MONTGOMERY VAMC	JACKSON	MS	39216	1	17	5
GREENVILLE VA CLINIC	GREENVILLE	MS	38701	0	8	NOT OFFERED
HATTIESBURG VA CLINIC	HATTIESBURG	MS	39402	0	0	0
KOSCIUSKO VA CLINIC	KOSCIUSKO	MS	39090	0	0	NOT OFFERED
NATCHEZ VA CLINIC	NATCHEZ	MS	39120	0	0	0
BENJAMIN CHARLES STEELE VA CLINIC	BILLINGS	MT	59102	0	60	NOT OFFERED
BUTTE VA CLINIC	BUTTE	MT	59701	0	0	NOT OFFERED
DAVID THATCHER VA CLINIC	MISSOULA	MT	59808	0	0	NOT OFFERED
FORT HARRISON VAMC	FORT HARRISON	MT	59636	0	54	0
GLASGOW VA CLINIC	GLASGOW	MT	59230	0	0	NOT OFFERED
GREAT FALLS VA CLINIC	GREAT FALLS	MT	59405	0	74	NOT OFFERED
HAMILTON VA CLINIC	HAMILTON	MT	59840	0	0	NOT OFFERED
KALISPELL VA CLINIC	KALISPELL	MT	59901	26	13	NOT OFFERED

TRAVIS ATKINS VA CLINIC	BOZEMAN	MT	59715	0	78	0
CHARLES GEORGE VAMC	ASHEVILLE	NC	28805	1	49	0
DURHAM COUNTY VA	DURHAM	NC	27705	40	40	16
FAYETTEVILLE VAMC	FAYETTEVILLE	NC	28301	61	89	NOT OFFERED
FRANKLIN VA CLINIC	FRANKLIN	NC	28734	0	71	NOT OFFERED
GREENVILLE VA CLINIC	GREENVILLE	NC	27834	16	117	NOT OFFERED
HICKORY VA CLINIC	HICKORY	NC	28602	0	24	NOT OFFERED
JACKSONVILLE 4 VA CLINIC	JACKSONVILLE	NC	28546	62	40	0
KERNERSVILLE VA CLINIC	KERNERSVILLE	NC	27284	0	17	0
MSGT JERRY CRUMP VA CLINIC	FOREST CITY	NC	28043	8	32	NOT OFFERED
MOREHEAD CITY VA CLINIC	MOREHEAD CITY	NC	28557	0	147	NOT OFFERED
NORTH CHARLOTTE VA CLINIC	CHARLOTTE	NC	28213	0	40	NOT OFFERED
SOUTH CHARLOTTE VA CLINIC	CHARLOTTE	NC	28208	0	35	0
W.G. HEFNER SALISBURY VAMC	SALISBURY	NC	28144	0	41	0
WAKE COUNTY VA CLINIC	RALEIGH	NC	27603	68	73	NOT OFFERED
WILMINGTON VA CLINIC	WILMINGTON	NC	28405	0	40	0
FARGO VAMC	FARGO	ND	58102	14	44	0
GRAFTON VA CLINIC	GRAFTON	ND	58237	0	0	NOT OFFERED
GRAND FORKS VA CLINIC	GRAND FORKS	ND	58201	0	75	NOT OFFERED
JAMESTOWN VA CLINIC	JAMESTOWN	ND	58401	0	49	NOT OFFERED
GRAND ISLAND VAMC	GRAND ISLAND	NE	68803	0	28	NOT OFFERED
LINCOLN VA CLINIC	LINCOLN	NE	68510	3	30	0
OMAHA VAMC	OMAHA	NE	68105	0	41	37
MANCHESTER VAMC	MANCHESTER	NH	3104	4	68	NOT OFFERED
SOMERSWORTH VA CLINIC	SOMERSWORTH	NH	3878	0	39	NOT OFFERED
ATLANTIC COUNTY VA CLINIC	NORTHFIELD	NJ	8225	18	10	NOT OFFERED
CAPE MAY COUNTY VA CLINIC	RIO GRANDE	NJ	8242	0	19	NOT OFFERED
CUMBERLAND COUNTY VA CLINIC	VINELAND	NJ	8360	0	18	NOT OFFERED
EAST ORANGE VAMC	EAST ORANGE	NJ	7018	9	20	0
HOBBS VA CLINIC	HOBBS	NM	88240	0	30	NOT OFFERED
RAYMOND MURPHY VAMC	ALBUQUERQUE	NM	87108	8	68	0
IOANNIS LOUGARIS VAMC	RENO	NV	89502	31	57	42
NORTH LAS VEGAS VAMC	NORTH LAS VEGAS	NV	89086	7	14	0
SOUTHWEST LAS VEGAS VA CLINIC	LAS VEGAS	NV	89113	42	18	NOT OFFERED
BATAVIA VAMC	BATAVIA	NY	14020	0	0	5
BATH VAMC	BATH	NY	14810	0	0	NOT OFFERED
BINGHAMTON VA CLINIC	BINGHAMTON	NY	13901	0	33	NOT OFFERED
BROOKLYN VAMC	BROOKLYN	NY	11209	0	9	0
BUFFALO VAMC	BUFFALO	NY	14215	24	30	NOT OFFERED
CANADAIGUA VAMC	CANADAIGUA	NY	14424	0	30	0
CASTLE POINT VAMC	WAPPINGERS FALLS	NY	12590	15	2	NOT OFFERED
ELMIRA VA CLINIC	ELMIRA	NY	14901	0	0	0
ERIE WEST VA CLINIC	SYRACUSE	NY	13204	12	34	21
FDR HOSPITAL	MONTROSE	NY	10548	0	24	0
JAMES PETERS VAMC	BRONX	NY	10468	10	7	0
MARGARET COCHRAN CORBIN VA CAMPUS	NEW YORK	NY	10010	5	16	16
NORTHPORT VAMC	NORTHPORT	NY	11768	2	18	NOT OFFERED
ROCHESTER CALKINS VA CLINIC	ROCHESTER	NY	14623	0	29	0
SAMUEL STRATTON VAMC	ALBANY	NY	12208	0	27	0
SYRACUSE VAMC	SYRACUSE	NY	13210	4	NOT OFFERED	NOT OFFERED
WATERTOWN VA CLINIC	WATERTOWN	NY	13601	0	31	4
AKRON VA CLINIC	AKRON	OH	44319	12	12	NOT OFFERED
ATHENS VA CLINIC	THE PLAINS	OH	45780	0	0	NOT OFFERED
CAMBRIDGE VA CLINIC	CAMBRIDGE	OH	43725	0	17	NOT OFFERED
CANTON VA CLINIC	CANTON	OH	44702	6	18	NOT OFFERED
CARL NUNZIATO VA CLINIC	YOUNGSTOWN	OH	44504	0	16	NOT OFFERED
CHILLICOTHE VAMC	CHILLICOTHE	OH	45601	0	32	0
CINCINNATI VAMC	CINCINNATI	OH	45220	20	8	NOT OFFERED
DAVID WINDER COMMUNITY BASED CLINIC	MANSFIELD	OH	44906	0	12	NOT OFFERED
DAYTON VAMC	DAYTON	OH	45428	28	21	0
EAST LIVERPOOL VA CLINIC	CALCUTTA	OH	43920	0	20	NOT OFFERED
LAKE COUNTY VA CLINIC	WILLOUGHBY	OH	44094	0	15	NOT OFFERED
LANCASTER VA CLINIC	LANCASTER	OH	43130	0	30	NOT OFFERED
LORAIN VA CLINIC	SHEFFIELD VILLAGE	OH	44035	5	12	NOT OFFERED
LOUIS STOKES CLEVELAND VAMC	CLEVELAND	OH	44106	7	26	85
MIDDLETOWN VA CLINIC	MIDDLETOWN	OH	45005	0	29	NOT OFFERED
NEW PHILADELPHIA VA CLINIC	NEW PHILADELPHIA	OH	44663	0	13	NOT OFFERED

PARMA VA CLINIC	PARMA	OH	44129	0	36	0
PORTSMOUTH VA CLINIC	NEW BOSTON	OH	45662	0	26	NOT OFFERED
RAVENNA VA CLINIC	RAVENNA	OH	44266	0	15	NOT OFFERED
SANDUSKY VA CLINIC	SANDUSKY	OH	44870	0	22	NOT OFFERED
TOLEDO VA CLINIC	TOLEDO	OH	43614	19	31	0
WARREN VA CLINIC	WARREN	OH	44485	0	21	0
ERNEST CHILDERS VA OUTPATIENT CLINIC	TULSA	OK	74133	13	28	NOT OFFERED
LAWTON VA CLINIC	FORT SILL	OK	73503	0	18	NOT OFFERED
MUSKOGEE EAST VA CLINIC	MUSKOGEE	OK	74403	3	27	NOT OFFERED
OKLAHOMA CITY VAMC	OKLAHOMA CITY	OK	73104	3	16	0
PORTLAND VAMC	PORTLAND	OR	97239	19	28	0
ROBERT MAXWELL VA CLINIC	BEND	OR	97701	0	79	NOT OFFERED
ABIE ABRAHAM VA CLINIC	BUTLER	PA	16001	19	18	NOT OFFERED
ARMSTRONG COUNTY VA CLINIC	KITTANNING	PA	16201	0	0	NOT OFFERED
BERKS COUNTY VA CLINIC	WYOMISSING	PA	19610	0	65	0
CLARION COUNTY VA CLINIC	MONROE TOWNSHIP	PA	16214	0	0	NOT OFFERED
COASTESVILLE VAMC	COATESVILLE	PA	19320	0	10	63
MICHAEL CRESCENZ VAMC	PHILADELPHIA	PA	19104	24	24	0
CRANBERRY TOWNSHIP VA CLINIC	CRANBERRY TOWNSHIP	PA	16066	0	21	NOT OFFERED
CUMBERLAND COUNTY VA CLINIC	MECHANICSBURG	PA	17055	0	62	0
DUBOIS VA CLINIC	DUBOIS	PA	15801	0	15	0
ERIE VAMC	ERIE	PA	16504	0	1	0
HUNTINGDON COUNTY VA CLINIC	MAPLETON DEPOT	PA	17052	0	35	NOT OFFERED
INDIANA COUNTY VA CLINIC	INDIANA	PA	15701	0	69	0
JAMES VAN ZANDT VAMC	ALTOONA	PA	16602	4	18	35
JOHNSTOWN VA CLINIC	JOHNSTOWN	PA	15904	0	33	0
LANCASTER COUNTY VA CLINIC	WILLOW STREET	PA	17584	0	17	NOT OFFERED
LEBANON VAMC	LEBANON	PA	17042	10	34	0
PITTSBURGH VAMC	PITTSBURGH	PA	15240	12	32	0
STATE COLLEGE VA CLINIC	STATE COLLEGE	PA	16801	0	29	NOT OFFERED
WILKES-BARRE VAMC	WILKES-BARRE	PA	18711	17	18	NOT OFFERED
YORK VA CLINIC	YORK	PA	17402	0	53	NOT OFFERED
EURIPIDES RUBIO VAMC	PONCE	PR		0	38	NOT OFFERED
MAYAGUEZ VA CLINIC	MAYAGUEZ	PR		72	49	NOT OFFERED
SAN JUAN VAMC	SAN JUAN	PR		70	37	31
PROVIDENCE VAMC	PROVIDENCE	RI	2908	0	24	0
GOOSE CREEK VAMC	GOOSE CREEK	SC	29445	0	53	NOT OFFERED
DANA CORNELL DARNELL VA CLINIC	GREENVILLE	SC	29605	16	26	NOT OFFERED
MYRTLE BEACH VA CLINIC	MYRTLE BEACH	SC	29577	10	9	0
RALPH JOHNSON VAMC	CHARLESTON	SC	29401	2	21	0
WILLIAM JENNINGS BRYAN DORN VAMC	COLUMBIA	SC	29209	11	16	17
FORT MEADE VAMC	FORT MEADE	SD	57741	24	17	41
HOT SPRINGS VAMC	HOT SPRINGS	SD	57747	0	23	NOT OFFERED
RAPID CITY VA CLINIC	RAPID CITY	SD	57701	0	45	8
ROYAL JOHNSON VA HOSPITAL	SIOUX FALLS	SD	57105	3	21	NOT OFFERED
ALVIN YORK VAMC	MURFREESBORO	TN	37129	15	14	NOT OFFERED
CAMPBELL COUNTY VA CLINIC	LAFOLLETTE	TN	37766	0	127	NOT OFFERED
CHATTANOOGA VA CLINIC	CHATTANOOGA	TN	37421	29	68	0
CLARKSVILLE VA CLINIC	CLARKSVILLE	TN	37043	16	15	NOT OFFERED
JAMES QUILLEN VAMC	MOUNTAIN HOME	TN	37684	6	14	0
LTC LUKE WEATHERS JR VAMC	MEMPHIS	TN	38104	5	19	26
MORRISTOWN EAST VA CLINIC	MORRISTOWN	TN	37813	0	22	NOT OFFERED
NASHVILLE VAMC	NASHVILLE	TN	37212	44	15	0
WILLIAM TALLENT VA OUTPATIENT CLINIC	KNOXVILLE	TN	37919	0	32	0
ABILENE VA CLINIC	ABILENE	TX	79606	0	12	NOT OFFERED
AUDIE MURPHY VAMC	SAN ANTONIO	TX	78229	13	28	NOT OFFERED
AUSTIN VA CLINIC	AUSTIN	TX	78744	24	32	0
BEAUMONT VA CLINIC	BEAUMONT	TX	77707	0	49	NOT OFFERED
DALLAS VAMC	DALLAS	TX	75216	3	26	0
DORIS MILLER VAMC	WACO	TX	76711	11	23	0
EL PASO SOUTH CENTRAL VA CLINIC	EL PASO	TX	79905	1	24	NOT OFFERED
GEORGE OBRIEN JR VAMC	BIG SPRING	TX	79720	35	8	NOT OFFERED
HARLINGEN VA CLINIC	HARLINGEN	TX	78550	26	58	0
KERRVILLE VAMC	KERRVILLE	TX	78028	0	23	0
LUBBOCK VA CLINIC	LUBBOCK	TX	79415	10	18	NOT OFFERED
MCALLEN VA CLINIC	MCALLEN	TX	78501	0	41	NOT OFFERED
MICHAEL DEBAKEY VAMC	HOUSTON	TX	77030	19	66	1

NORTH WEST SAN ANTONIO VA CLINIC	SAN ANTONIO	TX	78251	27	35	0
OLIN TEAGUE VETERANS CENTER	TEMPLE	TX	76504	24	22	18
THOMAS CREEK VAMC	AMARILLO	TX	79106	3	10	NOT OFFERED
TOMBALL VA CLINIC	TOMBALL	TX	77375	0	45	NOT OFFERED
WICHITA FALLS VA CLINIC	WICHITA FALLS	TX	76306	0	66	NOT OFFERED
WILSON AND YOUNG MEDAL OF HONOR CLINIC	ODESSA	TX	79765	0	0	NOT OFFERED
GEORGE WAHLEN VAMC	SALT LAKE CITY	UT	84148	30	26	NOT OFFERED
OGDEN VA CLINIC	SOUTH OGDEN	UT	84403	0	64	32
FREDERICKSBURG 2 VA CLINIC	FREDERICKSBURG	VA	22408	0	66	NOT OFFERED
HAMPTON VAMC	HAMPTON	VA	23667	26	20	20
HARRISONBURG VA CLINIC	HARRISONBURG	VA	22801	0	40	NOT OFFERED
MASSAPONAX VA CLINIC	FREDERICKSBURG	VA	22407	0	85	NOT OFFERED
NORTON VA CLINIC	NORTON	VA	24273	0	1	NO
RICHMOND VAMC	RICHMOND	VA	23249	41	48	26
SALEM VAMC	SALEM	VA	24153	0	41	76
BURLINGTON LAKESIDE VA CLINIC	BURLINGTON	VT	5401	0	1	NOT OFFERED
NEWPORT VA CLINIC	NEWPORT	VT	5855	20	0	NOT OFFERED
WHITE RIVER JUNCTION VAMC	WHITE RIVER JUNCTION	VT	5001	0	27	NOT OFFERED
AMERICAN LAKE VAMC	TACOMA	WA	98493	13	12	5
SEATTLE VAMC	SEATTLE	WA	98108	4	35	16
VANCOUVER VAMC	VANCOUVER	WA	98661	28	40	0
BARABOO VA CLINIC	BARABOO	WI	53913	0	0	NOT OFFERED
CLEMENT ZABLOCKI VAMC	MILWAUKEE	WI	53295	41	25	51
TOMAH VAMC	TOMAH	WI	54660	0	30	NOT OFFERED
WAUSAU VA CLINIC	ROTHSCHILD	WI	54474	0	9	NOT OFFERED
WILLIAM MIDDLETON VETERANS HOSPITAL	MADISON	WI	53705	8	23	0
BECKLEY VAMC	BECKLEY	WV	25801	0	45	0
HERSHEL WOODY WILLIAMS VAMC	HUNTINGTON	WV	25704	0	26	0
LOUIS JOHNSON VAMC	CLARKSBURG	WV	26301	0	27	0
MARTINSBURG VAMC	MARTINSBURG	WV	25405	0	40	0
PETERSBURG VA CLINIC	PETERSBURG	WV	26847	0	63	NOT OFFERED
CHEYENNE VAMC	CHEYENNE	WY	82001	0	80	0
SHERIDAN VAMC	SHERIDAN	WY	82801	0	28	0

Questions for the Record

Department of Veterans Affairs (VA) Questions for the Record
From a Hearing Titles
"Connections to Care: Improving Substance Use Disorder Care for Veterans
in Rural America and Beyond:
Committee on Veterans' Affairs
United States Senate

June 14, 2023

Questions for the Record from Senator Kyrsten Sinema

Question 1: 1 in 10 veterans in Arizona use substances to cope with trauma, depression, and anxiety. Staffing shortages have implications for the quality and timeliness of care we are able to provide. As staffing shortages, particularly in rural areas, continue, how is VA prioritizing timely care for mental health services in situations where staffing is slim?

VA Response: Of the more than 550,000 Veterans currently receiving substance use disorder (SUD) care from the Veterans Health Administration (VHA), VA treated a total of 124,275 rurally located Veterans with alcohol use disorder (AUD) and 66,439 rurally located Veterans with drug use disorders through the second quarter of fiscal year (FY) 2023. Historically, most SUD care was provided in person. Highly rural and rural patients adopted clinical video health for SUD treatment at higher rates pre-pandemic. In FY19, rates of clinical video telehealth visits for a SUD diagnosis ranged from 1-6% for urban, rural, and highly rural patients. The COVID-19 pandemic led to rapid and sustained increase in use of clinical video telehealth for SUD care in urban, rural and highly rural settings. In both FY21 and FY22, overall use of clinical video telehealth in visits for a SUD diagnosis was between 22-24% regardless of rurality. SUD funding is currently supporting telehealth-delivered SUD services in rural settings through attachment of SUD positions to several clinical resource hubs (CRH) and local VA medical center (VAMC) telehealth initiatives.

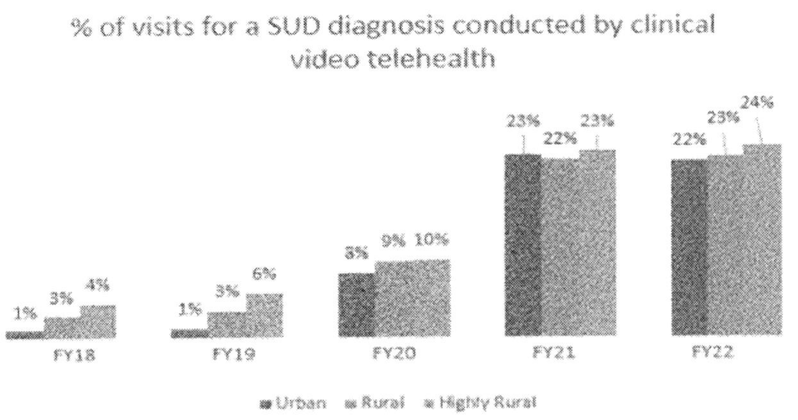

Regarding rural hiring efforts, VA relied on locally assessed need for clinicians across the enterprise. Hiring clinicians for telehealth positions (including at CRHs) helps ensure that care is available regardless of geography, either via video-telehealth or phone alone. Of the over 1,100 positions approved as part of SUD expansion, 149 are rural positions, of which 68 are onboard as of June 13, 2023. In addition, SUD funding supported 43 telehealth positions with a focus on serving Veterans who had challenges accessing face-to-face care (including rural populations). Of those 43 positions, 29 are onboard.

VA's Office of Rural Health (ORH) supports national SUD treatment initiatives. In FY 2023, ORH provided more than $5.3 million to support telehealth services for Veterans with SUDs. These telehealth services were provided through 48 VAMCs. ORH is providing more than $6.3 million to enhance access for Veterans experiencing SUD who live in rural areas with Clinical Pharmacist Practitioners (CPP). CPPs increase patient access, improve quality of care and decrease provider burden through the delivery and optimization of comprehensive medication management services for rural Veterans. This program connects Veterans to timely and appropriate care with 64 CPPs at 52 facilities hired to provide SUD care within the CPP Rural Veteran Access (CRVA) Project. VA has completed 129,078 SUD visits by CPPs in rural health projects.

The CRVA Mental Health Rural Expansion Access and Coordinated Health Efforts in SUD Project will extend on past efforts and integrate CPPs into Primary Care Mental Health Integration and Behavioral Health Interdisciplinary Program areas beginning in FY 2024. This project will seek to achieve the quintuple aim of access, quality, patient satisfaction, provider experience and health equity and is dedicated to expanding care to rural Veterans.

<u>Question 2</u>: While a long waitlist undoubtedly discourages veterans from seeking help in our VA facilities, there are many other social and institutional factors that may be preventing veterans from seeking the care they need. What can Congress and VA do to ensure veterans are made aware of the benefits available to them?

VA Response: VA has undertaken its largest outreach initiative in its history in support of the Sergeant First Class Heath Robinson Honoring our Promise to Address Comprehensive Toxics Act of 2022 (P.L. 117-168), which was enacted on August 10, 2022. This has included specific outreach to eligible—but not yet enrolled—Veterans through earned, owned and paid media efforts. Our messaging is focused on the expanded eligibility for health care and other benefits among new segments of the Veteran population. Each VAMC continues to stage multiple outreach events this year, including a special effort during July 2023 (more than 130 local events), to reach Veterans in specific zip codes where there is a high presence of these non-enrolled Veterans. VA's paid advertising campaign communicates to Veterans, their families and influencers broadly through TV, radio, social media, search and digital means, and includes special marketing toward Veterans of color, Tribal Veterans, women Veterans, homeless Veterans, LGBTQ+ and Veterans with other-than-honorable discharges. For example, there were events in Tucson and Page, Arizona where staff assisted Veterans applying for benefits, completing toxic exposure screenings and enrolling in VA health care. VA is also reaching out to eligible Veterans individually through a direct marketing campaign (email and mail) during June and July 2023.

To further ensure VA can reach every eligible Veteran, Congress could continue to fully support VA's appropriations request. VA is grateful for the support of Congress and appreciate Congressional staff's involvement with offsite events and the Committee's side-by-side relationship.

Question 3: We know that substance use and mental health disorders are often co-occurring. In situations where treatment may require shared decision-making, how is VA approaching holistic treatment that considers all medical and non-medical factors, and how can the VA improve this approach to minimize relapses?

VA Response: VHA Directive 1160.04, *VHA Programs For Veterans With Substance Use Disorders*, includes requirements pertaining to treating Veterans with co-occurring SUD and mental health disorders, as well as a shared decision-making approach to SUD care. Care is not time-limited, and treatment for co-occurring mental health, medical and psychosocial concerns is provided regardless of the current status of the Veteran's SUD diagnosis or current substance use.[1]

All specialty SUD programs and services are designed to meet the needs of Veterans with a SUD diagnosis, particularly those Veterans with new onset, unstable, severe or complex SUD conditions (e.g., co-occurring mental health and medical conditions). As such, specialized SUD programs must have the capacity to offer harm reduction services, identify co-occurring conditions, provide concurrent treatment and arrange appropriate follow-up care when indicated.

[1] https://www.va.gov/vhapublications/ViewPublication.asp?pub_ID=10070.

VHA Directive 1160.04 identifies shared decision-making (SDM) as a formal communication process for consensus building between a VA health care provider and patient when multiple evidence-based treatment alternatives exist to treat the patient's condition or problem. The provider and patient jointly participate in the process to arrive at a clinical decision or treatment plan. SDM requires the following three components: 1) clear, accurate and unbiased medical evidence about reasonable alternatives, including no intervention and the risk and benefits of each; 2) clinician expertise in communicating and tailoring the evidence for individual patients; and 3) patient values, goals, informed preferences and concerns, which may include treatment burden.

In addition, VHA is transforming from a traditional disease-based model to a system focused on empowering and equipping Veterans to take charge of their health and well-being and live their life to the fullest. The Whole Health model of care is a shift from episodic points of clinical care, primarily focused on disease management, to one that is based on a partnership with Veterans across time focused on whole health. This approach expands upon the traditional medical model to include a comprehensive continuum of care, suicide prevention services and other resources to empower and equip Veterans to take charge of their own health and wellbeing in support of their personal goals.

Department of Veterans Affairs
July 2023

Statements for the Record

FORGE VFR

Statement of Record

Forge VFR

Connections to Care: Improving Substance Use Disorder Care

For Veterans in Rural America and Beyond

It is clear that Substance Use Disorder (SUD) has a direct correlation with Veteran suicide. The 2022 National Veteran Suicide Prevention Annual Report, reporting numbers from 2020, shows that while between 2001 and 2020 the overall trend in Veteran suicide among individuals with a *known* SUD is down, we see the rate per 100,000 increased between 2019 and 2020[1]. This trend is alarming, as it is well understood by those who serve Veterans that the *known* SUD diagnosis is not an accurate representation of SUD among the Veteran population. Alcohol use in the military is engrained in our culture. We use alcohol to celebrate, to mourn, to commemorate and to reward. It would be naive to suggest that this alcohol use disorder doesn't lead to other substances, including cannabis, opioids and hallucinogens. Furthermore, we need to understand the separation from service for failing drug tests does not always result in a dishonorable discharge or legal involvement. There are Veterans who were separated from service for substance use who are eligible for VA health benefits, and there are separated service members who do not have VA benefits with a SUD. Those who suffer from a SUD continue to do so upon separation from service, even if undiagnosed prior to separation.

Substance Use Disorders among Veterans are often associated with other health conditions. Substance use can be used as a coping mechanism for those suffering from Post Traumatic Stress, those that suffered from Military Sexual Trauma, as well as those suffering from physical pain stemming from service-connected

[1] Office of Mental Health and Suicide Prevention, 2022 National Veteran Suicide Prevention Annual Report, pg 26 § (2022).

FORGE
VFR

injuries. Substance use diagnosis among "recent veteran users" rose from 27.9% in 2001 to 41.9% in 2020. [2] We know this, and even have a term for this, "self-medicating." The issue we face is how to alter this state of self-medication. And the answer to that must be access to care.

Under the MISSION ACT of 2018, current access standards for behavioral health care services, including substance use treatment, require the VA either provide an appointment within 20 days of request for care, and that this appointment be at a facility within 30 minutes of average drive time. Unfortunately, these standards are not equally met in all facilities, resulting in Veterans reporting wait times upwards of 30 days or more to begin needed treatment. Additionally, the MISSION ACT leaves room for Veterans to agree to waiting beyond these limits, without requiring the Veteran be made aware of their rights to care in the community.[3] When given no alternative offer, Veterans will often accept the appointment being offered beyond these standards under the impression that there is no alternative available. Finally, the Veteran has the right to request care in the community when it is agreed that it is in the best medical interest of the Veteran to receive community care, however the process for determining what is in the best medical interest of the Veteran is not specified, leading to different processes implemented in VAs around the country. We have all heard the saying "If you've seen one VA, you've seen one VA." While this colloquial saying helps diffuse contentious discussions, it does nothing to enforce uniformity in regulation among VA locations, leaving Veterans to have aggressively different experiences from VA to VA, and even from provider to provider within the same VA. Without frequent reporting on the usage of the Community Care Network (CCN), we are unable to determine trends in CCN referrals among facilities and the impact these referrals can have on wait times for Veterans, which was one of the primary intentions of the MISSION ACT.

---

[2] Office of Mental Health and Suicide Prevention, 2022 National Veteran Suicide Prevention Annual Report pg 27 § (2022).
[3] "VA Launches New Health Care Options Under Mission Act," VA News, June 6, 2019, https://news.va.gov/press-room/va-launches-new-health-care-options-under-mission-act/.

FORGE VFR

Veterans, as a population, are often resistant to reaching out for care, especially for behavioral health care. When Veterans do finally reach out, it is often at a time near crisis, or in crisis. While emergency care is available, and actions such as the COMPACT ACT work to increase access to emergency care, preventative care continues to be a difficult level of care to access. Getting a Veteran into an outpatient or intensive outpatient level of care is more cost effective for the VA and can prevent a SUD from becoming a crisis. The right care, at the right time, at the right place needs to be the standard practice implemented to prevent crisis from occurring. Emergency care is an important tool but should not be the primary focus.

Additionally, the MISSION ACT authorized the "Anywhere to Anywhere" telehealth approach for the VHA. This allows for the VA to utilize any and all internal providers for care via telehealth, regardless of location to the client. The same way that Veterans are a community within the community, regional differences can make care difficult at times. By choosing to utilize providers outside of the Veterans local community in lieu of utilizing the CCN, Veterans are forced into a telehealth treatment with an individual that may not understand their local culture. This ability to cross state lines for care is unique to the VA, and circumvents state laws that restrict the private sector, without the states having control.

Substance Use Disorder remains prevalent among active-duty service members and continues when service members separate. Access to care for behavioral health treatment can prevent an active SUD from becoming a crisis. This rings true in densely populated urban areas as well as rural and highly rural areas. The location in which a Veteran life should not impact the quality of care they have access too. Getting access to culturally competent, local care in a timely manner can prevent Veteran suicide. Ensuring this standard is equally implemented throughout the VHA system needs to remain of the utmost importance.

FORGE VFR

Eric Golnick
CEO- Forge VFR

Dalton McLaughlin
Government Relations Manager

Casey Lancaster
Policy Analyst

June 12, 2023

Members of the Senate Veterans Affairs Committee,

Thank you for taking the time to read this personal statement in relation to the hearing discussing substance use disorders in military veterans and at the request of the HunterSeven Foundation. I cannot speak on behalf of the entire veteran community, but I can share my personal, painful, experiences. I wrote this in my "sobriety journal," which is hundreds of pages of moral injury, stories of overdosing in bathrooms, attempts at suicide, and the painful reality we face daily. Written in 2018, I was 32 years old.

I am a Special Missions Unit veteran,
I am a wounded, combat veteran,
I am a father, I am a son,
I am an **addict**.

The first time someone tried to kill me, I felt many emotions. I felt fear. I felt anger. I was worried about my teammates. Then there was confusion. I was not expecting to be *confused*. My confusion was surrounded by motivated hate. The longer you spent downrange, the more determined you became to get home. **Amidst all the confusion and fear, I also felt alive.**

I felt wired because every moment you are being shot at, you are harmoniously, breathtakingly alive in the most barbarically instinctual way imaginable. You are introduced to a high you will **forever** chase. It is your first love; it's also your first **addiction**. Every single day something is blowing up. Every day your brain rips apart a little more. Gunshots tear up your memory, and IED blasts ruin your functioning. They chew holes into spots that used to be filled. That's where your identity used to be. You lose grip on your past, have trouble functioning in the present, and cannot fathom planning a future. Writing a sentence takes twice as long as I struggle to place this pen on the paper. Phone conversations send shards of metal piercing into my eardrum and deep into my brain.

I always thought I was crazy, but I have a ***broken brain***. I died at war. The old me left everything I knew to go to war. I never came home.

The son my parents knew, the brother my siblings knew, and the caring, passionate man my girlfriend knew... he never came home. Since I didn't die, what else would you call it? I liked the old me, but the old me died, covered in the blood of others. He died from the blasts, died staring down the barrel of my gun. The new me is crazy and anxious and can't remember. The new me lost all love; the new me runs, and the new me avoids. The new me remembers enough about the old me to miss him and resent the monster I've become. Those who miss the old me stand before the new me and feel my loss even though I am standing there. Everyone who knew the old me wants him back; they don't like who I've become, and no one wants to be around the new me... especially me.

Every day, I live with that. Over and over, the same smell, the same heat, the language, the women yelling in the streets, there is nothing sweet about it; it's all spoiled misery, and I was their unwelcomed company. For the most part, I was okay with it...

The static covers my brain. All I see is white... where am I? What is happening?

I am in the lead vehicle, dismounting to open the door to a skeleton. Or what is left of him. There are pieces of his skull, his torso fused to his plating; you can't hear anything besides the air zipping by your head, and you cannot see anything else but the misplaced chunks of hair and flesh tossed on the truck interior. You turn back to see the flames and flashes and hope that one accurately placed round will end your misery. Through the flashbacks, binge drinking, drug overdoses, addiction, and contemplating suicide attempts. WHAT IS GOING ON WITH MY BRAIN? Last night, I sat in my cot, and across the room, sitting in the chair, was a young girl covered in blood. Why is that farmer from the Hajj mart dead in my shower? Their eyes stay with me. They are all black. Their monstrous eyes pierce through my soul. No colors. Just black. I loved owning the night, but with the night came the darkness.

Like most, I felt most comfortable and in control in combat. You wake up and expect to die; you ***commit to death***, and punch your ticket before stepping off the objective for another mission. You ran the scenarios in your head, and once the rush was gone, you became a drunken, drug-abusing, narcissistic human being who could barely make it through the day. I didn't have much of anything going on, on the inside. So, I had to make up for it on the outside. I went from being a top performer on the team, and a respected professional, to becoming a nuisance and a burden who created more work and problems for everyone around me. It is a difficult concept for me to understand.

Simply, I exist from second to second. As I said earlier, there is no meaning to my past, my present is intolerable, and honestly, I don't expect my future to exist. When the sadness and brutal depravity of this world are laid at your feet and you find yourself sinking knee-deep, embedded within it rather than above, what hope do you really have?

All my shattered, spent, halfhearted actions have produced nothing but sadness, disappointment, and misery to those who I love. Do we endure? Do I endure? Do I tolerate this life I am plummeting into? Do we... do I let go of all things? I should remove my attachments. My Resentments. My Possessions. Even my loved ones. Should they do that so I can be free of pain and suffering? But what if I am already completely and utterly emotionally ***detached from this world***, I've invested in nothing. I am not even investing in myself. I should be steps away from freedom, right?

The old me is gone, and she hates the new me... *"Pull the damn trigger, end my life, end my misery... clean the goddamn walls and get on with your life."*

Deep down, I knew a part of her wanted to end it all, her stress, the drug abuse, end the nightmares. But no, I'm on my own. In the darkness, I own the night. I am **high up again**, much to her dismay. I am walking down into the basement. It's cold, damp, and dark but quiet—bone-chilling silence.

When it's dark, the darkness brings them back, I see them, I see their dark, black beady eyes. I hear their voices, their screams. I feel their blood. I sat there facing the wall, staring at the hole in the concrete. In an instant, I am back on the streets of Baghdad, the same hole from the blast that killed my brain. The darkness, the shadows, the numbing sound of silence, everything is quiet... except their voices. I don't know where I am. I can't tell if the smell is from freshly spilled blood in the heat of the night or leaking rusted pipes. I am holding the shotgun under my chin, the cold sensation of steel sending chills down my spine, familiar chills, chills from death, chills that know when death is near. Safety off, finger on the trigger. This is where I'll die, not in a firefight like Rabbit, not in an ambush like Top, not in the war, but in a dark, cold basement... buttstock on the ground, resting my head on the muzzle, hand gripping the barrel, thumb on the trigger.

...but I didn't pull the trigger.

And then I found myself here. Writing this to you. Writing about my pain. About my... addiction.

The darkness. The dark companion you'll always have, either assimilate or go absolutely bloody insane. I found love for Benzos in the teams; it took the edge off the steroids. Now a sudden, civilian navigating the system, I find myself in front of a VA doc who made it seem as if I was wasting his time. Rushing through a medication list he prints me off: *"In the morning: Adderall, Xanax, Gabapentin, Ropinirole, Pantoprazole, Tramadol for hypersensitivity, anxiety, nerve pain, restless leg, and acid reflux"*, with a blank stare, he continues on, *"in the afternoon, Xanax, Gabapentin, Ropinirole and Soma... you know what they are for,"* and then he finishes with, *"before bed take Trazodone to help you get to sleep, Xanax, Gabapentin and Ropinirole again, Zoloft and Prazosin for your nightmares..."* If I weren't going to kill myself, surely this chemical cocktail would kill me.

In 2018, that is where I was, full-speed, suicidal. Coming home to an empty house, everyone in my life had left, and only at the expense of myself, only I was to blame. I lost the brightness in my life, and I only had the darkness and the chemical cocktail to thank. I was angry and upset at those strangers around me for being disconnected from human life. They reminded me of preschoolers, kicking and screaming, running around with no purpose or motive while assuming they are the most important know-it-alls. Our American way of life is so disconnected that it is tough for me to find where I can connect into it all. We are a severely detached and divided nation, and for once, I actually missed Afghanistan. I missed the tribal feeling, the one-mission, one-goal those men and those women had. Their connections with one another are truly admirable. It sucks knowing you will never meet the caliber of men you met at war. **Never**.

But I was "home", and my "welcoming" came with a brutal hit to rock bottom. You'll either learn to cope, or you'll kill yourself. So, I decided to immediately cease the V.A. prescribed cocktail all at once. For I knew, the next bottom that I would hit would certainly be death.

This rock bottom came hard and fast, and I was alone. Quitting everything at once is something I'd never recommend to anyone. I laid in pain. Tossing and turning. Crying on the cold floor of an empty apartment. Changing my sweat-soaked clothes and shivering, vomiting, and keeping my Glock 19 nearby.

I don't know what physically pained me most, detoxing or the ***darkness***.

I suffered in pain for fourteen days. I cried for hours, over the guilt and the urge to escape came over me.

On the fifteenth day, I drove from New York to Jacksonville, Florida, to enter a private, inpatient rehabilitation facility for 30 days. If I didn't do this, I was going to die.

I moved to the oceanfront city to find "myself" again, to try and fix my broken brain. This time I wasn't alone. From meetings to working out, running the beach every morning, and learning new skills. I kept busy, but a purposeful busy.

Two years later, and I still hold to that. I am purposefully busy. I live by the values that encompass a stoic, virtuous man. I show up every day. I value myself. I have a renewed sense of purpose. Am I perfect? Hell no. But I continue to invest in myself. I set short-term goals and conquer them; for the first time in a long time, I have ambitions for the future. I own my time. I know that time is precious and limited.

I am sober.

I've found that when you love your flaws and imperfections, are entirely self-reliant, and depend on no one and especially no substance; you will create your own *'brightness.'* If anything I've written connects with you, I challenge you to follow that path. Just fight the urge to do it alone, and don't go cold turkey, but get sober. Find a therapist and a care team that will take you seriously, especially those actively finding ways to heal our TBIs, mental health concerns, and addiction. Exercise, do yoga to help with the pain, meditate, and find others who understand. Reach out to those that have already started that mission. You must be on a mission to heal yourself, your brain, and your soul, all together, holistically. I challenge you to find ways to build a new tribe, have fun, take action, create change, and always move to become a better version of yourself actively. We are leaders. Be heard when you aren't speaking. Be present when you aren't there.

In closing, I ask you to consider opening availability to my brothers and sisters in arms to seek substance use care and treatment where they are and when needed so they do not drive 15 hours to receive a holistic, whole-body approach to care.

In gratitude,

T. Paul Provenzano

Chapter 3

Invisible Wounds of War: Improving Mental Health and Suicide Prevention Measures for Our Nation's Veterans*

Committee on Veterans' Affairs

Wednesday, September 20, 2023
U.S. Senate, Committee on Veterans' Affairs,
Washington, DC.

The Committee met, pursuant to notice, at 3:41 p.m., in Room SR–418, Russell Senate Office Building, Hon. Jon Tester, Chairman of the Committee, presiding.

Present: Senators Tester, Murray, Brown, Blumenthal, Hirono, Sinema, Hassan, King, Moran, Boozman, Cassidy, Tillis, Sullivan, and Blackburn.

Opening Statement of Chairman Jon Tester

Chairman TESTER. We call this hearing to order.

September is Suicide Prevention Month. While we are all focusing on this topic today, it must be at the forefront of everything of what we do every day. Mental health is one of the biggest issues facing our country. It is certainly a big issue in my home State of Montana. It is certainly a big issue for our veterans.

That is why it is critically important VA does absolutely everything possible to connect more veterans with the mental health care and the suicide prevention that they need, regardless of where they live.

The latest data shows that 2020 had the lowest number of veteran suicides since 2006. That trend needs to continue. The data shows that more than 60 percent of the veterans who died by suicide in 2020 had no recent engagement with the Veterans Health Administration. That means the VA must work harder to get our veterans into the system.

---

* This is an edited, reformatted and augmented version of Hearing Before the Committee On Veterans' Affairs, United States Senate, Publication No. S. HRG. 118–227, dated September 20, 2023.

In: Supporting Our Veterans
Editor: Gina P. Sharpe
ISBN: 979-8-89530-504-1

In recent years, Congress has advanced critical legislation. I was proud to champion many of them, including the John Scott Hannon Veterans Mental Health Care Bill, Veterans Health Healthcare Improvement Act that I did with Senator Moran, and the STRONG Veterans Act of 2022.

These laws have helped the VA's mental health workforce and programs, including through alternative and local treatment options, but the fact is we have much more to do. That is why I recently introduced the Not Just a Number Act to require the Department to provide a more fully picture of the factors contributing to veterans suicide.

By making the Community Care for Veterans Act, would also strengthen veterans' access to life-saving residential treatment programs for mental health and substance abuse disorder.

Congress continues to do its part by giving VA the proper funding for mental health, and suicide prevention programs, and ensuring it has the tools to meet the veterans' needs. And while the VA has made progress, we still have work to do. The VA has been too slow in implementing the Hannon Act Telehealth Grants that would improve rural veterans' access to mental health care by increasing the number of locations that can provide VA Telehealth Services.

That is a particular concern of mine, given Montana has one of the highest rates of suicide in the Nation. A nearly 5-year implementation timeline is far too long. And I will expect an update on that initiative today.

I am also looking for an update on the Veterans Crisis Line. The STRONG Act included my reach for the Veterans Act to improve the Veterans Crisis Line oversight.

Last week, a new IG Report was released, raising more concerns about the Veterans Crisis Line. The Veterans Crisis Line is a life-saving resource for veterans, and it must be a top-performing entity within the VA. But as made clear by recent IG reports, it simply is not. I expect an update from the VA on how it is implementing the provisions from the STRONG Act, and how it is executing the IG's latest recommendations.

Finally, I was recently informed of the death, by suicide, of a longtime VA employee in Montana. That employee, like so many at the VA, was a veteran. VA employees deal with stressful topics and events each and every day, and they face a lot of the same challenges as the veterans they serve.

As the Department continues to improve its Mental Health Service for our veterans, I call on you to redouble efforts to care for its workforce across the enterprise. A workforce that feels understood and supported will be far better positioned to accomplish the mission of delivering vets the care and the benefits they have earned. Senator Moran is not quite here yet, so we will start with the first panel. And then I will yield to him when he gets here for his statement, if he so chooses to make it.

The first panel is: I would like to welcome VA's lead witness, Dr. Matthew Miller, the Executive Director of the Suicide Prevention at the Veterans Health Administration. He is accompanied by Susan Black, a Suicide Prevention Officer at the Outreach, Transition, and Economic Development Service of the Veterans Benefits Administration.

So we will start with you, Dr. Miller. You may proceed. You have got 5 minutes. Know that your entire written statement will be a part of the record.

Panel I: Statement of Matthew Miller

Dr. MILLER. Thank you, sir.

Good afternoon, Chairman Tester, Ranking Member Moran, and distinguished Members of the Committee. Thank you for the opportunity to discuss the Department's efforts to implement legislation related to veterans' mental health care, and suicide prevention.

I want to thank this Committee for its support and continued collaboration on reducing veteran suicide. This critical relationship is reflected in the resources that the Congress has repeatedly secured for VA.

In 2020, 44,298 adult Americans died by suicide, of those, 6,146 were veterans. These numbers are more than statistics; they reflect veterans' lives prematurely ended, which continue to be grieved by family members, loved ones, and the Nation.

Suicide is a complex problem with multifaceted and interweaving contributing factors. Suicide is not just a mental health issue, with no single cause; there is no single solution to suicide for veterans. Yet, one veteran suicide is one too many. VA cannot do this work alone. In order to address individual, relational, community, and societal risks, and protective factors, VA is collaborating with other Federal agencies, public and private partnerships, government at local, State, and national levels, veterans service organizations, and local communities.

Together, we are implementing a full-public-health approach as outlined in the White House Strategy, and VA's 10-year National Strategy for Preventing Veteran Suicide.

These guiding documents are operationalized through VA Suicide Prevention 2.0 Initiative, Suicide Prevention NOW, and emerging innovations combined with research and program evaluation.

Further implementation of new laws, including the STRONG Act, Hannon Act, COMPACT Act, and the National Suicide Hotline Designation Act, are all critical part of these efforts, as mentioned by you, sir, at the outset.

For example, Hannon Act Section 201 established the Staff Sergeant Parker Gordon Fox Suicide Prevention Grant Program, allowing the VA to provide grants to expand Suicide Prevention Services to veterans and their families, to reduce the risk of suicide.

In September 2022, VA awarded $52.5 million to 80 community-based organizations across 43 States, DC, and American Samoa. A second round of grant awards was announced today, ensuring reach to veterans across the Nation, not just those engaged in VA care or benefits.

Additionally, the STRONG Act contains more than two dozen sections that further support veterans' mental health care and suicide prevention, including further strengthening of the Veterans Crisis Line.

In July of 2022, the Veterans Crisis Line rolled out 988–PRESS–1. VCL prepared for the implementation of 988–PRESS–1, by hiring over 900 individuals, responders, to address increased demand, and to increase quality assurance, and program evaluation efforts. Since that launch, VCL has fielded over one million calls, texts, and chat messages.

On that note, and before I close, I want to acknowledge the recent OIG Report of a veteran's death by suicide following and in the context of a contact with the Veterans Crisis Line.

We, I, as a veteran, grieve the loss of this veteran. From the painful lenses of retrospective review we wish we could have done some things differently. It is our earnest desire and pledge to apply the wisdom gained through this review to strengthen processes as we continue to serve veterans who are at the center of all we do, even at this very minute as we answer calls.

Mr. Chairman, this concludes my remarks. My colleague, Dr. Black, and I are prepared to address any questions that you may have.

[The prepared statement of Dr. Miller appears on page 45 of the Appendix.]

Chairman TESTER. Dr. Miller, thank you for your testimony, and thank you for being here.

I will yield my time to the wily young veteran, former Chairman of this Committee, Senator Murray.

Senator Patty Murray

Senator MURRAY. Thank you very much, Mr. Chairman.

Let me just, first of all, thank you both for being here. But the fact that nearly a third of women veterans experience sexual assault or harassment while serving our country in uniform is really staggering. And unsurprisingly, we know that military sexual trauma is a significant cause of mental health issues for these women. In fact, women who are survivors of military sexual trauma are nine times more likely to develop PTSD than other women veterans. There was a 2018 VHA directive that requires all VA facilities to have a designated coordinator to help veteran survivors of military sexual trauma access mental health care and other resources.

But in my home State of Washington, the Puget Sound VA, which treats, by the way, more than 65,000 veterans, doesn't, does not have a full-time person in this position, which seems notable for a facility of that size, and a position that is so important.

So Dr. Miller, I want to ask you, what steps is VA doing and taking to make sure that all VA facilities, including Puget Sound VA, have enough resources to assist and reach out to survivors of military sexual trauma?

Dr. MILLER. Thank you for the question, Senator. I agree with you 100 percent, as does the VA and Suicide Prevention, that addressing military sexual trauma is critically important and a key component of suicide prevention. Exactly what you have said, there is increased risk with regard to suicide in this area.

We, at the national level, have a policy in place, requirements at the local level regarding the very points of contact that you mentioned. We receive regular reports on a quarterly basis regarding staffing, and then we work with local facilities through the VISN with regard to gaps or according——

Senator MURRAY. So is my VA facility going to get a coordinator or not?

Dr. MILLER. Your VA facility should be receiving a message stating, "Tell us what the plan is to fulfill this FTE 1.0."

Senator MURRAY. When will that occur?

Dr. MILLER. I don't know the exact timing of that vis-a`-vis the current date. I would imagine by the end of the quarter. or the start of the quarter, but I would be happy to check on this and then send this——

Senator MURRAY. If you can get back to me and tell me specifically when that is going to happen, I would appreciate it.

Dr. MILLER. Yes, ma'am.

VA Response: Per VHA Directive 1115 Military Sexual Trauma (MST) Program, each facility must have a designated MST Coordinator who is typically given at least 0.2 FTE of time specifically dedicated to the administrative responsibilities of the role. VA Puget Sound Health Care System has 2 MST Coordinators labor mapped 0.3 and 0.2 FTE; the current MST Coordinators' start dates were March 20, 2020 and July 19, 2021.

Senator MURRAY. Thank you. Let me ask about homelessness. There are 33,000 veterans experiencing homelessness in the U.S., 1,500 of them in my State, veterans who have experienced homelessness are four times more likely than other veterans to attempt suicide. And I know the VA has made progress in reducing the number of veterans who lack housing, but we also need to make sure that we are utilizing our knowledge of risk factors and engaging with these veterans to help prevent them from experiencing homelessness in the first place.

So Dr. Miller, what is the VA doing right now to reach out to veterans who are experiencing homelessness, and provide them with the mental health services that they need?

Dr. MILLER. I think that the answer to that question, ma'am, starts with identifying where are veterans at the highest risk for suicide within that particular situation. And what we have learned is that veterans are at the highest risk for suicide 30 to 60 days prior to homelessness status or losing their home. So a big part of the issue for us is identifying veterans who are at high risk.

Senator MURRAY. How do you do that?

Dr. MILLER. I think that it is an issue of measuring and monitoring through the Homeless Program Office at the local level, up to the national level.

Senator MURRAY. Is that happening?

Dr. MILLER. It is happening. I don't think that it is perfect, because it is very difficult to identify, 100 percent, who is at risk within 30 to 60 days. We had a situation that we faced this week where I assisted, along with some other colleagues, a veteran and his spouse who found out within 5 days that they were losing their home. We put them in direct contact with resources and assistance, but the timing can be very short. There are areas for improvement there, and we are committed to working on them.

Senator MURRAY. Okay. Well, Congress and the VA have been putting a lot of effort into reaching out to veterans with the message that it is okay for them to ask for help.

Dr. MILLER. Mm-hmm.

Senator MURRAY. That when they are feeling alone, when they are feeling depressed, there is people and resources available for them. So it is really concerning to see on the VA's website that the wait time for a mental health appointment at the Puget Sound VA Medical Center is over a month long. I have personally had veterans tell me that they have had to wait as long as 3 months just to get an appointment.

I know it is challenging. I know it is complicated. But what is the VA doing to make sure that veterans who are experiencing a mental health crisis access the care they need when they need it? Dr. MILLER. Same-day access is the first step that should be in place at every local facility regarding this, following same-day access, attending to staffing, and ensuring that staff can accommodate the demand.

Senator MURRAY. Okay, but it is not happening. So what do we do?

Dr. MILLER. Then we, from a national level, we consult, we offer consultation to the local level regarding where they are seeing barriers, where they are seeing impediments to access, and assisting them with constructing a plan, an action plan for following through and making improvements.

Senator MURRAY. Okay, can I get you to get in touch with the Puget Sound VA Medical Center and find out why these wait times are so long, and follow up on what we are going to do to fix it?

Dr. MILLER. Absolutely.

Senator MURRAY. Thank you.

VA Response

Current Average Wait Times for a New Mental Health Individual Appointment

- Includes appointments scheduled in advance over the past 30 days, including telephone appointments; however, does not include appointments made the same day
  - Seattle VA Medical Center–37 days
  - American Lake campus–11 days
- Includes all scheduled appointments, including those scheduled the same day, over the past 6 months; however, does not include telephone appointments
  - Seattle VA Medical Center–20.2 days
  - American Lake campus–22.5 days

Note: All eligible Veterans have same-day mental-health access at the American Lake and Seattle clinics with no pre-scheduled appointment necessary.

Chairman TESTER. Senator Moran.

Senator Jerry Moran

Senator MORAN. Chairman, thank you. I will forego my opening statement and maybe make a few comments at the end. But let me ask questions of Dr. Miller.

Dr. Miller, the Office Inspector General published a report last Thursday, September 14th, detailing deficiencies at the Veterans Crisis Line and how the Crisis Line staff failed to take appropriate action with the veteran who died by suicide that same night, the night that he contacted the crisis line. The report also details significant issues with the Veteran Crisis Line leadership and some staff. What are you doing, personally, to make certain that the deficiencies detailed in the Inspector General's Report are fixed quickly?

Dr. MILLER. Thank you for the question, Senator. We are better than what was depicted in that report. And we have to do better than what was depicted in that report. Personally, since you asked for that particular perspective, when I was first presented with the situation, with a call from OIG, directly, telling me about their concerns, I enacted pulling the responder from responder duties and initiating a full review of the work.

That became what you see with Responder 2 and 3 in the review and the report. From that time, we have been working very aggressively to make changes. Such that, to the point right now, there is 11 recommendations specific to the Veterans Crisis Line in this report. We have made significant progress on eight of the eleven. There are two that involve close collaboration with the Office of Information and Technology. There is one that involves new information from a personnel perspective that we are pursuing.

Senator MORAN. Dr. Miller, what would be your—why does it take an Inspector General Report for this to be addressed? What is not taking place at the VA to get this solved before this particular veteran committed suicide?

Dr. MILLER. There are aspects of this situation that involve standards and expectations that are new to the field of crisis call; for example, text retention. Text retention is not a standard for the National Suicide Prevention Lifeline, nor is it known how many even in the Lifeline engage in text retention. It also has significant challenges, from an OIT perspective, balancing privacy, security with retention.

We have been engaging for the last 2 years, even prior, to this particular situation, in what we would need to do to change our text platform to allow us retention. This report is not the first time we have thought about this and tried to move to this. The issue is finding a platform that OIT approves of that does not jeopardize veteran safety.

Senator MORAN. As you might expect, I think my staff and I will have additional questions, perhaps in writing, and maybe in a conversation.

Dr. Miller, let me follow on a different topic, within the John Hannon Act, there is the Staff Sergeant Fox program, it seems to be overly administratively burdensome and has significant, what I would call, excessive restrictions on the use of funding. Do you disagree with those broad conclusions? And what changes would you expect to alleviate—make to alleviate the concerns that I am raising, or the concerns that have been raised to me?

Dr. MILLER. Yes. Thank you, Senator. I appreciate that. We, as you are, are proud of the Fox Grant Program. I do not disagree, however, with your statement. I think that this is a developmental process. This is the first time that we have engaged in grants, and we are learning to walk that fine line between too much and too little, in terms of requirements and measurements.

I think that there is at least three things that I would be happy to talk with you at greater depth, that we are learning along the way about walking that proverbial fine line. But we are committed to learning, growing, adapting as we move forward.

Senator MORAN. There is a lot of things that are really pleasing to me in this legislation, and this grant program is one of them that I think gives an opportunity for community and personal engagement in veterans' lives.

Dr. MILLER. Yes.

Senator MORAN. That I think is really, really important, and I want to see it succeed. And if there is something, I would like to have the conversation, but also if there is something that is missing legislatively, congressionally, please make sure that I know that.

Dr. MILLER. I appreciate that. We will do so, sir.

Senator MORAN. Thank you.

Chairman TESTER. Senator Hassan.

Senator Margaret Wood Hassan

Senator HASSAN. Thank you, Mr. Chair, and Ranking Member Moran for the hearing. And Dr. Miller and Ms. Black, thank you as well for being here.

I was really glad to see that the VA has chosen a week next month, October 16th to 20th, to designate as the first official Buddy Check Week in which veterans conduct peer-to-peer wellness checks. As you know, Senator Ernst and I introduced and passed into law the bill to make this happen, our bipartisan legislation required the VA to build on what the American Legion had already started with the Buddy Check Week, by making it a nationwide VA initiative.

Can you talk about how the VA plans on conducting outreach to maximize the impact of the first nationwide VA Buddy Check Week?

Dr. MILLER. Yes, thank you for the question. We are really looking forward to the first Buddy Check Week; that is scheduled for October 16th to initiate. We are also hoping to, and targeting, pairing the release of our annual report with the initiation of Buddy Check Week as a call to action. We are currently engaged in the process of talking with our close partners, the VSOs, regarding Buddy Check Week and implementation.

One of the biggest concerns that we have with implementation is, making sure veterans feel equipped to engage in it constructively and helpfully. We have completed training, therefore, for Buddy Check Week, and we will be rolling that out within the next week.

Senator HASSAN. Great, thank you for that. I wanted to follow on Senator Murray's lead to talk a little bit about women veterans right now. Women veterans face unique hurdles to accessing VA health care and benefits, even though more than 30 percent of new VA health care users are women, and there have been—there has been a threefold increase in the number of women veterans accessing VA mental health services since 2005.

So I want to help raise awareness among women veterans about the Women Veterans Network, or WoVeN Program, which aims to develop peer support networks that are specific to the unique needs of this growing population of women veterans. What steps has the VA taken to address the unique mental health challenges that women veterans face? And how has the WoVeN Program been developed to help improve outcomes for the women who participate in it?

Dr. MILLER. Yes. Thanks for that question. And thanks for highlighting this as an example of an important program for women veterans. I agree with you. It absolutely is. What we are doing at the outset, in terms of broad messaging, is talking about the point that you made: that women veterans have unique risk factors, they have unique protective factors, and we need to be able to address those in a tailored way.

In terms of WoVeN—pardon me—in terms of WoVeN, we have made some significant, I think, program evaluation observations and adjustments after the initial implementation. I think two examples serve as important to know for that. Number one, we have developed a Train the Trainer Program. Number two, we have learned that we can go from a co-lead paradigm to a single individual leading. These two lessons learned and the implementation plan will, exponentially, increase in the next year our ability to implement more of these groups and opportunities.

Senator HASSAN. Okay. That would be really excellent. One of the things I continue to hear, especially in rural areas in New Hampshire, from women veterans, is how hard it is for them to know where the other women veterans are and to provide the kind of peer-to-peer support that is so important. So I would look forward to continuing to work with you on that.

A last question is about something I worked with Senator Cramer on: The bipartisan and bicameral push to enact the Solid Start Program. That directs the VA, as you know, to contact every veteran at least three times by phone in the first year after they leave active duty service, to check in and help connect them to the VA programs and benefits that they have earned and deserve. Last month alone, the VA contacted 23,479 veterans through the Solid Start Program. How does the VA tailor outreach through the Solid Start Program to veterans with mental health care concerns, and what have you done to ensure that those mental health concerns are being addressed as quickly and effectively as possible?

Dr. MILLER. Great question, not to be punny, but VBA is taking the lead on doing solid work in this. I defer to Dr. Black.

Dr. BLACK. Yes. And thank you for that question. So when you look at the Solid Start Program, that is one of the primary focuses, is ensuring that when we are making those contact with the veteran, that we are asking those questions. So all of our Solid Start representatives, they are trained in suicide prevention awareness; so when they are on those calls that is one of the topics that is discussed, that is a topic that is discussed.

And not only that, our Solid Start makes a priority for any veteran who was seen in mental health the year prior to separating from the service. We make that a priority, and we engage those individuals as far as suicide prevention and mental health topics. About 80 percent of those priority veterans, we have made those successful connections with, so that is definitely a priority.

Senator HASSAN. Okay, that is really, really helpful because obviously if they had had a mental health consult or issue during service, the confusion or unease during transition, which is just, from what veterans tell me, it can be a pretty confusing time, makes them even that much more vulnerable, right?

Dr. BLACK. Yes, and ensuring that we have—make that warm handoff from care to care is vital.

Senator HASSAN. Excellent. Well, thank you, Dr. Black and Dr. Miller.

Chairman TESTER. Dr. Cassidy.

Senator Bill Cassidy

Senator CASSIDY. Hello. This is an incredibly damning OIG Report, incredibly damning. And I am struck that the executive director, who apparently interfered with the OIG Report, was not fired. She is reassigned, I presume still getting a paycheck; I assume she is still building a pension, having demonstrated her lack of truthfulness in conversation with the OIG.

I am told that the Director of Quality and Training, or Training and Quality, is in the same position as this person was before. Now, we have passed accountability measures for people who don't do their job, and it sounds like interfering with an investigation of a suicide, which may have been inappropriately handled on a Veterans Crisis Line, is incompetence.

So it may be a decision above your pay grade, but can you tell us why the only accountability that has been had so far is that somebody moved over to the Secretary's Office?

Dr. MILLER. Dr. Cassidy, we agree 100 percent with the necessity of accountability and holding our staff and team members to the highest level of standards when it comes to serving our veterans. The Executive Director that you mentioned is not named in "interference", to use the term that you used; the individual who was listed as Director of Quality is discussed in that, the information that we had to that effect is new from the OIG evaluation in their review. It is not uncommon to receive new information——

Senator CASSIDY. Well, then maybe, "The Executive Director," I am quoting, "Reported that after completion of a quality assurance review, it was decided there is," quote, "Insufficient information for us to really move forward on a root cause analysis; however, leaders initiated the root cause analysis after the OIG notification of the inspection, although the text conversation had not been obtained."

Now, it sounds like somebody is asleep at the wheel, and the question is, was it just incompetence, or was it just a cover up? So is anything being done about it? What is this person earning? Are they earning less than they were before?

Dr. MILLER. No, sir. What you are referring to is an RCA in the context of reviewing the text exchange; this gets to the text retention issue.

Senator CASSIDY. Stop. I am not asking text retention. I am asking, were the people responsible for the failure of this system, and who did not initiate the appropriate follow-up, and/or apparently tampered with people, responder number one, have said things which may have influenced the way they responded to the OIG; how are they being held accountable?

Dr. MILLER. They are under review using an appropriate personnel, guidance policy, and subject matter experts.

Senator CASSIDY. And the person who was transferred, did they get a cut in pay? Are they making the same money; or are they making more?

Dr. MILLER. I am not aware of a person transferred, sir.

Senator CASSIDY. I thought somebody was transferred to the Secretary's Office out of the position they had. Am I right on that? That is correct. I am told that is correct.

Dr. MILLER. There is an individual who took a different job; there was not an individual that was transferred.

Senator CASSIDY. Okay, took a different job. Just voluntarily took it and everybody said, incredibly well qualified, and no stains upon the record?

Dr. MILLER. I can't speak to the hiring process that was engaged, sir.

Senator CASSIDY. And when did the process of review begin for each of these two individuals?

Dr. MILLER. The process of review began for the first situation with responder one, that is mentioned in the report, immediately. The process of review——

Senator CASSIDY. I am sorry. What is the date on that?

Dr. MILLER. The date would be November——

Senator CASSIDY. And I am sorry. And I don't mean of the root cause analysis.

Dr. MILLER. Oh.

Senator CASSIDY. I mean of the apparent attempt to influence how the OIG was spoken with.

Dr. MILLER. Right. We did not—we did not become aware of that till OIG gave us feedback to that effect, which was about a year after the answer——

Senator CASSIDY. And how long ago was that?

Dr. MILLER. That would have been in the spring of 2021—I am sorry, '22.

Senator CASSIDY. And so the spring of 2021, and so a person has been—'22, has been under review since then; has anything resulted from that review?

Dr. MILLER. That is different, sir. You are talking about the review with regard to responder one.

Senator CASSIDY. Mr. Miller, I feel like you know what I am asking, but you are deliberately dodging the question. I want to know when did the review begin, of the two people whom this report alleges interfered with the investigation and/or told folks how to respond differently than what apparently was the truth?

Dr. MILLER. The answers to your question, sir, require technical responses——

Senator CASSIDY. Okay. But tell me what day—what month did those investigations, of those two people began, by the VA?

Dr. MILLER. The investigation with responder one initiated——

Senator CASSIDY. And again, I am not speaking of the fact that the veteran died. I am speaking of the fact that the supervisor, apparently, shall we say, misbehaved. When did the supervisor's misbehavior begin to be investigated?

Dr. MILLER. That began when we learned of——

Senator CASSIDY. And what was the date of that?

Dr. MILLER. The draft report was received by the OIG, I want to say, maybe two, three months ago; that is when we first came to the information of the——

Senator CASSIDY. And so how long will this investigation take to still hold them accountable, if indeed, the OIG is correct, that their actions were as you described?

Dr. MILLER. I can't answer that question for you.

Senator CASSIDY. That veteran was ill-served, and there—as best as I can tell, an attempt not to hold people accountable. And my, gosh, that is a pattern. Thank you.

Chairman TESTER. Thank you, Senator. There is no doubt your line of questioning is appropriate. And your disgust with the situation is entirely appropriate. I think that we demand excellence from the people in the VA, and people need to be held accountable, and we are going to ensure that—I am going to be following up with the IG on this issue tomorrow, and I will download with you from his perspective.

With that, Senator Hirono.

Senator Mazie K. Hirono

Senator HIRONO. Thank you, Mr. Chairman.

I noted that Senator Murray, my colleague, mentioned the high incidence of military sexual trauma experienced particularly by women. Dr. Miller, would you consider that a factor? Experiencing sexual trauma in the military a factor in suicide?

Dr. MILLER. Absolutely, it is a risk factor, yes.

Senator HIRONO. So I would say that, as I read your testimony, and you know these various risk factors, I would suggest to you that you include sexual military trauma in this list that you have. I think that is really important to call it out because of the high incidents of women who experience MST. So in noting the number of—by the way, would you start doing that as you prepare testimony for these kinds of hearings?

Dr. MILLER. Are you are referring to the written testimony——

Senator HIRONO. Well, that you should put in that military sexual trauma is a factor in suicide.

Dr. MILLER. Yes.

Senator HIRONO. So when we look at the numbers that you noted in 2020, that seems to be the most recent numbers we have. I hope those numbers are relatively accurate and not vastly undercounted. But 6,146 were veterans who committed suicide. Do you know how many of this number were women?

Dr. MILLER. Yes, that is available within our report.

Senator HIRONO. What is it?

Dr. MILLER. Off the top of my head; I am sorry, I don't know. It is by count much lower than men. It is by rate, rising, and higher.

Senator HIRONO. I think that is what should concern us because as more and more women enter the service, their suicide numbers, sadly, are going up. And do you know how many of these suicides had—was associated with opioids?

Dr. MILLER. In terms of opioid overdose or prescribing——

Senator HIRONO. Yes. I would start that, opioid overdoses?

Dr. MILLER. Yes. We do have a report that is available for opioid deaths, overdose that is separate from suicide reporting.

Senator HIRONO. Oh. Thank you. So what would that number be?

Dr. MILLER. That is a report that is generated by the Substance Use Disorder Program Office within the Office of Mental Health. There is also a publication from 2019 that updates that information, but we can take that back.

[The publication referred to by Dr. Miller appears on page 103 of the Appendix.]

VA Response: VA's most recent reporting regarding Veteran overdose mortality is available in the following publication:

Begley MR, Ravindran C, Peltzman T, Morley SW, Stephens BM, Ashrafioun L, McCarthy JF. 2022. Veteran Drug Overdose Mortality, 2010-2019. Drug and Alcohol Dependence. 233:109296. doi: 10.1016/j.drugalcdep.2022.109296. Epub 2022 Jan 12. https://pubmed.ncbi.nlm.nih.gov/35219064/.

PDF also attached.

Per Table 3, in 2019, there were 229 opioid overdose deaths among women Veterans, and there were 3,197 opioid overdose deaths among all Veterans.

Per the Begley et al. paper, attached, which includes the following information:

Table 3. Veteran drug overdose mortality counts 2010–2019, overall and by drug category

	Overall 2010 Deaths	Drug	Overdose 2019 Deaths	Opioid 2010 Deaths	Overdose 2019 Deaths	Stimulant	Overdose
						2010 Deaths	2019 Deaths
All Veterans	3669	4865		1891	3197	612	2172
Sex							
Female	356	372		172	229	35	102
Male	3313	4493		1719	2968	577	2070

Senator HIRONO. So would you say that that is a significant number of opioid overdoses that involve veterans?

Dr. MILLER. Yes. Yes. That is a significant issue.

Senator HIRONO. So thank you for telling us that opioid overdoses are not counted as suicides, because I think that it would be enlightening. I would have thought that it would be a part of that information.

Dr. MILLER. May I add—may I add one caveat to that?

Senator HIRONO. Yes.

Dr. MILLER. It depends on what the medical examiner puts on the death certificate. If the opioid overdose is viewed as an accident, it is not a suicide.

Senator HIRONO. It is not. I understand. I do have a question about some of the categories or the—some specific populations that have a higher incidence of suicides. And in one of your reports, I noted that the rate of suicides among Asian-American, Native Hawaiian, and Pacific Islander veterans is higher. And as a part of a response to a question that I had asked of Secretary McDonough, he noted that there were demonstration projects related to tailored mental health outreach for specified veteran populations, including AANH veterans and women veterans.

So can you describe what you would consider a tailored outreach for women veterans? And a tailored outreach for AANHPI veterans?

Dr. MILLER. Yes. We have been working on this, and happy to talk about it. We have developed a partnership with the Rocky Mountain MIRECC to study suicide prevention in this particular area, and specifically dedicated upon it. One publication has thus far emerged from that on geospatial considerations and how it impacts our knowledge of this population and in turn our programs. And they are currently in active recruitment for individuals to participate in the next phase of research.

Simultaneously, we spent a couple of weeks this summer traveling to Guam and to the Mariana Islands to talk firsthand with important points of contact there, including Governor's Challenge teams.

Senator HIRONO. You are telling me, then, that you are specifically focusing on certain ideations relating to AANHPI veterans?

Dr. MILLER. Yes.

Senator HIRONO. I would like to find out more about what you are doing, what you are learning, and whether that informs some of the resources that you are providing toward outreach to these populations.

Dr. MILLER. Yes.

Senator HIRONO. And I am particularly interested also in your outreach to women veterans.

Thank you, Mr. Chairman.

Chairman TESTER. Senator Blackburn.

Senator Marsha Blackburn

Senator BLACKBURN. Thank you, Mr. Chairman, and thank you for being here. This is an area that we all have concerns about in Tennessee, with our clinics, with our large veteran's population that is there. We do hear a good bit about this. I want to ask you all this: If I were a veteran in crisis and I reached out on the 988 right now and asked to be seen by the VA, how long would my wait be?

Dr. MILLER. So—I want to give you a technical answer, but you don't want a technical answer. The real answer to that is, it depends on the local facility that you would be referred to through the——

Senator BLACKBURN. All right; I pulled some numbers.

Dr. MILLER. Yes.

Senator BLACKBURN. Out of our region 32 of the 33 VAs in our region, the wait time would be longer than a week. And the reason I looked at that is because we looked at the

National Library of Medicine Study that goes in and they do the surveys on those that are hospitalized because they attempted suicide. They did not succeed. Forty-eight percent of them said, within 10 minutes, from the time they thought about it to the time they made the attempt, that that was the amount of lapsed time.

Dr. MILLER. Yes.

Senator BLACKBURN. Now, if you want to look at some of these numbers. And this is what startled me, because these are individuals that are in crisis, we, as a Nation, a government, have promised these veterans healthcare. And then if you look at the—one of the clinics in Nashville, it is a seven-day wait; the Alvin C. York Veterans' Hospital over in Murfreesboro, eight days; sixty-six days at the Cookeville Clinic.

Dr. Black, you have been to UT, you know where that clinic is. And you know the Chattanooga Clinic, seventy-one days; Campbell County Clinic, ninety-six days. So this access issue is one that we have got to solve.

I want to switch topics to an IG report on a patient suicide following mismanagement of the Veterans Crisis Line, and it was on the 14th of September. I found it interesting that the Director of the Veterans Crisis Line did not define the patient's death as a "sentinel event". So what is the VA definition of a "sentinel event"? Because I would think that that mismanagement and that death would be classified as a "sentinel event".

Dr. MILLER. Yes. According to policy, and I feel badly, talking about policy and technical things in the context of a veteran who is—who is not with us and died by suicide. According to policy a "sentinel event" is defined as a death or near death, and can be reasonably associated with, from a causal perspective, to action or non-action on the part of last contact.

Senator BLACKBURN. Okay. But he committed—he took his life within 30 minutes of speaking to somebody on that line.

Dr. MILLER. Mm-hmm.

Senator BLACKBURN. And if someone were to text, how long does it take you to respond? What is the amount of time on the text? That it would take——

Dr. MILLER. Our response if someone text us, is immediate.

Senator BLACKBURN. Immediate?

Dr. MILLER. Yes. Now, the individual that we are texting with, it is not uncommon that their response is not immediate. There could be 15, there could be 20 minutes lag.

Senator BLACKBURN. Do they ever call that number that they are getting the text from, to make that personal contact? Or do they just sit there and text it?

Dr. MILLER. Yes. Our policy is that if the risk assessment indicates, we need to switch them to phone from text, and that was one of our—that was one of the things that we did wrong in this situation.

Senator BLACKBURN. Okay. I do have some additional questions. My time is running out, but I am wanting to look at your staffing levels—I will submit this to each of you for writing—and the way that you are utilizing community care to help ease the burden on that staffing. I also want to know what kind of training you are doing to individuals that are Crisis Line responders; what kind of training they are receiving?

Thank you, Mr. Chairman.

Chairman TESTER. So Senator Blackburn, we will put that into the record, and get a response for those. So thank you.

Senator BLACKBURN. Yes.

Chairman TESTER. Senator Blumenthal.

Senator Richard Blumenthal

Senator BLUMENTHAL. Thanks, Mr. Chairman.

I want to just return to the exchange you had with Senator Hirono on drug overdoses.

Dr. MILLER. Mm-hmm.

Senator BLUMENTHAL. Those are not counted as suicide?

Dr. MILLER. Drug overdoses that the coroner, or the medical examiner determines on the death certificates are accidental, are not the official CDC definition of suicide, so they are not coded as a suicide. Those do not come to us for the suicide report.

Senator BLUMENTHAL. So it depends on the local coroner?

Dr. MILLER. Yes.

Senator BLUMENTHAL. So the definition that you gave me earlier, or you gave to Senator Blackburn, or you gave us earlier, about in effect, the causal link, how does that factor into what you count as a suicide by overdose?

Dr. MILLER. You know, that is getting into a question of—it is more in the areas of the medical examiner or the coroner. Usually, and very generally speaking, there needs to be indication of motive. Motive can be indicated by the means, motive can be indicated by a letter, or artifacts left behind, as two examples.

Senator BLUMENTHAL. I think what you are telling us is that the numbers of suicide may, in fact, be far greater than what you have tabulated, and what you have given to Congress year after year, because this local coroner, I mean, I am a former State official, lots of coroners have different definitions, different way of applying that, what you called a technical definition.

And I am a lawyer and I can't repeat the way you put it, essentially, it is causal connection. And I don't know how a coroner makes that determination, which then determines the VAs reporting to the United States Congress. I think those numbers are probably tremendously incomplete.

Let me ask you a more general question. You know, according to you: Suicide is a complex problem with a multifaceted interweaving of potential contributing factors; that is true. Would you say that we have really made significant progress over the last 10 years?

Dr. MILLER. I think there the two areas that my mind would go to, to answer that question. Two questions really, have we advanced on understanding and treating or improving the ''why''? And have we advanced on improving the ''how''?

Senator BLUMENTHAL. Well, have we advanced on the numbers?

Dr. MILLER. We have not advanced on the numbers.

Senator BLUMENTHAL. We have not advanced on the numbers, so I don't know how you could tell me we have made progress on this problem. If the same numbers are dying, if the rate of suicide is 1 in 17, 1 in 20, 1 in 21; I don't even know the most current figure, how it depends on the numbers of veterans, not the numbers of suicides, but the numbers of suicides are basically unchanged. How could you tell us that we have made progress?

Dr. MILLER. Because we have seen certain areas of higher risks or risk where we have seen improvements and decreases; for example, veterans who are in VHA care and diagnosed with PTSD, there has been a 30 percent reduction in suicide rate over the last 20 years. Veterans in VHA care diagnosed with a depressive disorder, there has been a greater than 20 percent reduction.

Senator BLUMENTHAL. Well, those are veterans in VHA care?

Dr. MILLER. Mm-hmm. And veterans——

Senator BLUMENTHAL. What about the total number?

Dr. MILLER. And veterans not in the——

Senator BLUMENTHAL. I think our Nation is judged, not by the numbers who are in VHA care, they are bound to be lower, I would hope they would be lower, but the numbers overall. If you were judging our Nation, those numbers are unchanged. I mean, I think we need to face the fact, and I am encountering constituents every day who say: Why can't we make progress?

Dr. MILLER. My answer to that sir, it is the "how," 70 percent of veterans die by firearms. That is the number that hasn't changed, and has only gone up. And until we make a significant improvement in that area, we probably will not see a significant decrease in veteran suicide.

Senator BLUMENTHAL. So my time is expiring, but have you advised the leadership of the VA that it should issue a warning to veterans and their families that firearms should be removed from their homes. And they should support red-flag statutes, and emergency risk protection orders in States where they are not now? And I have been probably one of the leading advocates in the Senate for separating people from guns when they say they are going to kill themselves and kill others? Shouldn't the VA be much more aggressive in advocating for those statutes?

Dr. MILLER. We provide technical consultation on everything that comes our way from you and back up through the chain. I just flew here from Denver where I was partnered with someone from your State, sir, and the President of NSSF, to address firearm manufacturing industry regarding what we can do together and collaboratively, to message exactly what you are saying.

Senator BLUMENTHAL. My time has expired. Thank you, Chairman.

Chairman TESTER. Yes. Thank you. Before I get to Senator Tillis, I would just say that, I believe you are on Armed Services, I think Senator King is Armed Services, and Senator King knows this because we have talked about it, the transition between active military and the VA, we need to do some work on, because I really think that is a huge driver for the suicides.

Senator Tillis.

Senator Thom Tillis

Senator TILLIS. Yes, starting with the fact that two-thirds of those who are taking their lives every day are not connected to the VA, we have got to figure out a way to get them better connected. Dr. Miller, and Dr. Black, thank you both for being here. You know, the exchange that you had with Senator Cassidy about, maybe a mistake, and it may very well be that somebody who was in a position to where they could have gotten the consult done, intervene, save a life. But it could have also, and more likely be related to a breakdown of a process and staffing, and a number of other things. I just can't imagine that somebody working in that position would actually not care about trying to save that veteran's life.

Dr. MILLER. Senator——

Senator TILLIS. But it is what it is. And to the extent that they failed to follow processes they obviously need to be disciplined.

Dr. MILLER. Yes, sir.

Senator TILLIS. I just believe in my heart of hearts it has got to be something more fundamental. The OIG analyzed, I guess, the analysis of consults for PTSD, military sexual trauma, or couples therapy, submitted from November 1st, 2020, through June 2022. They found 39.3 percent of psychotherapy, 39.5 percent of PTSD, 27 percent of military sexual assault, and 67, almost 68 percent of couples therapy consults, did not meet the required time of 30 days from the patient indicated date.

This sounds to me like a—and I guess as a part of the OIG Report, they said it looked like staffing issues, backlogs, the Clinical Research Hub no longer available to Hub staffing concerns. Do you agree with the OIG's assessment, or the information they receive from mental health leaders that you do have staffing backlog issues that are a problem? And if you do, how are they being addressed?

Dr. MILLER. Yes, sir. To answer your question accurately, to make sure I am thinking of the same OIG Report, are you referring to the one from North Carolina and Asheville?

Senator TILLIS. Yes.

Dr. MILLER. Yes. Okay. Yes. From my review of what I know of that OIG Report, there was concurrence to all the recommendations that were provided. I also believe that if we were to look at it today, that that facility has made some meaningful progress regarding mental health hiring. I do know that the Chief of Mental Health is today sitting at a training program for BHIP, which was also mentioned in that particular report, so they are making advancements on that as well.

Senator TILLIS. Just moving on to other information that was included in the OIG Report, one thing that stuck out at me is—look, I know I talk with a lot of veterans, I talk with a lot of veterans service organizations, and they all like the brick-and-mortar presence of the VA, about when they can get an appointment, and when they can get the care they need. In the behavioral health space, we do not have enough in the VA or in the general community of the general population.

But can you speak to some of the passages in the OIG Report that said that people within the VA were really discouraging community care referrals for behavioral health; why they would do that?

Dr. MILLER. So I think that from that, and specific to the situation, from my understanding of it, there were discussions about exactly what we have said in here, which is VA care works, and let us capture as much of that as we can through appropriate mental health staffing. I think that there may have been interpretations of that that led to then believing that it was a black and white and then discouraging community referrals. I believe in the response to that OIG, the facility attempted to clarify that, and one of the recommendations that they are engaging is staff-wide training on that very issue, sir.

Senator TILLIS. Yes. I think it is critically important——

Dr. MILLER. Yes.

Senator TILLIS [continuing]. For anyone in the VA. And I am a big supporter of the VA. I like to think of myself as a cheerleader, I very seldom flog you all in these open hearings but—very seldom—but for something like this, we have got to have balance. This is about providing care.

Dr. MILLER. Mm-hmm.

Senator TILLIS. And unless you think you are knowingly providing a community care referral to somebody who is not competent to provide the care, refer the case.

Dr. MILLER. Yes.

Senator TILLIS. And then build a capability and serve more within the VA, but that particularly in behavioral health crisis situations, days and minutes matter.

Dr. MILLER. Yes.

Senator TILLIS. And I think that anyone who, in the VA, is guilty of saying: Well, you know, we just need to keep them in the mix, a few more days, a few more weeks. First, you are playing, potentially, with somebody's life, and you are—the person who is saying that is running counter to what I have heard from everybody in the VA: Get the care, quality care as quickly as possible, in the VA if possible, but in the community when necessary.

Dr. MILLER. That is all that matters. I agree with you 100 percent. You would know this better than I do, sir, but I believe specific to that region and your constituents, community care, mental health care is in short supply. It seems difficult to come by.

Senator TILLIS. It is, and that is why we are—And Mr. Chair, I just want to mention this for future consideration. I met with Secretary McDonough when he was in Charlotte, about a month ago, and I was talking to him about the Bipartisan Safer Communities Act, and so it made me think about it when Senator Blumenthal spoke up, that is one of the single largest investments in behavioral health that this Congress has made in modern history.

One of the things I asked Secretary McDonough is, have we tuned it right to where—if you think about Eastern North Carolina, think about between Fort Bragg and Camp Lejeune, is there someplace down there where maybe we have something that we haven't had before? Collaboration with the VA, collaboration with the Army, collaboration with the private sector, to stand up a behavioral health capability that does really exist, it is scaled down in that area.

So I would like for us, if we could, I have talked to Denis about it, but I would like to see if the plain text as we passed it, facilitates that sort of thinking. Or if we need to open it up and potentially consider that in areas where I think it could be helpful.

Dr. MILLER. And improve telehealth in those areas. Yes, sir.

Senator TILLIS. Yes. Thank you. Thank you, Mr. Chair.

Chairman TESTER. Senator King.

Senator Angus S. King, JR.

Senator KING. Thank you, Mr. Chairman.

Dr. Miller, nice to see you in person, we talked last week. One of the main issues that seem to be motivating suicides is financial, and financial distress, and I think the data is four times—veterans with incomes below $50,000 who have financial problems are four times as likely to have ideation of suicide. What about a pilot in the helpline, of the Crisis Line, of having some financial expertise that could be referred? Are you having a financial problem, here is somebody you can talk to.

Dr. MILLER. Yes.

Senator KING. Is that something we could work on?

Dr. MILLER. Yes, is the short answer. What you are getting at though, sir, is an important point in terms of instead of having maybe the referral from the Veterans Crisis Line go to mental health, maybe it would be more appropriate for it to go to a financial counselor, in which case then there is a ripple effect in capacity with mental health. You save by putting people in the right place at the right time. Yes.

Senator KING. So is this something that you don't need legislation; is this something you could pilot for, in one VISN, for example?

Dr. MILLER. Yes. What we can pilot is, we are starting a new Veteran Center for Financial Empowerment. That center will offer, through VBA, and services that are available with VBA, referral to free consultation for financial issues. That will allow us to get some initial data on demand and need and be able to report that back to you for next steps.

Senator KING. I would appreciate it. I think that is an important step. Let us see what the data shows us because it does appear to be one of the causation factors. Workforce, it seems like every hearing that we are at, we talk about workforce, and I keep hearing about the difficulty of onboarding people.

For example, if you want to bring on a new therapist, it may be a therapist, it may be a clinical social worker, it may be a psychologist, you have got to do three different—three different job descriptions and go through a long process. And in fact, I have heard of mental health directors who are spending 20 hours a week on administrative functions of onboarding people. How do we crack that problem? It just seems to be a problem throughout the agency.

Dr. MILLER. Yes. I feel your pain and theirs. We hired 900 Veterans Crisis Line responders in the last year, a-year-and-a-half, and a significant portion of my time is paperwork to help move those issues in hirings along. I think that we are taking a good step in this area through the Under Secretary's initiatives that are informally called "Tiger Teams". There are at least six key areas, suicide prevention is one, but another one is hiring and retention and workforce management optimization. Watching how that group is able to progress with the targeted goals and outcomes will be important.

Senator KING. Well, I would hope something, and this isn't for you necessarily, but for the VA generally, instead of this iron hand of control from Washington, why shouldn't the local VA facility be able to hire the people they need? Washington can give them guidelines; here are the standards, here are the minimum standards, and those kinds of things. But somebody in Maine, if they need somebody, they ought to be able to reach out into the community and try to find them, and not go through all the steps that appear to be in this process.

I don't expect you to answer that, but I think that is something, Mr. Chairman, we ought to talk to the Agency about. There arejust—I keep hearing about the administrative burden of bringing people on board, and then we just—we need them.

Final question, I think it was the Chairman who used the term "better connected," about getting people connected into the system. One of the ideas that I am working on is that an active-duty service member can pre-enroll in the VA while still in active duty as part of the TAP process. Do you have a reaction to that?

Dr. MILLER. Yes. I think that would—personally, I think that would be extremely helpful in terms of streamlining the process. Currently, what can be done is a transitioning service member can preregister; they cannot pre-enroll. The reason why they cannot pre-enroll is because, by law, they have to be a veteran by the legal definition of a veteran to enroll.

Senator KING. Fortunately, laws are the business that we are in here.

Dr. MILLER. Yes, sir.

Senator KING. Great. Well, I think that is something I would like to see us work on. Thank you, Mr. Chairman.

Chairman TESTER. Senator Boozman.

Senator John Boozman

Senator BOOZMAN. Thank you, Mr. Chairman. And thank you and Senator Moran for having such an important hearing. You know, with all the rancor that is going on around here, but this Committee really does work in a very, very bipartisan way, and because of that, in the last couple of congresses we got an awful lot done.

We all know that suicide is really complex; it is a complicated crisis, there is no single solution. We also know that if people are in the VA system, they are less likely to commit suicide. Most of the people that are committing suicide are outside of the system. So one of the things that we have worked on, and most of the Committee has worked on, is trying to make it such that we could capture those folks that are outside of the system, get them some help in the community, and then ultimately bring them into the VA where they can get even additional help. Dr. MILLER. Mm-hmm.

Senator BOOZMAN. Dr. Miller, I appreciate you highlighting the Staff Sergeant Parker Gordon Fox Suicide Grant Program in your testimony. When we wrote the grant program, we intended to provide Federal resources to organizations in the community that coordinate Suicide Prevention Services outside of a clinical setting. I have met with many grant recipients and heard incredibly positive feedback on the program.

After one year of this program being in effect, what are the biggest lessons that you have learned? And have you identified ways to improve for the future? So this has been going on for a while; you have got these grant programs out there. What are you finding with them?

Dr. MILLER. Yes. I think one thing that we are learning is, it is written into the law the importance of screening for risk, and ensuring that the services are going to those who are at higher risk. But we are learning, as part of that process, that one of the many beauties of this grant is the services that a lot of the grantees are providing, are what we may call ''upstream'' in nature. So it is a bit contradictory for them to be, necessarily, screening for risk, and screening out those who aren't high risk, when a lot of the work they are doing is moving upstream before these individuals become high risk.

So resolving that I think—discrepancy, I think is a challenge for us that we are committed to working with you and this Committee together. I think the second thing I would say is we are learning a lot about how to screen for risk in ways when you are not a licensed mental health professional, and it just feels out of your normal flow of what you do to pull out a survey, a questionnaire, and say: I have some questions here that I need to ask you.

So I think we are taking a close look at the screener tool that we have implemented as part of this, and wanting to take a look at: is there a better way to meet the requirements of the screen without necessarily asking grantees to slip into a role that feels very unnatural for them as part of their service.

Senator BOOZMAN. Yes. And this follows up on your comments, and then question—comments that Senator Moran had, but it does appear that when you visit with people, you know, that are involved, that there is just something about government that makes things pretty complex. And I am part of government; I understand that. But, you know, providing increased flexibility in that area, and, you know, the whole process, I think, would really be helpful. Dr. MILLER. Absolutely; I think that would—I would want that to be an open discussion between us, because how I may define increased flexibility, I may have a blind spot then in terms of what you were intending with the law and the applications of the law. So I think it is really important we continue our open and collaborative dialogue so that we are fully capturing your intentions with the law.

Senator BOOZMAN. No. I agree, and I think something would be helpful if we could discuss with you, but also get some providers in, you know, to help us realize some of the unintended consequences. We all want the same thing.

Dr. MILLER. Mm-hmm.

Senator BOOZMAN. That may be, you know, a requirement, or whatever; just makes it a little bit more difficult.

Dr. MILLER. Yes. I am looking forward to Panel Two. I think it will give us some good insights and steps forward.

Senator BOOZMAN. Thank you.

Dr. MILLER. Thank you.

Chairman TESTER. Senator Sinema.

Senator Kyrsten Sinema

Senator SINEMA. Well, thank you, Chairman Tester, for holding this hearing. And thank you to our panelists for being here, and for the critical services you provide for America's veterans. I will focus my questions on mental health resilience for veterans and for their community. But first I want to address a time-sensitive issue. Much of what we discussed today centers around access to care for veterans, and part of that access is transportation to the point of care, like a VA hospital or a clinic. The VA is currently implementing a rule that decreases veterans' access to ambulance services, particularly in rural parts of the country, like Northern Arizona.

So I commend Senators Tester and Moran for their quick bipartisan work drafting and introducing the VA Emergency Transportation Access Act to address this issue, as well as a related amendment to the appropriations bill that I hope to vote on in the near future. I look forward to working with the Committee and the VA to protect veterans' access to life-saving ambulance services.

Since coming to the Senate, I have led bipartisan efforts to help service members and veterans build supportive resilient communities; first, by earning broad support and passing my Sergeant Daniel Somers Veterans Network Act into law, and more recently by introducing the Military Suicide Prevention in the 21st Century Act. As we know, networks of support for our veterans are vital to their well-being.

So my first question is for you, Director Miller. National Community Health Partners, which is based in Southern Arizona, has recently launched a project called "The Best Is Yet to Come" funded through the Staff Sergeant Parker Gordon Fox Suicide Prevention Grant Program; one of three such grantees in Arizona. Can you speak to the importance of these grants to community organizations?

Dr. MILLER. Yes. Absolutely, I think there is a few things that come together under the heading of our community-based Suicide Prevention Plan that reinforce your points exactly. The community- based Suicide Prevention Plan focuses on the fact that suicide prevention is not just clinical; it does not just occur in the room between a patient and provider, it occurs in the community. And as such, we have the Governor's Challenge, we have the development of community coalitions and collaborations, and then we have the Fox Grants.

Arizona is leaning forward in each of these areas, and what we have seen out of States like, and such as Arizona is the importance of, at the State level, at the county level, forming veteran suicide prevention plans for the community that are informed and built by the community. And then we are able to come in and support, through the Governor's Challenge, we are able to come in and support through the Fox Grants. The fact that you see that with the Fox Grants is evidence of the strength of that in Arizona.

Senator SINEMA. Mm-hmm. Thank you. I still hear from my Veterans Advisory Committee in Arizona that the lack of a cohesive network creates challenges for veterans. So what additional resources do veterans have to find a community after their service? Dr. MILLER. I think that that is a critically important consideration because one thing that we know, and I think we are going to see this more and more in the data, there is a relationship between connection, lack of connection, and suicide, particularly for veterans. So in terms of creating a community, I think one important step is the Solid Start. To that I will defer to Dr. Black.

Dr. BLACK. And thank you, Senator. Yes, the Solid Start Program is that first critical year after separation from the Military. So those calls at 90, 180, and 365 days it is helping to connect to the community, so when our Solid Start representatives are making that call that is some of those questions as asked, and helping connect them to their local VSOs, is one of the things that they will do.

If that is something that is an issue for the veteran it is based— those calls are based on the veteran need. So if they are saying: Yes, I am having a hard time, you know, finding community connections. That is something that will be addressed in those calls. Senator SINEMA. And are there any metrics that we can use to gauge the growth and strength of these types of support networks?

Dr. MILLER. I think that the metrics that are associated—the first thing that comes to mind is the metrics that are associated with the Governor's challenge and the work that we are doing there. So the practical application of that would be: What is Arizona seeing in terms of the number of community collaborations that have been built, implemented, maintained. That would be an important indicator. Nationwide we just reached 1,500. How is that relative in Arizona? Is it growing? What lessons are we learning?

Senator SINEMA. I see my time has expired. Thank you, Mr.

Chairman, for holding this hearing on such an important topic.

Chairman TESTER. Thank you, Senator Sinema.

So you heard my opening statement, and I think you are fully aware that 60 percent of the veterans who commit suicide don't have any engagement with the VA. Senator King has a bill that will enroll the service member before they get out of the service, in the VA. I want your opinion. Is that a solution?

Dr. MILLER. So there is the answer that I could give which is, we will review that through our Technical Consultation Team and experts and we would happy——

Chairman TESTER. Except I want your opinion.

Dr. MILLER. My opinion is that when you look at engaging preregistration, and the percent that we are able to do with that, and then you look at how that converts to pre—or how that converts to enroll enrollment, there is a gap. So the short answer is, if you can cut that gap down between preregistration and enrollment, and make it all the same, that just makes sense to me. But that is just Matt Miller talking.

Chairman TESTER. Well that is right—we are in front of this Committee though. Okay? If you were a ''nobody'' you wouldn't be here, all right. So Dr. Miller the STRONG Veterans Act includes the silent monitoring requirements of the Veterans Crisis lines.

Dr. MILLER. Yes.

Chairman TESTER. The IG was critical of that too in his report. What assurances can the VA—can you provide—can the VA provide to this Committee that Veterans Crisis Line responders are receiving the appropriate amount of silent monitoring today?

Dr. MILLER. Yes. A few things; and I think that is really important, because that is one of the keys to rebuilding trust, I think, in this situation. Number one, if you look at our staffing levels in January of '21 when this tragedy occurred, we were about 550 responders. We have since added 900-plus responders.

Why does that matter? That matters because the context of this situation is we were using someone in an overtime role who wasn't regularly a responder. My point is, we don't have to do that anymore to answer any call. So that is one step that has been necessary here.

The second step is, two forms of silent monitoring that must occur on a monthly base and be reported, 90 percent supervision, or supervisor performance monitoring, 80 percent silent monitoring. We report that on a monthly basis, as I said, and as part of the OIG recommendations we are going to be reporting that and our progress to OIG. We will not be able to close that recommendation until we reach a level that they are satisfied with.

That said, I know for a fact, because I looked at it today, we are at over 90 percent for both the supervision silent monitoring, and the silent monitor silent monitoring, two forms.

Chairman TESTER. All right; you answered my second question with that answer. So in Section 701 of the Hannon Act, and by the way this law was passed—was signed in a law in 2020; it implements new telehealth access grants, the VA doesn't expect to be able to give awards out until 2025, not to beat this, but 2020 is when it was signed into law, we are not going to get any grants after 2025, telehealth is really important in a rural State, I think it is important in an urban State too, quite frankly. What can you guys do to expedite that roll out? Or are you happy with that timeline?

Dr. MILLER. We are not happy with that timeline.

Chairman TESTER. Okay.

Dr. MILLER. I think that in talking to those who are leading this particular effort my understanding and perception is that we are not happy, we have looked at options to expedite, there has been some consultation that is needed to occur with OGC, and OGC has found themselves needing to fill in some details toward enactment. And the impression that I got in talking with them is, it is better to measure twice, cut once, than to do it wrongly, legally.

Chairman TESTER. I got it.

Senator KING [continuing]. In months.

Chairman TESTER. Yes.

Senator KING. That is a standard I——

Chairman TESTER. That is a very good point, Senator King. I would also point out that that we are—if it takes us 5 years to do a telehealth grant to get them out the door, we have got no hope to ever get electronic medical records done. We have just got no hope.

Dr. MILLER. We were, I think, very quick and efficient with Staff Sergeant Parker Gordon Fox, so I think there is hope.

Chairman TESTER. Okay. The last question, because we have got another panel, though I will defer to the Ranking Member if he has another question; and maybe even to Senator King, but it had better be a damn good one.

Recently, we introduced the bipartisan Not Just a Number Act, Senator Boozman was just here, we introduced it together, it requires a VA to examine association between veterans' use of VA benefits and suicide. I think you could also bring in the point that Senator King talked about, about financial difficulties.

Dr. MILLER. Mm-hmm.

Chairman TESTER. Dr. Miller, how could Outreach do an analysis of veterans who use VBA programs help? Do you think it would?

Dr. MILLER. Let me give you——

Chairman TESTER. Do you think it would be worth the time spent to look at them?

Dr. MILLER. Yes, sir. Let me give you an example to illustrate. REACH VET is considered a leader, nationwide and internationally, in risk prediction for suicide. REACH VET is based primarily on clinical factors pulled from the medical chart. We know that from looking at the data the majority of veterans who die by suicide by firearm don't show up in the top 50 percent of risk for REACH VET. They show up in other areas that are outside of the clinical. So then the short answer founded upon that is, yes, sir.

Chairman TESTER. Okay. Senator Moran.

Senator MORAN. Thank you, Chairman. I will use my time of my opening statement that I didn't give, to just ask a couple of clarifying questions. First of all, Senator Tillis, in Asheville, your answer to him involved that—and the question that I want to raise is about the lack of suggestion, or recommendation, or appointment to community care. And your answer was that we think that there was a policy in place that we were trying to keep our patients within the VA, we believe we provide better service. And you indicated, I think, Dr. Miller, that the Asheville staff was being retrained or trained to get this right; is that—did I make that up, or that is what you said?

Dr. MILLER. I think the only thing that I would suggest modification on, is I don't know that there was a policy in place. I think that there was a communication about the general spirit of VA provides great care, let us provide great care.

Senator MORAN. And the point I was—that is what you said. The point I want to make is that the directions, though, were given to the hospital at Asheville, not more broadly within the VA?

Dr. MILLER. Yes. In this particular OIG, all——

Senator MORAN. Because OIG pointed this out?

Dr. MILLER. Yes.

Senator MORAN. I would say that it is happening across the country, that that is not a policy, but this belief that the VA provides the best service, and therefore community care is often not suggested to a veteran. I hear about it consistently at home, I hear about it from my colleagues, and it is not what the MISSION Act says. The issue there is that you can have community care, if your wait time is too long, or if it is in the best interest of the patient, the veteran, determined not by the VA, but by the veteran and his or her provider.

Dr. MILLER. Yes. Well——

Senator MORAN. I am restating what the law is, but it is not, ever been clear to me that the VA is interested in making community care that widely available, and I think it is particular important in this hearing, where mental health services are rare, hard to find, within the VA, and sometimes outside the VA, we don't have enough providers anyplace. But it is also important because it can be a life and death circumstances, and the failure to suggest community care is one of those life and death circumstances.

It, again, is not in compliance with the law as we wrote it and I wish that your answer would have been, the VA is now providing direction to all VAs, all VISNs, all hospitals, all providers that community care is an option in the circumstance, particularly when a veteran cannot get an appointment within the VA.

Let me ask a more technical question. I think you have said that if you are suggesting ideation of suicide, you can get an appointment within 24 hours; did I hear that? Or is that true?

Dr. MILLER. That is not what I meant to say in that particular context. What I think I was talking about was same-day access that any veteran should be able to request and there should be an option for it at the VA facility, or the community-based outpatient clinic. Now, with that said, yes, there should be immediate access for any veteran who is experiencing suicidal thoughts.

Senator MORAN. The point I want to try to make sure I understand is, I think you said: we could get an appointment within that time frame. And does ''get an appointment'' mean you are seen by a provider? Or does ''get an appointment'' mean you are scheduled to be seen by a provider?

Dr. MILLER. No. In this case, in a crisis, if we are talking about— and we are not even talking about an appointment; let us say we are talking about an encounter, an engagement, you go and do the appointment after the fact, just to make sure that it is logged into the system. That is what should occur with same-day access, and with the certain——

Senator MORAN. Same-day access is different than getting an appointment. Same-day access is same day access, getting an appointment is something that is written on a piece of paper and——

Dr. MILLER. Yes.

Senator MORAN. All right.

Dr. MILLER. What you are highlighting is a nuance that I think is important, and that is that there are different dimensions of access. There is emergency access, there is routine first appointment, and there is follow-up episode of care. What we need to do in the VA, is be carefully watching, providing for, and monitoring all three types of access.

Senator MORAN. You are talking VA health care broadly; or VA health care as it relates to mental health and suicide?

Dr. MILLER. Well, I would argue broadly. However, mental health specifically is unique somewhat in that you commonly see the need for emergency first appointment routine follow-for episode of care.

Closing Statement of Senator Jerry Moran

Senator MORAN. And now for my closing statement Mr. President—Mr. Chairman, which was the opening statement: I had a veteran from Kansas visit my office today, this morning, and this is her story, she shared that after the beginning of mental health treatment at a Kansas VA Medical Center. She was referred to a local Vet Center because of staffing shortages at the VA Health Center. When she reached out for an initial appointment with the counselor at the

Vet Center she was told their case load was already full, unless she was experiencing suicide ideation they would not be able to prioritize her.

Six weeks later the veteran received a follow-up call from the Vet Center saying: We will not be able to help you at all. We don't have the staff. I think was the point. That is now months ago, and she has had no follow up, no effort to re-engage, never met with a counselor.

And unfortunately, I don't think this is an isolated circumstance. And so this is an example, and I heard this with Senator Murray in her conversations about the number of days. I heard it with Senator Blackwell. And the number of days for care and treatment for an appointment, for attention for—and so the other point that I make is not one time, this veteran said, did she ever hear anything about the possibility of going to the community, because both the hospital and the Vet Center failed her for lack of capability of seeing her due to staffing shortages.

It is why my support for community care is not at all based upon any bias against the VA, it is that too many veterans fall through the cracks when there is, the reason that we created community care in the MISSION Act, was a result of their lack of capabilities of a hospital in Phoenix meeting the needs of our veterans, and so we gave all—initially Choice and then the MISSION Act, we gave an option to try to solve the staffing shortages.

They still exist, and the law says a veteran is entitled to, in many circumstances, care in the community but they don't know it if the VA doesn't tell them, and if the VA doesn't make it available for them. What am I missing?

Dr. MILLER. Nothing, sir. Message heard.

Senator MORAN. Thank you.

Chairman TESTER. And that was at a CBOC in Wichita?

Senator MORAN. It was at a hospital in Kansas.

Chairman TESTER. A VA hospital?

Senator MORAN. A VA hospital in Kansas.

Chairman TESTER. Okay. Yes. Look, thank you guys very, very much. I appreciate you being here Dr. Miller. I wished to let Dr. Black speak more, but you did—you did a fine job answering the questions. We appreciate you both being here.

I think as the Ranking Member said to me a bit ago, we have had so damn many hearings on mental health, and it doesn't seem like anything has changed. And there is no doubt in my mind that you want to do the best for our veterans, and you are trying to do the best for your veterans, and this was really frustrating for me to say, but we have got to do better. We have just got to do better. This is just—this isn't saleable. It is keeping people out of our military when we need more people in our military. It is ruining lives. It is ruining families. And so we all need to work together to make sure this happens, and please know that this Committee would probably give you anything you ask for when it comes to mental health. We just need to make sure that what you are asking for is something that actually will make a difference. Thank you.

Senator MORAN. Mr. Chairman, the legislation that we are talking about, John Hannon——

Chairman TESTER. Yes.

Senator MORAN [continuing]. It is a result of your leadership. I chaired the Committee when this legislation was passed. It was your piece of legislation named after a veteran in Montana.

Chairman TESTER. That is correct.

Senator MORAN. This matters to you, it matters to me.

Chairman TESTER. Yes.

Senator MORAN. And I want to be helpful to you. This Committee does want to work together with the Department of Veterans Affairs to save lives.

Chairman TESTER. Yes. Amen. And so we are all on the same page here. Okay. Thank you for your time. We are going to get the next panel going. Thank you.

I will start by welcoming our witnesses to the second panel. First up is going to be John Eaton, who is the Vice President of Complex Care at the Wounded Warrior Project.

John, I will tell you, earlier today I got to meet with some women from the Wounded Warrior's Project, and I will tell you that it was enlightening and beneficial for me, and I am glad you sent them over, if you did, or somebody did, but it was a nice conversation. Then we are going to hear from Gilly Cantor. And I am going to tell you, Gilly, you are the first "Gilly" I ever met. Okay. And it is good to have you here. You are the Director of Evaluation and Capacity Building for the D—D'Anielo—better yet—Institute for Veterans and Military Families, at the great University of New York, Syracuse. And it is good to have you here.

I would ask you to keep your comments to 5 minutes as with the previous panel. Please know that you are full written statement will be a part of the record.

We will start with you Mr. Eaton.

Panel II. Statement of John Eaton

Mr. EATON. Thank you, Chairman Tester, Ranking Member Moran, and the distinguished Committee members, for this opportunity to speak.

Since 2003, Wounded Warrior Project has been working to transform the way America's injured Post-9/11 veterans are empowered, employed, and engaged in their communities. For the past 20 years, we have supported warriors through and beyond their transition to civilian life with services in mental health, physical health, peer connection, career counseling, and financial wellness. We currently offer these services to over 195,000 veterans across the country, and we are welcoming hundreds more every month.

Our vision to foster the most successful, well-adjusted generation of wounded service members in our Nation's history brings with it the responsibility to identify, address, and serve the mental health needs of the veterans who reach out for help. In our 2022 Annual Warrior Survey, nearly all respondents reported experiencing post-traumatic stress, traumatic brain injury, or other mental health injuries during their military service, 83 percent reported experiencing more than one.

Outreach and awareness-building have been critical parts of our mission because, sadly, many veterans don't seek the help they need due to fear of being negatively labeled, or they don't know the programs and services that are available to them. Wounded Warrior Project is here to help them, at no cost, get the specific type of mental health help they need to take the next step on their journeys to recovery.

Of course, we believe no single organization can meet the needs of our injured veterans. We also believe that evidence-based mental health treatment works when it is available and when it is pursued. However, the best results will be found when we embrace a public health approach focused on increasing resilience, improving psychological well-being, and building an aggressive prevention strategy. VA is our biggest and most important partner in that pursuit, and it is critical that we give them the tools they need to succeed.

Our written statement outlines several ways that Congress can help. But this afternoon, I will focus on five important steps that this Committee can take to help take the veterans suffering from the invisible wounds related to their service of our Nation.

First, we have to reduce wait times for accessing mental health. VA's access standard is reasonable on paper, but the practical experience for many veterans who ultimately seek care through Wounded Warrior Project indicates that many of them are being offered appointments well beyond the target, without any clear discussion with their provider about how care may be found more quickly in the community.

In addition, the lack of a consistently applied access standard for residential rehabilitation care for mental health, has essentially resulted in no true access standard for care. Fortunately, both the Making Community Care Work for Veterans Act, and the Veterans Health Act offer solutions to both of these problems and improvements over the status quo.

Second, we have to acknowledge and respond to the fact that access to care issues at the VA are a symptom of a larger challenge of needing more mental health providers. Recent HHS research indicates that 164 million Americans live in areas with mental health professional shortages, and so it is no surprise that VA is facing several shortages in psychology, psychiatry, and social work in many of its facilities.

To address these problems, we call on Congress to pass the VA Careers Act and the Mental Health Professionals Workforce Shortage Loan Repayment Act, the first of which would help VA recruit and retain more mental health providers, while the latter would address the fact that mental health isn't just a veteran problem; it is an American problem, and we simply need to get more providers in the field.

Third, we should to continue encouraging VA to leverage telehealth as a means of making care more accessible. Veterans who share their stories with us through surveys and action, often prefer telehealth for its convenience; however, those preferences should not be assumed, and veterans should be provided with clarity and transparency when telehealth is available as an alternative to in-person care. We believe that telehealth should satisfy access standards only when a veteran has agreed to it, with a clear understanding of their options.

Fourth, we continue to support investment in VA grants and partnerships within the community to provide upstream suicide prevention services. We remain hopeful that the Fox Grant Program will become a permanent fixture in VA's public health strategy. However, we believe that attention should be given to how service eligibility determinations are made and how clinical care can be responsibly provided before the program is made permanent.

Fifth, and finally, we encourage this Committee to take care in understanding that brain health is not always synonymous with mental health, and that there are steps we can take to improve the quality of life and mitigate factors for suicide among those who have suffered traumatic brain injury. A growing body of research is showing a greater association between TBI and suicide. And while TBI often co-occurs with a mental health diagnosis, we encourage stronger support and long-term care to address the care and financial stressors that can affect those with moderate to severe TBI.

To that end, we urge Congress to pass the Elizabeth Dole Home Care Act, and Expanding Veterans' Options for Long-Term Care Act, which would collectively serve the long-term needs of younger veterans who need this care earlier in life.

In closing, I want to thank this Committee for the invitation to testify. And welcome your questions.

[The prepared statement of Mr. Eaton appears on page 54 of the Appendix.]

Senator MORAN. Thank you. Gilly Cantor.

Statement of Gilly Cantor

Ms. CANTOR. Thank you, Mr. Chairman, Ranking Member Moran, and Members of the Committee. Thank you for this opportunity to testify.

I am Gilly Cantor. I serve as the Director of Evaluation and Capacity Building at the D'Aniello Institute for Veterans and Military Families at Syracuse University.

Our contribution to this conversation is rooted in upstream approaches to suicide prevention. For 10 years, we played a key role in building and evaluating networks of health and community- based social service organizations, originally those are part of our AmericaServes Initiative, which is in 18 communities across the country.

These collaborative models have demonstrated that helping veterans navigate to the full scope of services and resources they need beyond clinical interventions alone is an integral component of suicide prevention. At the same time, we have witnessed unprecedented effort from this Committee, and Congress, and the VA, to better integrate communities into suicide prevention strategies. It is the strong belief of the IVMF, and on behalf of our partners, that we must not give up on the promise of these efforts, but rather ensure that they live up to their potential.

So today, I would like to reinforce why communities remain essential to effective suicide prevention, and I would like to demonstrate that establishing transparency and accountability between the VA and communities, at scale, is both achievable and necessary.

There are three findings I want to highlight from a study that we did with the VA Center for Health Equity Research and Promotion. We looked at collaboration between AmericaServes networks, and VA medical centers and their communities.

First, we found high overlap between AmericaServes and VA data, even in communities with low levels of partnership. In other words, many veterans enrolled at the VA are, unquestionably, also receiving services in their communities.

Second, veterans served by both the VA and the community were comparatively younger. They included more Black, Hispanic, and women veterans, and they had more health-related social needs, like housing and food security. So in other words, communities are reaching the most marginalized veterans experiencing the most hardship.

And third, when partnerships were strong, veterans receiving healthcare from the VA and services in the community, were more likely to have those needs successfully met. So when we work together, the stressors impacting veterans' well-being can be more effectively addressed.

Broader research shows, and this was talked about earlier, that these economic, social, and interpersonal circumstances increase the risk of suicide. Imagine what more we could do if non-health data like this was examined regularly and shared. We must support legislation like the Not Just a Number Act, and bring all the data the VA and communities have to bear on this issue.

Additionally, we know from our own evaluation of AmericaServes in Pittsburgh, that hundreds of veterans are formally referred between the VA and the community each year, because this data is meticulously tracked, the VA has full access to this information. This level of transparency is also happening in other places, such as North Carolina and Texas, but it is not happening everywhere. Finally, I would like to share opposing accounts we heard during our roundtable with 11 of our partners who are recipients of the Staff Sergeant Fox Suicide Prevention Grant Program. In one community, the Suicide prevention coordinator sat shoulder-to-shoulder with the grantee. They streamlined enrollment into the VA for those who screened eligible due to the risk.

In other communities, suicide prevention coordinators were hardly aware of the program, and the ability to facilitate that enrollment was not happening. We need to make these successful communities the rule and not the exception.

We have submitted a full brief as a statement for the record on that roundtable, and encourage the Committee and the VA to consider its findings. And we are happy to talk about it as much as they would like.

If there is one message that I would like to leave you with, in light of some of the tragic things that have happened, again, focusing upstream, it is this: We think there is more to be hopeful about than there is to criticize. We are all here because the stakes remain high and the consequences of failure are quite, literally, existential. But we have collectively taken meaningful action and effective steps toward our shared goal.

We simply need to monitor our progress and have the courage to adjust course along the way if necessary. Thank you.

[The prepared statement of Ms. Cantor appears on page 70 of the Appendix.]

Chairman TESTER. I want to thank you both for your testimony, and I want to start by commending you both for the work that you and your organizations do. I will tell you, I like the optimism of saying that we have more to be thankful for than we do to be critical of. You know, if this was an easy issue, we would have had it settled a long, long time ago. The human mind is a hard thing to try to figure out how it works, and there is proof around this place all the time, so it is an interesting situation.

I am going to start with you, Mr. Eaton. As I indicated in my introduction of you, this morning some women from the Wounded Warrior's Project came to my office, and I talked about a lot of things, including a survey that Wounded Warrior's Project just did about women veterans. Could you give me an idea on what that survey said about mental health, if it said any—I haven't had a chance to read the documents they gave me, okay, but if it said anything about mental health, could you talk about that? And if there are solutions, talk about those too?

Mr. EATON. Yes, thank you, Mr. Chairman. And thank you for meeting with the women warriors from Wounded Warrior Project. Just yesterday, we released the report, so the 2023 Women's Warrior Report; and it was based on surveys, as you mentioned, from 5,000 women warriors from our alumni, as well as in-person focus groups across the country, to really collect qualitative and quantitative data.

The findings across multiple areas, you know. To name a few: access to care, transition from military to civilian life, as well as financial wellness. With respect to the mental health area, anxiety and depression were the top two health challenges reported by women warriors. And research shows that women are more likely to show moderate to severe symptoms, as well as PTSD symptoms, than our male warriors.

Also, a higher percentage experienced loneliness and isolation compared to men as well, which is hugely detrimental, as we know and have discussed today, to our overall mental health.

There is good news that came out, one of which women were found to score higher on resiliency measures, and eight out of ten women warriors reported—have accessing professional help at least 12 times over the last year. So we are, as a population, very resilient and engaged in their mental health and wellness, which is a really good finding.

And so what can we do? You know, what we have taken away is really the opportunity to focus on transition, and how do we ease the stress and foster better connections to other veterans and support networks and after service, as well as making the VA a more desirable place for care by making it easier to access with appointment times and gender-specific care; and finally, additional research that can be done to understand the whys behind how men and women are experiencing trauma, and thus, seeing the results of the survey.

Chairman TESTER. Was there any sort of conversation around how well the VA is doing?

Mr. EATON. So that is a topic we discussed with veterans across all of our alumni, and over 90 percent of our alumni report using the VA for their services. When we think about access to care, we hear the same feedback from our female warriors as we do male warriors, and you know, long wait times perhaps, and how that affects, you know, it is really important when we are at the moment of readiness to really capture that momentum, and oftentimes without that, we are seeing poor health outcomes, both mental, physical, family, and relational issues as well.

Chairman TESTER. So Gilly, this next question is for you. The Not Just a Number Act is a bill that we have—and Senator Boozman, I appreciate your mention of it—because I think suicide goes way beyond just mental health practices. This bill would also look at things like disability compensation, education, employment benefits, home loans, foreclosure assistance, housing assistance programs.

From your seat, how could you—from your seat, tell me your analysis of veterans who use VBA programs and how this bill could improve VA suicide prevention efforts?

Ms. CANTOR. Sure, I don't know a lot about exact likelihoods, or things like that, but I do know of a recent Brown University Study that looked at Vietnam veterans, specifically, and their usage of disability compensation, and it was directly associated with certain improved health outcomes, which just tells you that there is a lot more to look at there.

And I think that if we can't look at that data regularly, then we are doing something wrong. And I think that in order to make that possible, it wouldn't surprise me if it there is sort of some underlying infrastructure problems, technology-wise, and gets into the weeds, and it is boring data stuff. But I really think that part of it has to do with how different agencies, including within the VA, track data, and it doesn't line up.

We have seen it between DoD and VA, it is even within VBA to VHA. It is really hard to match things up and to look at things really clearly and get an understanding of what is going on without taking years to do a research project. And that is a problem.

Chairman TESTER. Okay. Thank you both very, very much.

Senator MORAN.

Senator MORAN. Senator King, I would be happy if you would like to go next.

Senator KING. I will go after you.

Senator MORAN. Let me start with you, Mr. Eaton. Thank you very much for being here today. Thank you for your work on behalf of Wounded Warrior's Project. I appreciate very much your remarks in your testimony, and your written testimony about the Veterans Health Act. It reflects an effort by Senator Sinema and I on a topic that we have been trying to be prevalent on and relevant on today.

Could you discuss in detail, more detail how the VA's current misinterpretation of access standards set forth in the MISSION Act are having a consequence on veterans' access to care?

Mr. EATON. Yes. And thank you for the question. You know, we discussed in our written statement, so the VA's MISSION Act, you know, standards that do not exist around the critical mental healthrehabilitation programs. So instead, veterans and advocates are left to really interpret that VHA directive, and in our experience, it provides little predictability on acceptance of referrals, length until a decision; and other really important factors when we know that time is of the essence.

What we are seeing in our C3, our Complex Case Coordination Program, works with the most in-need warriors who are experiencing mental health concerns, and oftentimes an RRTP is an indicator for their care. And so what we are seeing, though, you know, local policy variations that are, again, unpredictable referrals, lengthy wait times, and really not a formally calculated way to be consistent about how we are understanding those options so we can advocate for the veteran. And what also comes as a result is that alternative treatment options that could result in a community referral or an inter-VA referral aren't taking place.

And so, you know, in totality, that really just shows that, you know, what we are seeing is veterans are not accessing the care they need when they need it, and delays in finding that appropriate care really enable our opportunity to capitalize on the momentum and the willingness to get that treatment, which often-times is years in the making and really important.

Senator MORAN. Mr. Eaton, from time to time I am told that the reason that the VA is not making referrals for community care is the lengthy wait times in the community. Is that anything that you hear, and what is the reality there when we know there are wait times also at the VA?

Mr. EATON. Sure. And that is a great point. I think as we talk about mental health shortage, it is obviously something that is not only seen within the VA. And so it is very regional-specific, and that is why our team looks at all options, the primary, working with the VA within that program to establish their holistic care within that system of care. What I know is that we have a very cultivated group of partners from RRTP programs that are part of the Community Care Network, and it would be our experience that we have very quick response times for when those needs arise.

For example, we serve over 6,000 warriors a year with outpatient mental health services, with wait times less than 14 days for a first appointment, and generally in most cases. And so I think, depending on the region, it could be a better choice, whether it is VA or a Community Care Network. But ultimately, we really feel the veteran should have more visibility into that conversation.

Senator MORAN. Thank you for that answer.

Ms. Cantor, you, in your testimony, talk about the recent convening of 11 organizations who are Hannon Fox grantees. This takes me back to my first question earlier: Would you elaborate on the need for the VA? You talk about the screening issues remain a barrier, elaborate on the need, or what the VA could do to open up the eligibility standards to meet the needs of veterans who we are trying to reach and better serve.

Ms. CANTOR. Sure. So one of the issues that came up was around who is eligible, and then also on which services are eligible at which points. And I really appreciated how Dr. Miller described the tension that is going on between trying to get it to be the right people and the right things. And I think that what we are seeing andwhat the communities are saying is that depending on which screeners—individuals screen for risk, some, not others, and it depends on the person, that that can cause people to screen ineligible. And so they are looking for more flexibility in which screeners they use, or the possibility of making sure that as long as they are screening on one, even if not the other, that that constitutes enough of a risk for someone to get—to be eligible to be enrolled. They are also hoping that they can increase which services are eligible for coverage under the program so that they can try to do better outreach and get more people in the door in the first place, access to transportation, being able to provide food, making it a more welcoming environment for people to come in and connect with others, and address isolation, and then hopefully ask for help.

Senator MORAN. Any ways for the screening—to streamline the screening and make it more friendly?

Ms. CANTOR. They expressed a need to make it more conversational, that was one thing that came up repeatedly, and that the forms that accompany the screeners that they have to fill out would also need to be tailored to accommodate that style where, right now, it is difficult for them to do those intake screenings and then have to populate other things. And so there is sort of this extra barrier during the screening process, just for them to make sure that those conversations Dr. Miller referred to, as trying to ensure that they are not clinical conversations because the goal of this is to take the clinical element out and get more people, get more of the ten people who die by suicide that are not connected to the VA, comfortable, screened, and connected.

Senator MORAN. Any suggestion that this help from these organizations that receive the Hannon Fox grants that that would help us get to those who are not engaged with the VA?

Ms. CANTOR. I think—this is me speaking—I think it would. I think that most of them—you know, I mentioned the study we did, 70 percent of this doesn't apply to all those partners, but for those that it does apply to, 70 percent of the people that are veterans that they work with showed up in VA data. But that means that 30 percent didn't. And that is just from the veterans, they also serve family members, they also serve caregivers, et cetera. So there is—I see at least a 30 percent opportunity there for people that they are talking to every single day.

Senator MORAN. Ms. Cantor, I never thought about, when we wrote the Hannon Act that these grants to community organizations might increase the population of who is served. But your testimony, your conversation with me, that kind of a light bulb went off that, I don't know whether it is true, but it sure seems kind of commonsense to me that one way to serve more veterans, those veterans who are not engaged in the VA today, can be through a community organization.

Ms. CANTOR. Thank you for that comment. I fully agree.

Senator MORAN. Okay. Senator King.

Senator KING. I want to start with two general comments. Number one, you may wonder where everybody is. At this very moment; there is a Classified All-Senators Briefing on the conflict in Ukraine. And that this is one of the most dedicated committees in the Senate. But I just want you to understand that sometimes we have these inevitable conflicts in terms of time. So that is what— that is where everybody is right now.

Senator MORAN. Senator King is pointing out that he and I are supposed to go as well.

[Laughter.]

Senator KING. Yes. Yes. Okay, second, in these hearings we always are talking about how we can improve things, we can do better, and they often turn into somewhat negative about the VA. I think I can tell you from the point of view of what I hear from my veterans in Maine, they really like the care that they are getting from the VA. They are impressed by the personal qualities of the people that they meet with, and they get—they get great care.

Now, one of the issues is access. The question is when do you get the care? And that is a larger issue. We have got an enormous shortage in this country of mental health professionals. In fact, we have got an enormous shortage of just about everything. One of our major hospitals just told me recently they are short 800 nurses. I mean, that is what we are up against.

So I think we need to understand that it is not for lack of trying that the VA is short-staffed, that this is a nationwide problem, in and around the VA, but just generally.

So the question is, I think, what tools can we provide to the VA that they can more effectively compete in the workforce market? And I don't expect you to answer that, but if you have any thoughts, Ms. Cantor? I want to get this——

Ms. CANTOR. That is a really—no, that is a really hard—I mean, that is a great, that is a great idea, Senator. I think one of the things that this is not necessarily helping with mental health specifically, but it is a model that could be applied. There is a great program out of New York City called "PROVE", that is a peer-to-peer model, and they train their social workers in their social work program through—to work with veterans. And thereby, in addition to helping a peer-to-peer model, which can, again, be upstream from other challenges and help people feel connected on campuses. It is training a new workforce of culturally competent social workers. And I think that models like that could be applied outside of the social work space. It is something that could be done. I know that—I don't know the number, but it is my understanding that a huge percentage of physicians are partially trained at the VA because of the high-quality care that—and program and education that can be offered there.

It is surprising to me that it is not a more competitive and interest—and place to work that people would be interested in working.

Senator KING. Well, I do think this is something we need to think about.

Ms. CANTOR. Yes.

Senator KING. If this is a competitive marketplace, we are going to have to—for example, I learned recently, no one in the Federal Government is allowed to be paid more than the President. That is $400,000 a year. Try hiring a cardiologist for $400,000. I mean, that is the kind of thing that we need to discuss, we need to talk about waivers, and to be sure that we have access to the professionals that we need.

Telehealth, Mr. Eaton, you mentioned that, and I don't know if you are aware of the answer to this question. I probably should have asked it of the prior panel, but do we have licensure issues with telehealth? If you have got a VA facility in Augusta, Maine, can a veteran go there and get counseling from a counselor in Kentucky? Do you know?

Mr. EATON. I am not aware of the VA's approach and what they are able to do across State lines, but I do know through PSYPACT, there is a growing number, an overwhelming majority of States that are able to have cross-state service through psychology. And we leverage that within our Warrior Care Network as well as our outpatient.

Senator KING. Clearly, that is something we need to do. And in my talking with veterans and others, mental health, and behavioral health lends itself to telehealth. A lot of people are even more comfortable talking to a screen, and they don't have to wait in a doctor's office and worry about stigma, and who is in the—who is sitting in the chair next to them. And you mentioned they have got to understand their options, but I think telehealth is an opportunity to provide the care nationwide that perhaps might not be available, particularly in a rural area.

Mr. EATON. Well, a hundred percent agree. And that is what we have seen, you know, when we——

Senator KING. I like that on the record. "A hundred percent agree." I appreciate that.

Mr. EATON. During our survey with our warriors, of those that were offered telehealth services, 90 percent accepted that. And those that were not offered, only 40 percent said that if they were offered, they would not have elected that service. So we see it as, again, increasing access, increasing capacity, and it is a positive experience for veterans.

Senator KING. And one of the other, in terms of the providers, what I am told is, there is a much lower level of missed appointments; there is a better—they are getting to the appointments, which is better for the providers. So I do think that is something that we have got to—we have got to work on.

Ms. Cantor, your thoughts on telehealth?

Ms. CANTOR. I agree. I think that it makes sense for many people. I think that, similar to what we were talking about with community care, that it comes down to patient choice; and that if that is something that they are willing to do, that that makes a lot of sense. And I think, missed appointments, in particular, is a missed opportunity, and it also, with telehealth, addresses the transportation problem that is a huge cause of that for in-person visits.

Senator KING. Particularly in rural areas?

Ms. CANTOR. Particularly in the rural areas.

Senator KING. Great. Well, thank you all very much for your testimony, and I appreciate the work that you are doing. And we are in a learning mode here, so if there are suggestions, ideas, that is what we want to hear, ways that we can try to fix things, whether it is—it could be a law change, but it could also be something that we can work with the VA administratively, that doesn't involve a law change.

If there are things, and we have talked about earlier, you heard us talking about the onboarding, and the barriers to bringing new people in. So share your thoughts; we are in the idea business around here. Thank you.

Thank you, Mr. Chairman.

Senator MORAN. Senator King, thank you. Thank you for your full, lengthy participation today.

Senator KING. Sure.

Senator MORAN. Mr. Eaton, Ms. Cantor, thank you very much for your testimony. Thanks for joining us today.

The Members of the Committee will have one week to submit written questions, and we would ask the witnesses to respond to them as quickly as possible.

The Committee is now adjourned.

[Whereupon, at 5:42 p.m., the hearing was adjourned.]

Appendix. Prepared Statements

Statement of Dr. Matthew Miller, Ph.D., MPH, Executive Director, Suicide Prevention, Office of Mental Health and Suicide Prevention Veterans Health Administration Department of Veterans Affairs Before the Committee on Veterans' Affairs, U.S. Senate "Invisible Wounds of War: Improving Mental Health And Suicide Prevention Measures For Our Nation's Veterans" September 20, 2023

Good morning, Chairman Tester, Ranking Member Moran and distinguished Members of the Committee. Thank you for the opportunity today to discuss the Department's efforts to implement recently enacted laws related to Veterans' mental health care and suicide prevention, including P. L. 116-171, the Commander John Scott Hannon Veterans Mental Health Care Improvement Act of 2019 (Hannon Act) and Division V of P.L. 117-328, the STRONG Veterans Act of 2022 (the STRONG Act) included in the Consolidated Appropriations Act, 2023. Accompanying me today is Dr. Susan Black, Suicide Prevention Officer, with the Outreach, Transition and Economic Development Service in the Veterans Benefits Administration.

In 2020, 44,298 adult Americans died by suicide. Of those, 6,146 were Veterans. These numbers are more than statistics—they reflect individual lives prematurely ended and they continue to be grieved by family members, loved ones and the Nation as a whole. More work remains to amplify Veteran suicide prevention efforts alongside each of you at the national, state and local levels.

Suicide is a complex problem with a multifaceted interweaving of potential contributing factors. In addition to mental health risk factors for suicide, we must look at a broader array of other contributing factors such as sociocultural risk factors and health related social needs that are also associated with suicide ideation and attempts.

Unemployment, chronic pain, insomnia, relationship strain and the death of a loved one are examples of individual factors outside the specific frame of mental health which may play a role in suicide. International, national, community and relational factors also impact suicide risk (e.g., inadequate access to care, global health concerns, war, economic crises or homelessness).[1] With no single cause, there is no single solution, and we must be comprehensive in our approach to prevent Veteran suicide.[2]

Every death by suicide is a tragedy and we will not relent in our efforts to end Veteran suicide. We know that suicide is preventable. It is a national public health issue that affects people from all walks of life, not just Veterans. Eliminating Veteran suicide is a top VA priority, and we continue to work diligently across the Department and with Federal, tribal, state and local governments to advance a public health approach to suicide prevention. The VA suicide prevention strategy is guided by the National Strategy for Preventing Veteran Suicide 2018-

---

[1] Turecki, G., & Brent, D. A. (2016) Suicide and suicidal behavior. *Lancet, 387*, 12271,227–39.

[2] Zalsman, G., Hawton, K., Wasserman, D., van Heeringen, K., Arensman, E., Sarchiapone, M., Carli, V., Höschl, C., Barzilay, R., Balazs, J., Purebl, G., Kahn, J. P., Sáiz, P. A., Lipsicas, C. B., Bobes, J., Cozman, D., Hegerl, U., & Zohar, J. (2016). Suicide prevention strategies revisited: 10-year systematic review. Lancet Psychiatry, 3(7), 646–659.

2028 and is in full alignment with the President's 2021 National Strategy for Reducing Military and Veteran Suicide.[3] More specifically, the VA suicide prevention strategy advances a comprehensive, cross- sector, evidence-informed public health approach with focal areas in lethal means safety (LMS); crisis care and care transition enhancements; increased access to effective care; addressing upstream risk and protective factors; enhanced research coordination; data sharing; and program evaluation efforts.

VA's public health approach requires a focus on evidence informed clinical and community initiatives. This means maximizing prevention efforts that cut across all sectors in which Veterans may interact and collaborating with Veterans Service Organizations, state and local leaders, medical professionals, criminal justice officials, private employers and many other stakeholders. VA's public health strategy combines collaborations with communities to implement tailored, local prevention plans while also focusing on evidence-based clinical strategies for intervention. We focus on both what we can do now, in the short term and over the long term, to implement VA's National Strategy for Preventing Veteran Suicide, through the following:

- Suicide Prevention (SP-2.0) Community-Based Intervention for Suicide Prevention (CBI-SP) model; and
- SP 2.0 Clinical Telehealth model which is a clinical approach focusing on broad dissemination of evidence-based psychotherapies.

The Suicide Prevention Now Plan (NOW) aims to develop and deploy interventions that are deemed to reach Veterans at high risk for suicide within 1 year. Led by staff in VA's Suicide Prevention Program and key VA partners, the plan includes targeted mental health and suicide prevention strategies to support Veterans, Veterans Health Administration (VHA) providers and the community. The five priority areas of the Now plan are as follows: (1) LMS, which promotes secure storage of firearms so that someone at elevated risk for suicide is less likely to use the firearm to attempt suicide; (2) suicide prevention in at-risk medical populations; (3) outreach to and understanding of prior VHA users; (4) suicide prevention program enhancements; and (5) educational media campaigns.

Through CBI-SP, 50 States and 5 territories are participating in the VA Substance Abuse and Mental Health Services Administration Governor's Challenge and more than 1,500 community coalitions have been formed across the country, working together towards ending Veteran suicide. The goal is to equip communities to help Veterans get the right care delivered whenever, wherever and however they need it.

The SP 2.0 Clinic Telehealth Program was implemented through a partnership between VA's Suicide Prevention and the VHA National Clinical Resource Hub leadership team to stand up national telehealth capability to provide the following evidence-based practice treatments (EBP):

- Cognitive Behavioral Therapy for Suicide Prevention;
- Problem-Solving Therapy for Suicide Prevention; and

[3] Department of Veterans Affairs (2018). National Strategy for Preventing Veteran Suicide. https://www.mentalhealth.va.gov/suicide_prevention/docs/Office-of-Mental-Health-and-Suicide-Prevention-National-Strategy-for-Preventing-Veterans-Suicide.pdf.

- Dialectical Behavior Therapy, as well as the Safety Planning Intervention.

Currently, there are over 100 clinical staff serving through SP 2.0 Clinical Telehealth. These providers are trained to offer EBPs for suicide prevention to Veterans with a recent history of suicidal self-directed violence. This service is available through all 18 Veteran Integrated Service Networks. As of September 18, 2023, since the program launched in April 2021, SP 2.0 Clinic Telehealth Program has completed over 7,000 mental health intake sessions.

According to the 2022 National Veteran Suicide Prevention Annual Report, when it comes to comparing Veterans and U.S. adults who died from suicide in 2020, guns were more commonly involved among Veterans (71.0%) than non-Veterans (50.3%).

The NOW Plan facilitated the Keep It Secure LMS media campaign, which launched in September 2021 and ended in June 2023 and garnered over 2.8 billion impressions, over 1.7 billion video completions and over 26 million website visits. This campaign targeted and reached a diverse audience of Veterans and their concerned others. By increasing time and space between lethal means and individuals at risk for suicide, suicide is reduced.

VA continues to innovate in this area and in February of 2023 VA announced the 10 winners of Mission Daybreak, a $20 million grant challenge aimed at developing innovations to reduce Veteran suicide. During this challenge, VA received more than 1,300 innovation submissions from Veterans, Veteran Service Organizations, community-based organizations, health technology companies, startups and universities – with solutions ranging from lethal means safety concepts and targeted virtual care programs to other promising suicide prevention solutions that offer healing and recovery to Veterans. Mission Daybreak is the largest cash Federal incentive prize since the establishment of the Prize Authority.[4]

Hannon Act

The Hannon Act was built upon this comprehensive approach, and we are pleased to report on VA's progress in implementing the Hannon Act since our last hearing on this topic in 2020. Broadly, the Hannon Act prioritized staffing expansion, targeted suicide prevention efforts, and research, establishing best practice models for mental health care delivery and providing critical oversight and accountability for mental health programs. We look forward to discussing VA progress in these areas.

Suicide Prevention

Regarding suicide prevention efforts, the Hannon Act has expanded access to critical mental health care resources. Section 201 of the Hannon Act established the Staff Sergeant Parker Gordon Fox Suicide Prevention Grant Program (SSG Fox SPGP), allowing VA to provide grants to eligible entities to expand suicide prevention services to eligible individuals and their

---

[4] Department of Veterans Affairs (2023). Winners Revealed in VA's $20M Mission Daybreak Grand Challenge to Reduce Veteran Suicides. https://news.va.gov/press-room/winners-revealed-in-vas-20m- mission-daybreak-grand-challenge-to-reduce-veteran-suicides/.

families to reduce the risk of suicide. In September 2022, VA awarded $52.5 million to 80 community-based organizations in 43 States, the District of Columbia and American Samoa. These organizations provide or coordinate the provision of suicide prevention services, thereby significantly expanding services provided to Veterans in the community. In March 2023, VA prepared for the second round of grant awards by publishing a Notice of Funding Opportunity for renewal grants and new organizations to apply for grants worth up to $750,000. The application period opened March 2, 2023, and closed May 19, 2023. The review and award process are underway. Awards will be announced by September 30, 2023, for services in fiscal year 2024. In July 2023, VA held its third in-person technical assistance event for the SSG Fox SPGP grantees. This two-day event included: LMS training; program guidance and implementation strategies; and the opportunity to share grantee success stories and examples of innovative suicide prevention services from among the cohort.

The Hannon Act provided VA the opportunity to review established suicide prevention processes to identify opportunities to enhance implementation. Several clinical initiatives identified in the Hannon Act have also been implemented across VHA as part of the SP Now plan. A few examples of these initiatives include increased hiring of mental health staff in Specialty Care clinics with Veterans at high risk for suicide, the Recovery Engagement and Coordination for Health-Veterans Enhanced Treatment (REACH-VET) Program and Safety Planning in the Emergency Department (SPED).

These initiatives are having a significant impact on patient safety. As of August 8, 2023, more than 54,500 VHA prescribers, representing all VHA facilities, have prescribed naloxone to over 477,500 Veterans with over 4,210 reported opioid overdose reversals. VA also implemented REACH-VET, which uses predictive modeling to identify Veterans at highest risk for suicide and then works to outreach and engage Veterans in care. REACH-VET has been associated with increased attendance at outpatient appointments, a greater proportion of individuals with new safety plans and reductions in mental health admissions and emergency department visits and reduction in suicide attempts. VA is exceeding benchmarks for all five REACH-VET metrics.

SPED is an evidence-based practice shown to reduce suicidal behaviors by 45%.[5] SPED promotes safety planning with Veterans who present to the emergency department with suicidal ideation, providing follow-up contact until treatment engagement occurs. Through technical assistance and individualized consultation, VA is exceeding SPED performance expectations, and the new White House strategy focused on reducing military and Veteran suicide is now looking to implement the practice in non-VA community hospitals.

Mental Health Services

VA provides mental health care services through a stepped-care model to promote mental health treatment at the least intensive level of care appropriate. Services include a full range of inpatient, residential and outpatient specialty and general mental health services available in VA and through community partners. Veterans may receive mental health care through primary

---

[5] Stanley, B., Brown, G. K., Brenner, L. A., Galfalvy, H. C., Currier, G. W., Knox, K. L., Chaudhury, S. R., Bush, A. L., & Green, K. L. (2018). Comparison of the safety planning intervention with follow-up vs usual care of suicidal patients treated in the emergency department. *JAMA Psychiatry*, *75*(9), 894–900.

care, self-directed options such as mobile apps and online programming, or through tele-mental health services.

The demand for mental health care continues to grow. The number of Veterans seen by mental health providers has doubled since 2006. VA employs 17,000 licensed mental health providers to address ongoing demand and expanding health care eligibilities; ensuring appropriate staffing levels are maintained is essential. VA is committed to not only hiring critical mental health staff, but also enhancing opportunities to train and develop mental health care professionals to address the national shortage. VA is committed to the mental health staffing model outlined in Section 501 of the Hannon Act. The VA has experienced tremendous mental health staff growth over the last 2 years. The Secretary and Undersecretary for Health are committed to hiring efforts targeting mental health staff and leveraging the staffing model developed in response to the Hannon Act. While at the early stages of the initiative, VA recognizes staffing efforts must continue to enhance access to care for underserved and rural areas of the Nation. To enhance hiring opportunities, VA continues to build on the occupational series for Licensed Professional Mental Health Counselors and Marriage (LPMHC) and Marriage Family Therapists (MFT). Since 2019, the number of LPMHCs and MFTs working in VA has more than doubled, and we are excited to continue to expand staffing across the enterprise.

Finally, recognizing the availability of mental health staff across the Nation is limited, the Hannon Act created opportunities to "grow our own" through educational scholarships. Hannon Act Section 502 authorizes Readjustment Counseling Services (RCS) to provide scholarships to individuals seeking mental health related advanced degrees in psychology, professional counseling (LPMHC), marriage and family therapy (MFT) and social work (MSW). The individual recipients will be required to work at a Vet Center for 6 years after graduation. RCS has completed the required regulatory process and partnered with the associated VA scholarship program offices have awarded the initial 29 scholarships for the fall semester 2023. These scholarships include tuition, book vouchers and monthly stipends and priority was given to Veteran applicants (17 awards). RCS is moving to a rolling application period with ongoing review and award for future semesters. RCS is continuing targeted outreach to universities in hard to recruit areas including rural and tribal communities. In addition, RCS is also engaging with professional organizations such as the American Psychological Association. These actions are designed to increase application submission from all professions.

Mental Health and Suicide Prevention Research

Opportunities to expand research to increase our understanding of suicide risk factors is a critical component of the Hannon Act. For example, VA is funding a study of the relationship between altitude and suicide among Veterans. This work is being led by a team of investigators from the Durham VA Medical Center in North Carolina working in collaboratively with investigators from the Department of Energy and using the supercomputer resources of the Department of Energy. The study began June 1, 2021, and is on track for completion within the Congressional timeline.

To expand our understanding of medical risk factors associated with suicide risk and increased mortality, VA initiated a contract with the National Academies of Sciences Engineering and Medicine (NASEM) in September 2022 that will continue through September

2024. The purpose of the contract is for NASEM to "to evaluate the effects of opioids and benzodiazepine on all-cause mortality of Veterans, including suicide." In the coming months, we anticipate the investigators will be presenting their independent analyses to the NASEM Committee, and the Committee will continue to meet in 2024, review the data analyses and prepare their final report.

The Hannon Act addressed opportunities to enhance health care practices through new and updated systematic practice reviews and in establishing tool kits for VA and community health care providers. Recognizing the critical importance of Clinical Practice Guidelines (CPG) for the treatment of serious mental illness, VA established two distinct workgroups of national experts to review best practices in the management of bipolar disorder and in psychosis. In 2023, VA and the Department of Defense (DoD) published new CPGs for bipolar disorder and for first-episode psychosis and schizophrenia. Additionally, the workgroup updating the VA/DoD CPG for Assessment and Management of Patients at Risk for Suicide (2019)[6] is actively engaged and on track for publishing the updated CPG in 2024. The Hannon Act also directed VA to assemble a provider toolkit and training materials for treating mental health comorbidities in collaboration with DoD. This toolkit is an assembly of publicly accessible resources for managing a wide array of mental health conditions, including violence and anger, cognitive disorders, moral injury, obsessive compulsive disorder and mood disorders, among others.

Strong Act

The STRONG Act contains more than two dozen sections that bolster VA's efforts to support Veterans' mental health and supports Veterans' equitable access to VA's life-saving resources by expanding mental health outreach to traditionally underserved Veterans, developing and delivering the most effective treatments, better equipping VA's workforce to provide care and further strengthening VA's Veterans Crisis Line (VCL). The STRONG Act requires VA to update training for the VA workforce and VCL staff, implement pilot programs, expand access to mental health care, conduct analysis and research and provide outreach to Veterans regarding mental health resources.

The STRONG Act aligns with VA's top clinical priority of preventing Veteran suicide and connecting Veterans with the best care through the expansion of culturally competent mental health and suicide prevention services to traditionally underserved Veterans and increased staffing and staffing across mental health disciplines.

VA has already successfully met the requirements of 3 of the 27 substantive sections contained in the law. Two of the completed sections are in title II of the Act, which focuses on VCL quality improvement action. The VCL is a national call center with trained responders available to any Veteran, Service member, or their loved ones 24/7/365. Launched in 2007, the VCL started with 14 trained responders working out of a call center in Canandaigua, N.Y. To date the VCL has responded to over 6 million calls, chats and texts and issued over 1 million referrals to local Suicide Prevention Coordinators. Beyond the call, VCL initiates the follow-up with caring letters, an evidence-based intervention found to reduce the rate of suicide death,

---

[6] Use Department of Veterans Affairs (2019). VA/DoD Clinical Practice Guidelines for Assessment and Management of Patients at Risk for Suicide, https://www.healthquality.va.gov/guidelines/mh/srb/.

attempts and ideation (Reger, et al. 2019). VCL services are enhanced by the Peer Support Outreach Call Center, providing outreach by certified peer specialists to support hope and recovery-oriented services after the initial call to VCL.

Through Congressional legislation and a Federal Communications Commission directive, VCL partnered with the Substance Abuse and Mental Health Services Administration and the 988 Suicide and Crisis Lifeline to establish 988. After the 988 roll out July 2022 through September 7, 2023, VCL demand has increased by the following amounts across phone, text, and chat services:

- Phone-based demand increased by 12.77% compared to the same time from the previous year.
- Text-based demand increased by 43.34% compared to the same time from the previous year.
- Chat-based demand increased by 10.78% compared to the same time from the previous year.

VCL is actively expanding operations to maintain the quality crisis intervention and mental health support services it provides. Since February 2021, VCL has grown from 877 full time employees (FTEE) to 1,812 FTEEs. In addition, VCL currently has 1,082 FTEE crisis responders, compared to 541 FTEEs in February 2021 . The implementation of title II and all the remaining sections is ongoing through collaboration with internal and external stakeholders.

Economic Factors Related to Veteran Suicide

Some Veterans report difficulty in transitioning to civilian positions and difficulty translating military-related skills to higher-paying civilian jobs. Unemployment and poverty are correlated with homelessness among Veterans. Financial hardship and economic stressors are major predictors of Veteran suicide. The Veterans Benefits Administration (VBA) provides a variety of benefits and services upstream which can help reduce or eliminate risk factors associated with suicide and promote protective factors for some Veterans. Programs such as Solid Start, Disability Compensation, Pension, Veteran Readiness and Employment and Education/GI Bill assist Veterans with transitioning to civilian life, connecting with benefits, establishing and achieving educational, vocational and career goals and supporting financial well-being.

VA Solid Start (VASS)

The first year after separation from military service poses challenges for recently separated Veterans that can make it difficult to adjust to civilian life and, for some, increase their risk of suicide. To provide added support during this critical period and to support VA's efforts to address Executive Order 13822, Supporting our Veterans During Their Transition from Uniformed Service to Civilian Life, VBA launched VASS in December 2019. VASS provides early and consistent caring contact to newly separated Veterans at least three times during their critical first year of transition from the military (0-90 days, 91-180 days and 181-365 days post-discharge from active duty). Specially trained VA representatives address issues or challenges identified by Veterans during these calls and assist them with accessing benefits, services, health care (including mental health care), education and employment opportunities. After each successful connection, the Veteran receives a comprehensive follow-up email from the VASS representative that provides information on all issues discussed and lists connections for additional support and assistance. This email specifically provides contact information for service organizations and connections to state Veteran resources, based on information provided by the Veteran as to where they currently or intend to reside.

For fiscal year 2023 (through August) VASS has connected with 186,301 (71.3%) eligible Veterans. VASS also provides priority contact to individuals who had a mental health care appointment during the last year of active duty, supporting a successful transition to VA mental health care treatment.

Outreach, Transition and Economic Development (OTED) Service

In addition to VASS, OTED provides the Transition Assistance, Military to Civilian (M2C) Ready Framework, Financial Literacy, Economic Development Initiatives, Outreach and Personalized Career Planning Guidance. The M2C Ready Framework is a joint VA and DoD codified transition period beginning 365 days prior to separation and extending 365 days post-separation. It ensures successful and holistic interagency support for Service members and Veterans as they transition from military to civilian life. These programs also provide understanding of and easy access to VA benefits and resources to ensure Service members have a smooth and successful transition to civilian life. In addition, transitioning Service members, Veterans and their families are educated about employment opportunities, special hiring authorities and career support resources. Financial empowerment information and tools through partnership with the Department of Labor, DOD and Prudential is also offered. Additionally, outreach events focused on raising awareness of suicide prevention and available resources such as information on VCL and the new Dial 988 then Press 1 for the VCL is shared.

Providing support to Service members during their transition, both prior to and following their separation, is critical to preventing suicide in Veterans and transitioning Service members. Collaboratively, VHA and VBA utilize several programs to provide benefits and services aimed at helping reduce or eliminate risk factors associated with suicide while increasing protective factors for Veterans.

Conclusion

We appreciate the Committee's continued support and collaboration in this shared mission. Mr. Chairman, this concludes my statement. My colleague and I are ready to answer any questions you and the committee may have.

Wounded Warrior Project
Statement of John Eaton, Vice President for Complex Care on "Invisible Wounds of War: Improving Mental Health and Suicide Prevention Measures for Our Nation's Veterans"
September 20, 2023

Chairman Tester, Ranking Member Moran, and distinguished members of the Senate Committee on Veterans' Affairs – thank you for inviting Wounded Warrior Project (WWP) to submit this written statement for the record of today's hearing on mental health and suicide prevention. We share your commitment to easing the pain of veterans who are suffering from invisible wounds and appreciate the opportunity to offer our perspective on potential congressional action to improve post-9/11 veterans' access to mental health care and suicide prevention measures.

For 20 years WWP has been dedicated to our mission to honor and empower wounded warriors. In addition to our advocacy before Congress, we offer more than a dozen direct service programs focused on connection, independence, and wellness in every spectrum of a warrior's life. These programs span mental, physical, and financial domains to create a 360-degree model of care and support. This holistic approach empowers warriors to create a life worth living and helps them build resilience, coping skills, and peer connection. Our organization has grown alongside the warriors we serve, and we strive to tailor our programming to the evolving needs of a post-9/11 generation of warriors that has become increasingly diverse. Our reach extends to more than 195,000 veterans who are being served in various ways across the United States.

In this context, assisting warriors with their mental health challenges has consistently been our largest programming investment over the past several years. In Fiscal Year 2022, WWP spent more than $82 million in mental and brain health programs – an investment consistent with the fact that more than 7 in 10 respondents to our 2022 Annual Warrior Survey self-reported at least one mental health condition, and nearly the same amount (66.3%) reported visiting a professional in the past 12 months to help with issues such as stress, emotional, alcohol, drug, or family problems.[7]

As diagnoses of post-traumatic stress disorder (PTSD), depression, and anxiety have consistently ranked among the top five most self-reported conditions across previous editions of our Annual Warrior Survey, our Mental Health Continuum of Support has matured over the last decade and now allows us to engage each individual based on their unique needs.[8] WWP supports warriors by providing accessible and innovative solutions to mental health support including four programs focused specifically on mental health: Warrior Care Network, WWP Talk, Project Odyssey, and Complex Case Coordination. Each of these programs are designed to support and empower post-9/11 veterans and their families in building resilience and overcoming the challenges before them. Through these four programs in Fiscal Year 2022 alone, WWP provided warriors and their family members with nearly 55,000 hours of treatment for mental health conditions, including PTSD, traumatic brain injury, substance use disorder, and other mental health conditions.

---

[7] WWP's 2022 Annual Warrior Survey can be viewed at https://www.woundedwarriorproject.org/mission/annual-warrior-survey.

[8] More information on WWP's Mental Health Continuum of Support can be found at the end of the document.

Of course, WWP believes that no one organization can meet the needs of all wounded, injured, or ill veterans alone. Partnerships with and investments in other military and veteran support organizations help guide collaboration that allows WWP to amplify the effects of our efforts. For purposes of today's hearing, we will focus on our largest and most significant partner in meeting the needs of post-9/11 wounded warriors: the Department of Veterans Affairs (VA). The perspectives that follow are intended to identify and discuss what we believe to be among the most critical areas of concern related to mental health and suicide prevention as viewed through access to care, workforce, long-term care, financial wellness, and research perspectives.

Access to Care

- Ensure adherence to access standards and promote transparency in community care network wait times
- Improve timely access to residential rehabilitation treatment programs
- Encourage use of telehealth to remove barriers to care
- Prioritize evaluation of SSG Parker Gordon Fox Suicide Prevention Grant Program

More than 9 in 10 (91%) warriors who responded to the 2022 Annual Warrior Survey use VA for their health care needs. Only a segment of these respondents rely exclusively on VA for care however, and many use a variety of sources for mental health support – to include WWP programs and services. When dealing with stress, emotional challenges, or mental health concerns, WWP warriors report that they most often turn to: talking with family and friends (65.5%), talking with another veteran (60.6%), prescription medication (59.0%), services at VA medical centers (55.3%), and physical activity (54.6%). By offering peer support and a variety of programs tailored to address stressors across physical, mental, and financial domain, WWP is able to capture an informed perspective on why veterans seek care and why they turn to WWP.

Access to Mental Health Care

Currently when a warrior reaches out to WWP for mental health support, their first step to finding care is a conversation with our Triage team. The Triage team conducts screenings of a warrior's mental health history, provides the warrior with information about our various mental health offerings, and refers the warrior to the most appropriate mental health program within WWP or an external resource. In FY 22, our Triage team received 12,610 referrals to find warriors appropriate treatment, placed 10,634 referrals for mental health support (including 5,630 referrals to external outpatient care providers), and made their first connection with interested warriors an average of 1.04 days later.

A common point of feedback from warriors seeking care and support through WWP is that VA wait times for mental health are offered at future dates that exceed VA's access standard of 20 days for mental health care. Appointments that are many weeks – if not months – away erode trust in VA's ability to provide care at reasonable intervals. Appointment cancellations that result in even more delay can further discourage health seeking behavior or push veterans toward finding care independently. And when group therapy is offered in place of individual counseling to expedite care delivery, a veteran patient may feel that they are getting a lesser service or be turned off by the idea entirely. Options for seeking care in the community are rarely discussed in detail and more often left to the veteran to navigate (and enforce) their path to receiving care sooner. Instances like these allow organizations like WWP to step in and fill the need for rapid access to care that is tailored to meet individual needs and desires.

To this end, WWP supports taking additional congressionally directed measures intended to make community care more accessible for veterans seeking mental health care. WWP is pleased to support both the Making Community Care Work for Veterans Act (S. 2649) and the Veterans' Health Empowerment, Access, Leadership, and Transparency for Our Heroes (HEALTH) Act (S. 1315) and their respective embrace of addressing disparities on VA's adherence to access standards. While there are distinctions discussed in more detail in the sections that follow, both bills would recognize that the current access standards for mental health have been deemed appropriate across two Administrations – and that the key to success will be ensuring that they are clearly communicated and adhered to.

Access to Residential Rehabilitation Treatment Programs

The access standards contemplated by the VA MISSION Act (P.L. 115-182 § 104) and memorialized in the Code of Federal Regulations (38 C.F.R. § 17.4040) do not, in practice, extend to mental or substance use disorder care provided in a residential setting. VA has maintained adherence to access standards for this type of care through Veterans Health Administration (VHA) Directive 1162.02, which establishes a priority admission standard of 72 hours and, for all other cases, 30 days before a veteran must be offered (not necessarily provided) alternative residential treatment or another level of care that meets the veteran's needs and preferences at the time of screening.

Due to this approach, veterans seeking mental or substance use disorder care provided in a residential setting are not subject to the access standard protections assigned under law. VA is not required to inform these veterans of their expected wait time. See P.L. 117-328, Div. U, § 122. Veterans are not guaranteed the soonest possible starting time before a community referral must be made. See P.L. 117-328, Div. U, § 121; 38 U.S.C. § 1703(d)(4). The access standards used are not applicable to community care network providers who receive referrals for these veterans' care. See P.L. 117-328, Div. U, § 125; 38 U.S.C. § 1703B(f).

Most importantly, if appropriate community-based providers are identified and available to provide treatment, veterans waiting beyond VHA's policy-backed access standards have no dependable, clear, and consistent recourse to be referred for that care. VA has presented data suggesting that only 38% of veterans meeting priority admission criteria were admitted to VA within 72 hours, and that the average wait time before admission among all veterans receiving Mental Health Residential Rehabilitation Treatment Program (MH RRTP) care was 24 days – just 6 days less than the 30-day access standard and among a population where 53% were admitted within 14 days. Although information on admissions within 30 days was not provided in the presentation where this data was cited, we believe it reflects that many veterans have waited more than 30 days for admission to care.

We are excited to see a number of bills that are aimed at improving access to mental or substance use disorder care provided in a residential setting or VA's MH RRTP. There are currently three pieces of legislation seeking to address this issue in different ways. The first, the Making Community Care Work for Veterans Act (S. 2649) would require VA to update the policies and operational guidance for the MH RRTP program. VA would also be required to standardize the referral, screening, and admission process and complete the screenings and admission decisions within 72 hours for veterans who meet priority admission standards.

Additionally, an appeals process would be established for any veteran denied entry to the program or not offered a timely placement and VA would be required to update and conduct training for VA providers and care coordinators regarding these changes.

Next, the Veterans' HEALTH Act (S. 1315) would incorporate MH RRTP with the existing extended care services access standard (30-minute average drive time/20 days). This approach would remove the "non-institutional" qualification around extended services but would expressly exclude nursing home care. Lastly, the Veteran Care Improvement Act (H.R. 3520) would create a new access standard for alcohol and drug dependence MH RRTP (30-minute average drive time/10 days) and VA would be required to consider a veteran's eligibility within 72 hours of receiving their request.

While each of these bills address the issues we are seeing in terms of access to mental health and substance use disorder care in a residential setting in different ways, we believe they all represent an improvement from the status quo. We believe each approach would enhance accountability, transparency, and oversight on this critical provision of care and ultimately lead to better outcomes for veterans and ensure they are receiving the care they need in a timely manner.

Telehealth

Since the onset of the COVID-19 pandemic, VA has been a leader in embracing and providing telehealth. VA has seen a rapid rise in the numbers of veterans using telehealth to receive their care, and telehealth is similarly popular in the WWP warrior community. Among warriors who were offered a telehealth appointment in the last 12 months, 89.3% reported using telehealth during that period. Among those not offered a telehealth appointment, a majority (63.9%) said they would have used it if presented as an option. Telehealth is a cost-effective way to improve access to care for many warriors that may face barriers to care, including long driving distances, work schedules, and the need for childcare.

We are pleased to see that telehealth is addressed as an access to care issue in both the Making Community Care Work for Veterans Act (S. 2649) and the Veterans' HEALTH Act (S. 1315). Section 103 of the Making Community Care Work for Veterans Act would allow VA to offer telehealth appointments to veterans as means of satisfying access standards when the telehealth appointment is accepted by the veteran. Section 101(a) of the Veterans' HEALTH Act would omit telehealth appointment availability at VA from determinations of eligibility for community care network access; however, Section 105 would require VA to discuss telehealth appointment options with the veteran when it is available, clinically appropriate, and acceptable to the veteran.

While these two approaches are not in complete alignment, both hold potential to deliver better access to care than current practices. Generally speaking, veterans that seek mental health care through WWP express that options for care in the community are not clearly discussed with VA providers. As noted earlier in this section, the VA appointment is often the only option discussed in detail even when offered at a date that exceeds current access standards. Better outcomes can be achieved when options are clearly laid out, and in our experience, telehealth is often a preferred method for those we serve. However, these preferences should not be assumed, and veterans should be provided with more clarity and transparency when weighing their options for care. According to WWP's 2022 Annual Warrior Survey, of those WWP warriors who were not offered a telehealth appointment, 36.1% reported they would have said no to utilizing the appointment even if they were offered it (30.1% for women and 37.1% for male warriors). For that reason, WWP believes telehealth can met the access standards require only when a veteran has agreed to. Additionally, if a veteran choses to stop using telehealth in favor or in-person care, they should not be denied the right for in-person care and community care should be made available if VA is unable to meet the access standards.

Lastly, we should take additional steps to ensure better telehealth connectivity because access to broadband service benefits veterans in several important ways. Like all Americans, veterans benefit from strong and reliable internet access that can foster career opportunities through telework, access to online education, and more opportunities to participate in the digital economy. In addition, as the use of telehealth resources continues to expand, the access to a stable and affordable internet network is increasingly becoming instrumental in maintaining a veteran's physical and mental health and wellness.

Despite these benefits, veteran households subscribe to mobile broadband services at lower rates than households without veterans. 2.2 million veteran households lack either fixed or mobile broadband connections at home. The monthly cost of service or the cost of a computer is often cited as a key barrier to broadband adoption.[9] VA and Census Bureau data show that almost 7% of veterans live below the poverty level leading many to forgo home internet access and instead seek access in libraries or community centers.[10] This is especially pronounced in rural areas. Of the 4.4 million rural and highly rural veterans, 44% earn less than $35,000 a year and 27% do not access the internet at home.[11]

The Affordable Connectivity Program (ACP) is a Federal Communications Commission benefit program that helps ensure that households can afford the broadband they need for work, school, healthcare and more. The benefit provides a discount of up to $30 per month toward internet service for eligible households and up to $75 per month for households on qualifying Tribal lands. Eligible households can also receive a one-time discount of up to $100 to purchase a laptop, desktop computer, or tablet from participating providers if they contribute more than $10 and less than $50 toward the purchase price. The ACP is limited to one monthly service discount and one device discount per household. To be eligible, a household's income must be at or below 200% of the poverty level ($60,000 a year for a family or $29,000 for an individual)

---

[9] *See* JOHN HORRIGAN and MAEVE DUGGAN, PEW RESEARCH CTR., HOME BROADBAND 2015 4 (Dec. 2015), *available at* https://www.pewresearch.org/wp-content/uploads/sites/9/2015/12/Broadband-adoption-full.pdf; Colin Rhinesmith et al., Benton Inst. for Broadband & Society, *The Complexity of 'Relevance' as a Barrier to Broadband Adoption* (Jan. 2016), *available at* https://www.benton.org/blog/complexity-relevance-barrier-broadband-adoption.

[10] *See* U.S. DEP'T OF VET. AFFAIRS, *Veterans Poverty Trends Report* 3 (May 2015), *available at* https://www.va.gov/vetdata/docs/specialreports/veteran_poverty_trends.pdf (noting an 8.7% increase in veterans living in poverty in the 2010- 2012 time period, compared to the 2005-2007 time period).

[11] *Rural Veterans*, U.S. DEP'T OF VET. AFFAIRS, https://www.ruralhealth.va.gov/aboutus/ruralvets.asp (last visited Sep. 18, 2023).

or participating in certain government programs including veterans' pension or VA survivor benefits.

To date, over 600,000 veterans have signed up for the ACP; however, funding for the program is expected to run out by late Fiscal Year 2023 or early Fiscal Year 2024. The ACP was appropriated $14.2 billion in the Infrastructure and Jobs Act (P.L. 117-58, Div. J, Title IV) and WWP supports a reauthorization of funding for 1-2 years until the program can be made permanent.

Suicide Prevention Grant Program

Section 201 of the Commander John Scott Hannon Veterans Mental Health Care Improvement Act (P.L. 116-171) authorized the launch of the Staff Sergeant Parker Gordon Fox Suicide Prevention Grant Program, an innovative new approach to bolstering VA partnerships and enhancing collaboration on community-based suicide prevention strategies. In Fiscal Year 2022, the first year of this three-year pilot program, VA awarded $52.5 million to 80 organizations that provide or coordinate a range of suicide prevention programs for veterans and their families.[12] WWP was an early supporter of this initiative, and we remain committed to its success.

While metrics and impact are in the earliest stages of review, our feedback to date is largely anecdotal and based on our organizational experience. We agree that no one organization – and no single agency – can fully meet all veterans' needs. We recognize that empirically supported mental health treatment works when it is available and when it is pursued, but the best results will be found by embracing a public health approach focused on increasing resilience and psychological well-being and building an aggressive prevention strategy. In this context, we offer two important considerations for the Committee.

First, organizations WWP has worked with have expressed concern that the application and compliance requirements can be onerous. Although expectations were clearly laid out by VA,[13] some participants have shared with WWP that aligning a veteran's eligibility with delivery of specific services can be challenging. A veteran must meet definitions set out at Section 201(q)(4) of the Hannon Act, which includes consideration of a myriad of health, environmental, and historical risk factors for suicide. While acknowledging these predispositions are important in early and direct conversations about suicide, approaching such considerations without a foundation of trust can sometimes discourage veterans from being honest with their responses or willing to accept and engage in services. Allowing some time to foster a relationship enables engagement in difficult conversations that stem from place of care and compassion, rather than obligation. Navigating discussions in such a way can foster more immediate connect to services that mitigate their risk for suicide and reduce emergent needs while also making the delivery of those services ineligible for grant purposes. Others have noted that the high volume of veteran assessments required can induce incentives (like providing small gifts) for completion that may skew the quality of data gathered and what practices are sound under the premises of the grant. We encourage more investigation into how

[12] Matthew Miller, *VA grant funding helping prevent Veteran suicides*, U.S. DEP'T OF VET. AFFAIRS (Aug. 15, 2023), https://news.va.gov/122642/va-grant-funding-help-prevent-veteran-suicides/.

[13] Funding Opportunity: Staff Sergeant Parker Gordon Fox Suicide Prevention Grant Program, 87 Fed. Reg. 22630 (Apr. 15, 2022).

administrative practices can better align with the intended purpose of connecting more veterans with support.

Second, the provision of clinical care under this grant program should be more grounded in practical considerations for delivering veterans evidence-based mental health care. Currently, when grantees are treating eligible individuals at risk of suicide or other mental or behavioral health conditions, the grantee must refer that individual to VA for follow-on care. If they do not, any care given is at the expense of the grantee.[14] However, some veterans are not comfortable receiving care at VA for a variety of reasons. This puts the grantee in a difficult situation where they are forced to stop providing care or provide care at their own expense, something many programs may be unable to afford. Additionally, if a grantee is a part of VA's Community Care Network, they are still required to get additional VA authorization to provide a veteran follow-up care. We would ask the Committee to consider if there are ways this process can be improved so that more veterans at risk of suicide can be connected to care they know and trust as soon as possible.

Mental Health Workforce

- Provide support for VA to recruit and retain high quality mental health providers
- Advance policies that promote a stronger mental health and substance use treatment provider base across the United States

Currently we are facing a dire shortage of mental health providers, both in VA and in the community. The Health Resources & Services Administration estimates that 164 million Americans live in areas with mental health professional shortages.[15] They estimate over 8,000 providers are needed to fill this need.[16] Within VA there is a similar story. While VA has made good progress on filling vacancies, a recent report from the Office of Inspector General (OIG) found severe shortages in a number of critical areas. The OIG found that 91 VHA facilities identified psychology as a severe shortage occupation, 73 VHA facilities identified psychiatry as a severe shortage occupation, and 33 VHA facilities identified inpatient mental health registered nurse (RN) staff as a severe shortage area.[17] These shortages are directly impacting veterans' access to care, increasing wait times for mental health treatment, and putting veterans' lives in danger.

Wounded Warrior Project urges Congress to take urgent action to invest in a more robust mental health workforce. One way to do this is by passing the VA CAREERS Act (S. 10). This legislation would help to address the current mental health workforce shortages at VA by giving them additional tools to recruit and retain providers. It would modernize VA's pay system for physicians and high-level clinicians, allow VA to pay for licensure exam costs for future clinicians that are participating in VA scholarship programs, expand eligibility for health care

[14] *Id.*

[15] HEALTH RES. AND SERVS. ADMIN., U.S. DEP'T OF HEALTH AND HUMAN SERVS., HEALTH WORKFORCE SHORTAGE AREAS (Sep. 18, 2023), https://data.hrsa.gov/topics/health-workforce/shortage-areas.

[16] *Id.*

[17] OFF. OF INSP. GENERAL, U.S. DEP'T OF VET. AFFAIRS, OIG DETERMINATION OF VETERANS HEALTH ADMINISTRATION'S SEVERE OCCUPATIONAL STAFFING SHORTAGES FISCAL YEAR 2023 (Aug. 2023).

staff that can be reimbursed for professional education costs, and improve VA's workforce data reporting systems so they are able to better track hiring and onboarding. While this legislation's scope exceeds mental health, it can build upon momentum from previous legislation focused on mental health like the STRONG Veterans Act (P.L. 117-328, Div. V) which expanded the Vet Center workforce (§ 102), created more paid trainee positions in mental health disciplines (§ 103), and offered more scholarship and loan repayment opportunities for those pursuing degrees or training in mental health fields (§ 104).

To help address the shortage outside of VA and for those veterans who utilize VA's Community Care Network, Congress should pass the Mental Health Professionals Workforce Shortage Loan Repayment Act (S. 462/H.R. 4933). This bill would provide up to $250,000 in eligible student loan repayment for mental health professionals in substance use disorder treatment who pursue employment in Mental Health Professional Shortage Areas. With increasing numbers of veterans specifically seeking treatment for substance use disorder, passing this legislation will allow additional providers into this space, resulting in better access to care for veterans and shorter wait times for treatment.

Traumatic Brain Injury and Long-Term Care

- Remove barriers to care that can impede quality of life and promote better mental health

For many post-9/11 veterans, brain health is a crucial factor in overall quality of life. Brain trauma, specifically traumatic brain injury (TBI), has been referred to as a "signature injury" for post-9/11 veterans, and this remains true for many we serve. 37% of WWP warriors self-report experiencing TBI as a result of their military service. Research shows that TBI can have a serious impact on a veteran's mental health. Some of the most common symptoms reported from warriors after a brain injury include feeling anxious or tense, problems with sleep, and irritability. Of warriors who self-reported experiencing TBI, 72% visited a mental health professional within the last 12 months to help with issues such as stress, emotional, alcohol, drug, or family problems and 60% presented with moderate to severe symptoms for two or more mental health conditions. Warriors who self-reported experiencing TBI are also more likely to report suicidal thoughts in the past 12 months than warriors who did not report experiencing TBI, more likely to have suicidal ideations, and have a higher rate of needing aid and assistance from another person.

Other research has studied the relationship between TBI and suicide finding that the risk of suicide was 2.19 times higher for those with TBI than those without.[18] The risk was even greater for those with moderate to severe TBI.[19] Due to the elevated risk for this population, it is crucial that we support and create better programs and more options for veterans with moderate to severe TBI that can help to mitigate other compounding factors for this population like financial needs, caregiving needs, and access to care.

---

[18] Trisha A. Hostetter et al., Suicide and Traumatic Brain Injury Among Individuals Seeking Veterans Health Administration Services Between Fiscal Years 2006 and 2015, 35(5) J. HEAD TRAUMA REHAB. E1, E1-E9 (2019).

[19] Id.

One recent success in this area was the passage of the Long-Term Care Veterans Choice Act which was included in the Joseph Maxwell Cleland and Robert Joseph Dole Memorial Veterans Benefits and Health Care Improvement Act (P.L. 117-328, Div. U § 165) last year.

This law will allow veterans increased flexibility with their health benefits, authorizing VA to cover the cost of medical foster homes for veterans that are otherwise eligible for nursing home care. Not only will this result lower costs for VA, as the cost of a medical foster home is significantly lower than nursing homes, but veterans will also be given an option that allows them more independence and a potentially higher quality of life in a non-institutional setting.

Today, we urge Congress to take additional steps to increase options for care for veterans with TBI. One way to do this is by passing the Elizabeth Dole Home Care Act (S. 141/H.R. 542). This legislation would improve veterans' access to long term support services through provisions that would instruct VA to provide informal Geriatrics and Extended Care (GEC) program assessment tools to help veterans and caregivers identify expanded services they are eligible for. Other provisions would codify existing GEC programs and provide assistance to caregivers that are denied or discharged from the Program for Comprehensive Assistance for Family Caregivers into other VA provided support. These provisions will help to provide additional resources to veterans with complex needs, many suffering from the effects of TBI. We also urge you to include the important provision that would increase the non-institutional expenditure cap from 65% to 100% to help ease the economic burden that many of these veterans and their families face.

Another piece of legislation that will improve options for veterans with TBI is the Expanding Veterans' Options for Long-Term Care Act (S. 495/H.R. 1815). Like the new law allowing VA to pay for medical foster home lodging (with annual caps), this bill requires VA to implement a three-year pilot program that will assess the effectiveness of providing assisting living services to eligible veterans. This would allow veterans serious needs more flexibility and the option to live more independently. Lastly, the Innovative Cognitive Care for Veterans Act (H.R. 5002) would establish a pilot program at VA to partner with private organizations, nonprofit foundations, and other community support entities to provide veterans access to telehealth and other innovative technologies that slow the progression of cognitive disorders through interactive engagement and stimulation solutions. Given that TBI often results in cognitive issues, this program will give veterans with TBI access to new, innovative care that we believe will result in overall improved mental health outcomes.

While the above laws primarily focus on long-term care resources and the wellbeing of caregivers, it is not lost on WWP that the stressors impacting family members of those suffering from TBI can negatively impact the mental health wellbeing of the warrior.

Financial Wellness

- Foster financial security by advancing legislation that will provide economic empowerment
- Improve the standards for pursuing service-connected disabilities related to military sexual trauma

Another important factor that can have a considerable effect on a warrior's mental health is their financial well-being. According to our 2022 Annual Warrior Survey, 64% of WWP warriors reported that they did not have enough money to make ends meet at some point in the last 12 months. Amongst these warriors, 64% presented with moderate to severe depression symptoms, 57% presented with PTSD symptoms, 17% reported using recreational drugs within the past year, and 71% reported visiting a mental health professional in the last year.

The link between mental health and financial health is well established. Higher degrees of financial worries are significantly associated with higher levels of psychological distress.[20] Additionally, the Annual Warrior Survey found that warriors who reported moderate and high financial well-being were 4.6 times more likely to report having better mental health than the general U.S. population.

Financial Security Legislation

We believe that there are several important legislative paths Congress can take to improve veterans' financial security and with it, their mental health. The first is by passing the Major Richard Star Act (S. 344, H.R. 1282). This legislation would allow Chapter 61 retirees whose disabilities arose from combat-related activities, to receive both their Department of Defense retirement pay and their VA disability compensation concurrently. We believe these are two distinct benefits established by Congress for two different purposes and passing this legislation would give over 50,000 veterans the benefits, and improved financial stability, they have been unfortunately denied until now.

Additionally, we know that meaningful employment not only improves a veteran's financial situation but can also have a powerful impact on their overall mental health. There are currently several pieces of legislation WWP has endorsed to provide additional employment opportunities for veterans, a number of which leverage the vast number of opportunities with the federal government. The Get Rewarding Outdoor Work (GROW) for our Veterans Act (H.R.1786) would establish a two-year pilot program, administered by the Secretary of the Interior, to employ veterans in federal positions that relate to conservation, environmental protection, and resource management. The Veterans Border Patrol Training Act (S. 774) would establish a pilot program through the Department of Defense's SkillBridge program to train and hire transitioning Service members at the U.S. Customs and Border Patrol (CBP). And finally, the Employing Veterans to Feed America Act (H.R. 5014) would establish a pilot program to provide veterans employment at the Department of Agriculture, particularly in positions that would allow veterans access to the outdoors. In addition to the other benefits a veteran may receive from employment, these careers allow for other mental health advantages that have been found from being outdoors. A growing body of research has shown these to include reduced depression, improved physical and psychological well-being, social connection, and resilience.

Within VA jurisdiction, WWP also supports extending an important pilot to prepare veterans for careers in STEM fields. Congress can pass the VET-TEC Authorization Act (H.R. 1669) which would fund the Veteran Employment Through Technology Education Courses

20 Soomin Ryu & Lu Fan, The Relationship Between Financial Worries and Psychological Distress Among U.S. Adults, 44(1) J. FAM. ECON. ISSUES 16, 16-33 (2022).

(VET-TEC) program that offers eligible veterans training in high-demand areas including computer software, computer programming, data processing, information science, and media applications. VET-TEC participants have been more racially and ethnically diverse and more likely to have a service-connected disability when compared to the wider population of working- age veterans in the U.S. population.[21] At a time when wounded veterans continue to have challenges finding and maintaining employment, we believe that extending VET-TEC under this legislation will allow more veterans to prepare for and access better, higher-paying careers, allowing them to have reduced financial stress and improved outcomes.

Service Connection Related to MST

Lastly, Congress should pass the Servicemembers and Veterans Empowerment and Support (SAVES) Act (S. 1028/H.R. 2441). According to VA, 1 in 3 women and 1 in 50 men report experiencing military sexual trauma (MST) when they are screened by their VA provider.[22] However, we know that many instances of MST go unreported for a variety of reasons, including feelings of shame, fears of reprisal, and concerns that they won't be believed. Because so many instances of MST go unreported, it can be challenging to provide the necessary evidence when filing claims with VBA. This results in many individuals not being able to receive the benefits that they deserve, putting them in a more challenging financial position. The SAVES Act would expand the evidentiary standard for MST survivors applying for VA benefits by requiring VA to consider non-DoD evidence sources when reviewing MST claims. The legislation would also make other improvements to the MST claims process to ensure greater accuracy resulting in survivors having better support and resources moving forward.

Oversight and Research

- Protect veterans from the dangers of opioid prescriptions
- Improve reporting on veteran suicide

Protect Warriors from the Dangers of Opioid Prescriptions

Studies have shown that chronic pain is negatively associated with physical and mental health quality of life. Chronic pain may significantly reduce individuals' quality of life by causing functional, social, emotional, and socioeconomic changes, such as changes in sleep patterns, isolation, an increase in depression, and lack of productivity.[23] About three in four (75.8%)

---

[21] U.S. GOV'T ACCOUNTABILITY OFF., VETERANS EMPLOYMENT: PROMISING VA TECHNOLOGY EDUCATION PILOT WOULD BENEFIT FROM BETTER OUTCOME MEASURES AND PLANS FOR IMPROVEMENT 8 (Oct. 2022).

[22] Military Sexual Trauma, U.S. DEP'T OF VET. AFFAIRS, https://www.ptsd.va.gov/understand/types/sexual_trauma_military.asp (last visited Sep. 18, 2023).

[23] Bruno Saconi et al., The Influence of Sleep Disturbances and Sleep Disorders on Pain Outcomes Among Veterans: A Systemic Scoping Review, 56 SLEEP MED. REV. 101411 (2021); ARIEL BARIA ET AL., CHRONIC PAIN IN MILITARY VETERANS, FEATURES AND ASSESSMENTS OF PAIN, ANESTHESIA, AND ANALGESIA 225-234 (Academic Press, 2022).

WWP warriors responding to the 2022 Annual Warrior Survey scored in a range indicating moderate or severe pain. The overall average Pain, Enjoyment of Life, and General Activity (PEG) scale score among all WWP warriors was 5.3, which indicates moderate pain that interferes with activities and enjoyment of life.

For a number of reasons, it is concerning that over half of warriors (51.5%) responding to the Annual Warrior Survey are managing pain with prescription pain medication. Within an opioid epidemic that has touched countless lives across the country, drug overdose mortality rates among veterans increased by 53% from 2010 to 2019[24] resulting in over 42,000 deaths[25].

According to a 2019 study, nearly half of combat wounded veterans have reported misuse of prescription opioids.[26] VA's annual suicide prevention report revealed that the suicide rate for recent VHA users with a diagnosis of opioid use disorders rose by 35.4% between 2019 and 2020 (the highest rate of increase across all observed health diagnoses).

For these reasons, we encourage the Committee to provide veterans with more options to prevent addiction. First, we recommend oversight of VA's Opioid Safety Initiative. Launched in 2013, this initiative has led to many positive results including fewer veterans prescribed opioid use.[27] However, there may be other consequences worth exploring in consideration of statistics shared above. Second, new laws and approaches pursued outside of the VA health system may reveal best practices and research that can be tailored to VHA. For example, the Non-Opioids Prevent Addiction In the Nation (NOPAIN) Act (P.L. 117-328) addressed the prescription of non- opioid treatments used to manage pain in both the hospital outpatient department (HOPD) and the ambulatory surgery center (ASC) settings by expanding non-opioid options for patients.

With precedent as a guide, TRICARE may soon follow a similar path and implement a comparable policy.[28] We encourage the Committee to explore the possibility of extrapolating the framework implemented in the NOPAIN Act (P.L. 117-328) into VA's system.

Reporting on Veteran Suicide

To best address and prevent veteran suicide, it is critical that we have as much data about the issue as possible. The Not Just a Number Act (S. 928/H.R. 4157) will improve our understanding of what factors play a role in veteran suicide and what the most affective interventions are. First, the legislation will require submission of the "National Veteran Suicide Prevention Annual Report" before the end of September of each year. The legislation also requires VA to include essential data on not only veteran health care usage but also VA benefits usage such as VA home loans, GI bill benefits, and disability compensation. This will allow all

---

24 *Substance Use and Military Life DrugFacts*, NAT'L INST. DRUG ABUSE, SUBSTANCE USE AND MILITARY LIFE DRUGFACTS, https://nida.nih.gov/publications/drugfacts/substance-use-military-life (last visited Sep. 18, 2023).

25 Mark Begley et al., *Veteran Drug Overdose Mortality, 2010-2019*, 233 DRUG AND ALCOHOL DEPENDENCE 109296 (Apr. 2022).

26 Michelle Kelley et al., *Opioid and Sedative Misuse Among Veterans Wounded In Combat*, 92 ADDICTIVE BEHAVIORS 168, 168-92 (May 2019).

27 Press Release, U.S. DEP'T OF VET. AFFAIRS, VA Reduces Prescription Opioid Use By 64% During Past Eight Years (July 30, 2020) (*available at* https://news.va.gov/press-room/va-reduces-prescription-opioid-use-by-64-during-past-eight-years/).

28 *See* 10 U.S.C. §§ 1079(h), (j)(2).

stakeholders insight into not only what mental health practices impact veteran suicide, but also what additional benefits may play a factor. While each year's report includes important and illuminating data points, what is included in one year's report is not always included in the next year's report, which complicates our ability to track the overall issue and what interventions are most beneficial. The Not Just a Number Act will help to standardize the data that is collected and presented in each year's report.

Additionally, the legislation will require VA to report on what upstream programs and services at VA have the greatest impact on veteran suicide prevention and to provide recommendations on how these services and benefits may be expanded. It will require VA, along with the Centers for Disease Control and Prevention, to develop a publicly available toolkit for state and local coroners and medical examiners with the best practices for how best to identify and report veteran suicide deaths. Lastly, the bill will require VA to review and provide recommendations on whether the VA's Office of Mental Health and Suicide Prevention should be moved to the Office of Secretary level at VA. WWP believes this legislation will make necessary improvements to the VA's "National Veteran Suicide Prevention Annual Report" and will help the community learn how we can continue to best prevent veteran suicide. We urge Congress to pass this legislation.

Concluding Remarks

Wounded Warrior Project thanks the Committee and its distinguished members for inviting our organization to submit this statement. We are grateful for your attention and efforts towards addressing the critical issues of mental health and suicide prevention affecting our nation's veterans. We look forward to continuing to work with you on these issues and are standing by to assist in any way we can towards our shared goals of serving those that have served this country.

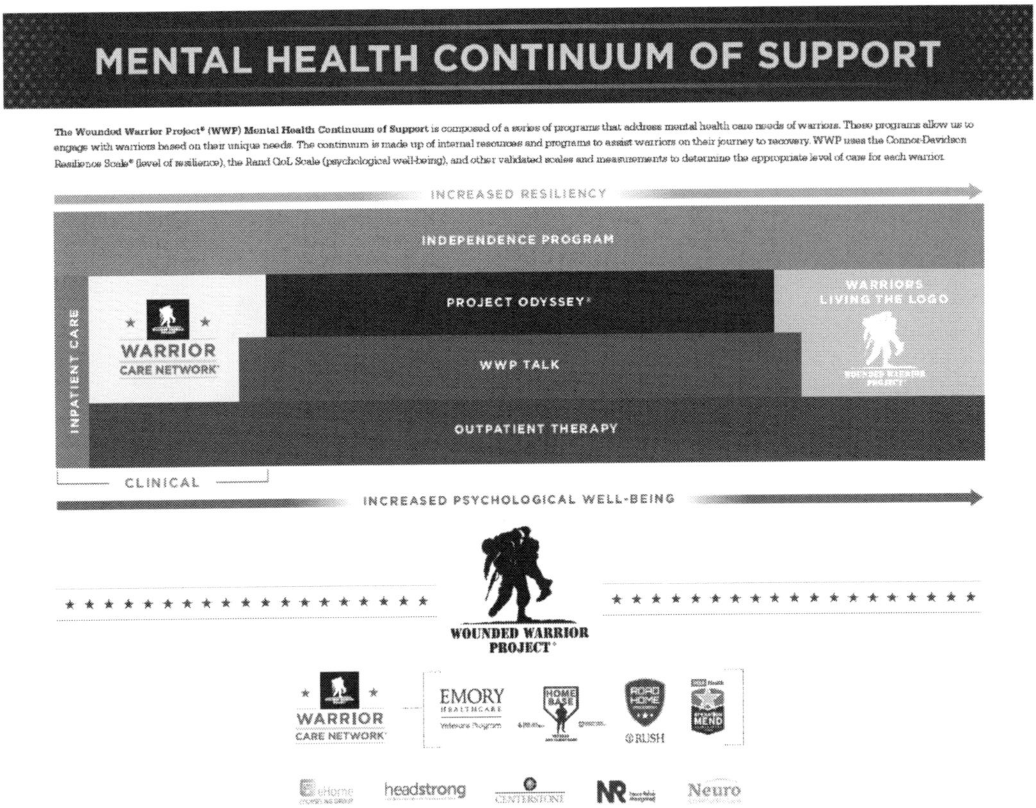

The continuum of support doesn't define an exact, prescriptive path to recovery, rather the individual needs of each warrior to determine the order and frequency of appropriate program engagement. For example, a warrior in acute psychological distress may be referred to a number of clinical intervention programs. Another warrior with less severe mental health issues may participate in only one or two programs. Subsequently, any warrior who has a setback may be re-evaluated and referred back to one or more programs for additional care. The goal is to provide the appropriate amount of care a warrior may need to get to his or her highest possible level of resilience, psychological well-being, and healing.

INPATIENT CARE
Clinical Intervention

Inpatient care is reserved for warriors in severe psychological distress who have exhausted all other resources. WWP may be able to fund inpatient services in order to stabilize warriors so that they can be engaged with other mental health programs in the continuum. The goal is to sustain and facilitate movement in the continuum through other programs.

WARRIOR CARE NETWORK
Clinical Intervention

To accelerate the development of advanced models of mental health care, WWP partners with four world-renowned academic medical centers to form Warrior Care Network®, leveraging our collective commitment and expertise. The Warrior Care Network treatment model delivers a year's worth of mental health care during a two- to three-week intensive outpatient program (IOP). This unique veteran-centric approach increases access to treatment and improves outcomes. Warrior Care Network provides a path to long-term wellness, improving the way warriors are treated today and for generations to come.

PROJECT ODYSSEY
Engagement Intervention

Project Odyssey is a 12-week mental health program that uses adventure-based learning to help warriors manage and overcome their invisible wounds, enhance their resiliency skills, and empower them to live productive and fulfilling lives. Based on their unique needs, warriors can participate in an all-male, all-female, or couples Project Odyssey. The program starts with a five-day mental health workshop, where warriors are challenged to step outside the comfort of their everyday routines. This opens them up to new experiences that help develop their coping and communication skills. After the workshop, participants work together with WWP to stay engaged, achieve their personal goals, and make lifelong positive changes.

★ PROGRAMS WITH MULTIPLE STAGES OF ENGAGEMENT ★

Within the continuum of support there are additional programs/resources that can be engaged at nearly any point in the continuum. These are WWP Talk and outpatient therapy. The Independence Program, which also encompasses multiple stages of engagement, is a unique component of the continuum. The resources provided by the Independence Program allow the most severely wounded warriors the ability to lead a full life at home instead of a long-term facility.

OUTPATIENT THERAPY • *Engagement and Clinical Intervention*

An additional clinical resource available to warriors across the stages of the continuum is outpatient therapy. Here WWP funds external partners to provide individual, family, or couples therapy delivered by a culturally competent therapist in the closest geographic location to the warriors as possible. With multiple funded clinical partners, warriors are able to engage in traditional outpatient sessions or, if in a remote location, engage in virtual therapy.

WWP TALK • *Engagement and Coordination Intervention*

WWP Talk is a telephonic emotional support program that breaks down the barriers of isolation and helps both warriors and family members plan an individualized path toward their personal growth. Participants work one-on-one with a dedicated team member during weekly emotional-support calls. Together, they set tangible goals and develop skills that lead to positive changes, like increased resilience and improved psychological well-being.

INDEPENDENCE PROGRAM
Engagement, Coordination, and Clinical Intervention

The Independence Program provides long-term support to catastrophically wounded warriors living with injuries such as: a moderate to severe brain injury, spinal cord injury, or neurological condition that impacts independence. The program is designed to support warriors who, without high-touch services, would struggle to live day to day due to the severity of their injuries. The Independence Program increases access to community services, provides rehabilitation through alternative therapies, and empowers warriors to achieve goals leading to a more independent life. Because every journey is different, we work as a team with warriors, their family members, and their caregivers to set goals to live a fulfilling life, at home, with their loved ones.

★ LIVING THE LOGO ★

WOUNDED WARRIOR PROJECT®

The WWP logo is much more than a trademark – it is what we see as the ultimate goal for all warriors engaged with the continuum of support to achieve. It is the collective goal of the continuum of support (through resources and teammates) to empower warriors to make it to this final phase and live our logo. The logo, one warrior carrying another warrior, represents a peer assisting a fellow veteran – in essence, carrying him through the recovery process until he can walk of his own accord (through heightened resiliency and psychological well-being). Eventually, as resiliency reaches the highest levels in the continuum, warriors are empowered to help carry fellow veterans, essentially becoming force multipliers as they are engaged as peer mentors.

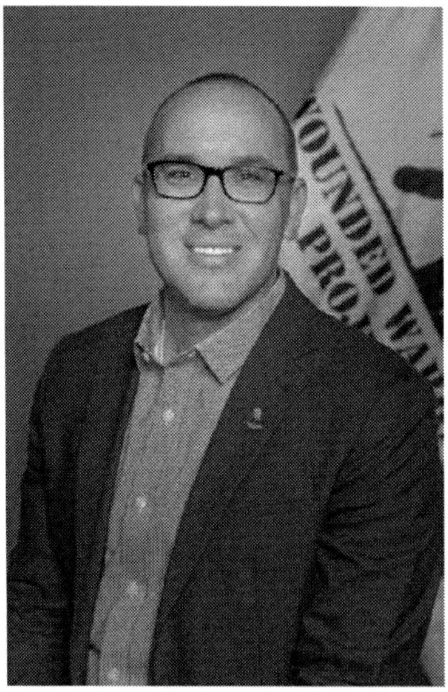

JOHN EATON
COMPLEX CARE VICE PRESIDENT

John Eaton serves as vice president, Complex Care at Wounded Warrior Project® (WWP). In this role, he is responsible for overseeing WWP's Mental Health Continuum of Support, to include C3 (Complex Case Coordination), Triage, WWP Talk and Project Odyssey.

Additionally, John serves as executive leadership for Warrior Care Network, a partnership between Wounded Warrior Project and four world-renowned academic medical centers, providing veterans and service members living with post-traumatic stress disorder, traumatic brain injury, military sexual trauma and substance use disorder with a path to long-term wellness.

Prior to this role, John has spent the last 18 years serving in healthcare leadership roles, most recently, as vice president of social and behavioral health at Flagler Health +. In this capacity, John was responsible for developing and operationalizing the Flagler Health+ behavioral health service-line to increase access, eliminate stigma and leverage innovation to address behavioral health and social health needs of communities across Northeast Florida.

Under John's leadership at Flagler Health +, Care Connect+ was established and has grown to include a network of more than 200 community-based organizations across Florida, with demonstrated success in advancing key health factors for veterans, such as homelessness, mental health, and social isolation.

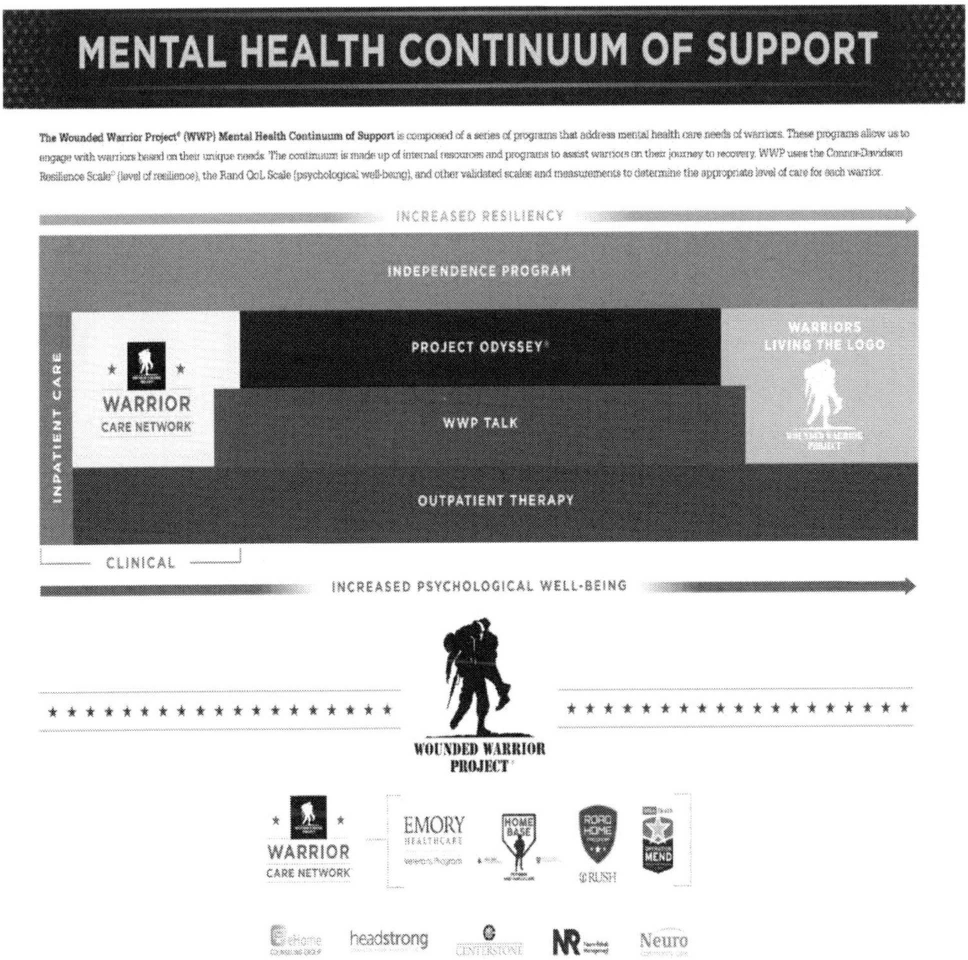

The continuum of support doesn't define an exact, prescriptive path to recovery, rather the individual needs of each warrior to determine the order and frequency of appropriate program engagement. For example, a warrior in acute psychological distress may be referred to a number of clinical intervention programs. Another warrior with less severe mental health issues may participate in only one or two programs. Subsequently, any warrior who has a setback may be re-evaluated and referred back to one or more programs for additional care. The goal is to provide the appropriate amount of care a warrior may need to get to his or her highest possible level of resilience, psychological well-being, and healing.

INPATIENT CARE
Clinical Intervention

Inpatient care is reserved for warriors in severe psychological distress who have exhausted all other resources. WWP may be able to fund inpatient services in order to stabilize warriors so that they can be engaged with other mental health programs in the continuum. The goal is to sustain and facilitate movement in the continuum through other programs.

WARRIOR CARE NETWORK
Clinical Intervention

To accelerate the development of advanced models of mental health care, WWP partners with four world-renowned academic medical centers to form Warrior Care Network®, leveraging our collective commitment and expertise. The Warrior Care Network treatment model delivers a year's worth of mental health care during a two- to three-week intensive outpatient program (IOP). This unique veteran-centric approach increases access to treatment and improves outcomes. Warrior Care Network provides a path to long-term wellness, improving the way warriors are treated today and for generations to come.

PROJECT ODYSSEY
Engagement Intervention

Project Odyssey is a 12-week mental health program that uses adventure-based learning to help warriors manage and overcome their invisible wounds, enhance their resiliency skills, and empower them to live productive and fulfilling lives. Based on their unique needs, warriors can participate in an all-male, all-female, or couples Project Odyssey. The program starts with a five-day mental health workshop, where warriors are challenged to step outside the comfort of their everyday routines. This opens them up to new experiences that help develop their coping and communication skills. After the workshop, participants work together with WWP to stay engaged, achieve their personal goals, and make lifelong positive changes.

★ PROGRAMS WITH MULTIPLE STAGES OF ENGAGEMENT ★

Within the continuum of support there are additional programs/resources that can be engaged at nearly any point in the continuum. These are WWP Talk and outpatient therapy. The Independence Program, which also encompasses multiple stages of engagement, is a unique component of the continuum. The resources provided by the Independence Program allow the most severely wounded warriors the ability to lead a full life at home instead of a long-term facility.

OUTPATIENT THERAPY • *Engagement and Clinical Intervention*

An additional clinical resource available to warriors across the stages of the continuum is outpatient therapy. Here WWP funds external partners to provide individual, family, or couples therapy delivered by a culturally competent therapist in the closest geographic location to the warriors as possible. With multiple funded clinical partners, warriors are able to engage in traditional outpatient sessions or, if in a remote location, engage in virtual therapy.

WWP TALK • *Engagement and Coordination Intervention*

WWP Talk is a telephonic emotional support program that breaks down the barriers of isolation and helps both warriors and family members plan an individualized path toward their personal growth. Participants work one-on-one with a dedicated team member during weekly emotional-support calls. Together, they set tangible goals and develop skills that lead to positive changes, like increased resilience and improved psychological well-being.

INDEPENDENCE PROGRAM
Engagement, Coordination, and Clinical Intervention

The Independence Program provides long-term support to catastrophically wounded warriors living with injuries such as: a moderate to severe brain injury, spinal cord injury, or neurological condition that impacts independence. The program is designed to support warriors who, without high-touch services, would struggle to live day to day due to the severity of their injuries. The Independence Program increases access to community services, provides rehabilitation through alternative therapies, and empowers warriors to achieve goals leading to a more independent life. Because every journey is different, we work as a team with warriors, their family members, and their caregivers to set goals to live a fulfilling life, at home, with their loved ones.

★ LIVING THE LOGO ★

The WWP logo is much more than a trademark – it is what we see as the ultimate goal for all warriors engaged with the continuum of support to achieve. It is the collective goal of the continuum of support (through resources and teammates) to empower warriors to make it to this final phase and live our logo. The logo, one warrior carrying another warrior, represents a peer assisting a fellow veteran – in essence, carrying him through the recovery process until he can walk of his own accord (through heightened resiliency and psychological well-being). Eventually, as resiliency reaches the highest levels in the continuum, warriors are empowered to help carry fellow veterans, essentially becoming force multipliers as they are engaged as peer mentors.

Written Testimony of Gilly Cantor, M.P.A., Director of Evaluation and Capacity Building, D'Aniello Institute for Veterans and Military Families at Syracuse University
Before the Senate Committee on Veterans' Affairs
September 20, 2023

Mr. Chairman, Ranking Member Moran, and Members of the Committee, thank you for the opportunity to testify on the topic of improving mental health and suicide prevention measures for our nation's veterans. My name is Gilly Cantor and I serve as the Director of Evaluation and Capacity Building at the D'Aniello Institute for Veterans and Military Families (IVMF) at Syracuse University.

The IVMF's contribution to this conversation is rooted in the research and practice related to upstream approaches to suicide prevention. For ten years, our institute has played a key role in creating, sustaining, and evaluating networks of health and social service organizations – originally as part of our AmericaServes initiative working alongside 18 communities across the country.

Mirroring a growing body of evidence in healthcare more broadly, these models have demonstrated that helping veterans navigate to the full scope of services and resources they need – beyond clinical interventions alone – is an integral component of suicide prevention efforts.

At the same time, we have witnessed unprecedented effort in recent years from Congress, the VA, and DoD through bipartisan legislation that better integrates communities into suicide prevention strategies, and we have observed both evidence of their success and opportunities to improve.

It is the strong belief of the IVMF and our partners that we must remain committed to bridging the gap between the VA and communities – between health and social needs. We must not give up on the promise of these efforts but rather ensure they live up to their potential.

To start, I'd like to make it clear why communities and accountable partnerships remain essential to effective suicide prevention solutions.

There are three findings I want to highlight from a recent VA-funded pilot study we conducted with the VA Center for Health Equity Research and Promotion. The study explored the extent and potential effects of collaboration between AmericaServes networks and local VA Medical Centers.

- First, we found a high percentage of overlap between AmericaServes and VA data, *even in communities with lower levels of formal partnership*. In other words, many veterans enrolled at the VA are unquestionably receiving services in their communities.
- Second, veterans served by both the VA and the community were comparatively younger; included more women, Black, and Hispanic veterans; and had more health-related social needs (such as stable housing, access to healthy food, etc.). In other words, communities are part of the system of care for *the most marginalized veterans experiencing the most hardship*.
- And third, when partnerships were strong, veterans receiving healthcare from the VA *and* social services in the community were more likely to have those needs successfully met. In other words, *when we work together*, the stressors impacting veterans' wellbeing are more effectively addressed.

Further, we know from research and data that establishing accountability and transparency between the VA and communities is both achievable and necessary if we want veterans to thrive.

- We know from research that economic, social, and interpersonal circumstances increase risk of suicide. Imagine what more we could learn and act upon if non-health data was examined regularly and transparently shared. We must support legislation like the Not Just A Number Act to bring all the data the VA has to bear on this issue. In fact, we should be looking beyond VA to DHHS, DoD, other health systems, and communities to ensure we have the fullest possible picture of veterans not currently served by the VA.
- From our evaluation of AmericaServes data in Pittsburgh, we know that hundreds of veterans are referred between the VA and the community annually. Because these cases are meticulously tracked, we know that individuals referred by the VA are most in need of household goods and transportation. We know that referrals are typically matched to an appropriate organization in under a day and successfully resolved the majority of the time. The VA has full access to this data. This level of transparency

and monitoring is possible – it is also happening in places like North Carolina and Texas, to name a few.

Finally, I'd like to provide one of several opposing cases we heard at a recent roundtable we hosted with 11 of our partners who are recipients of the SSG Fox Suicide Prevention Grant Program.

- In one community, the local Suicide Prevention Coordinator was willing to sit shoulder to shoulder with the Fox grantee to develop a dedicated protocol to streamline enrollment for veterans whose risk level made them eligible for the program.
- In other communities, however, local Suicide Prevention Coordinators were hardly aware of the program and their ability to facilitate enrollment in VA care remained unchanged.

We need to make the first community the rule, not the exception. Effective practices require enterprise implementation. We have submitted a full brief on this roundtable and encourage the Committee and the VA to consider incorporating its findings into this important program.

If there is one message to leave you with it is this: There is more to feel hopeful about than there is to criticize.

We are all here because the stakes remain high, and the consequences of failure are quite literally existential – but we have collectively taken meaningful steps toward our shared goal. The evidence bears out. We simply need to monitor our progress and have the courage to adjust course along the way if necessary.

Thank you for the opportunity to share this with you today, and I look forward to your questions.

Questions for the Record

Department of Veterans Affairs (VA)
Questions for the Record Submitted to
Dr. Matthew Miller, Ph.D., MPH
Executive Director, Suicide Prevention
Office of Mental Health and Suicide Prevention (OMHSP)
Veterans Health Administration (VHA)
Committee on Veterans' Affairs
United States Senate
"Invisible Wounds of War: Improving Mental Health and Suicide Prevention Measures for our Nation's Veterans"

September 20, 2023

Questions for the Record from Senator Marsha Blackburn

Question 1: What percentage of VA employees currently utilize remote teleworking at least one day a week? How many mental health (MH) professionals operate in a remote capacity (even in a temporary or partial status) for the VA?

VA Response: VA's Human Resources system, HR SMART, provides information about eligibility to telework, not the actual amount of time that an employee performs in a telework status. As of August 31, 2023, 25.9% of all VHA employees are eligible for telework of at least 1 day a pay period, with 36.9% of Mental Health (MH) professionals (Licensed Mental Health Counselor, Marriage Family Therapist (MFT), Peer Support, PT, Psychiatry, Psychology, Nurse (MH), Social Worker (MH)) eligible for telework at least 1 day a pay period.

Question 2: Does the VA currently have any staffing shortages for LPMHCs or MFT? What is the total number of LPMHCs that are employed by the VA as of September 20th, 2023?

VA Response: As of October 3, 2023, VHA has 815 LPMHCs onboard and 269 full-time equivalent (FTE) vacancies. There are currently 209 MFTs onboard and 62 FTE vacancies.

Question 3: What are the minimum qualifications to be qualified, and employed as a Veterans Crisis Line (VCL) Responder?

VA Response: VCL requires that all responders meet basic Federal Government hiring requirements; educational and/or experience requirements; specialized experience and/or education and demonstrate specific knowledge, skills and abilities. Basic Federal Government hiring requirements include U.S. citizenship (as outlined in VA Handbook 5005, Part II, Appendix G64, Social Science Specialist (Crisis Responder) Qualification Standards) and English language proficiency (as required by 38 U.S.C. § 7403(f)).

The following provides further details regarding the minimum qualifications to be qualified and employed as a VCL responder:

1. **Educational and Experience Requirements:** (must meet one) successfully completed a bachelor's degree or higher from an accredited college or university, the degree must be in behavioral health or social science field appropriate to the work of the position (e.g. psychology, social work, sociology, family counseling, mental health counseling, nursing, ministry and criminal justice); or 2 years of specialized experience as a first responder (e.g., Police, Medic, Emergency Medical Technician, Emergency Dispatch, etc.) or in a social science related field that included behavioral health crisis response; and 2 years of higher education (i.e., above the high school level) from an accredited college or university in a behavioral health or social science related field appropriate to the work of the position (e.g., psychology, social work, sociology, family counseling, mental health counseling, nursing, ministry and criminal justice); or successful completion of a bachelor's degree from an accredited college or university in any field and 1 year of specialized experience that included behavioral health crisis response or mental health counseling.

2. **Specialized Experience or Education:** Specialized experience, in addition to the basic requirements, must have 1 year of creditable experience equivalent to the GS-9 grade level, which is directly related to the position to be filled. Specialized experience is defined as: performing crisis intervention work in a clinical behavioral health setting; conducting risk assessments with contacts experiencing an emotional crisis and as a result, may harm themselves or others; coordinating with team members to initiate emergency services or create facility transportation plans, as clinically appropriate; and engaging multiple entities, including law enforcement, medical and mental health providers and third parties; or education can be a Ph.D. or equivalent degree from an accredited college or university in a behavioral health related field appropriate to the work of the position (e.g., psychology, social work, sociology, or family counseling.

3. **Knowledge, Skills and Abilities:** These must be demonstrated by applicants include the ability to provide an evidenced based crisis intervention through a variety of modalities (e.g., telephone interviews, chat/text services, or social media forums); the ability to carry out crisis management steps while withholding judgment on controversial behaviors and not imposing one's values during the contact; and the ability to effectively prioritize complex problems quickly and respond appropriately in a crisis situation.

<u>Question 4</u>: What training does a VCL Responder required to conduct to be qualified for the position?

<u>VA Response</u>: VCL has a robust training program that is accredited by numerous external agencies and provides responders the highest level of preparation to provide

crisis intervention. Specifically, VCL has maintained accreditation with the American Association of Suicidology (AAS) with its most recent re-accreditation in January 2023, as well as the Commission on Accreditation of Rehabilitation Facilities (CARF). The accreditation process for both AAS and CARF involve in-depth reviews of quality and training at VCL, including review of documents, policies, records and Standard Operation Procedures (SOP) related to training to ensure an effective program is in place. The qualified VCL Responders training program includes the following:

1. **Responders complete a total of 160 hours of classroom training:** Prior to completion of a competency test, VCL Responders complete training in the following subjects: Military Culture, post-traumatic stress disorder (PTSD)/Moral Injury, Hazardous Materials, Readjustment, Military Sexual Trauma, Engagement, Motivational Interviewing, Risk Assessment, Violence Risk Assessment Lethal Means Safety, Substance Use and Overdose Risk, Interaction Categorization Guidance, Crisis Intervention, Police Perspective, Medora (electronic record system), Documentation, Medical Records and Mock Workstation.

2. **Final Competency Examination:** Responder trainees are expected to complete a final examination to demonstrate competency at the end of the classroom period. Trainees who do not demonstrate competency are subject to review and potential discharge, as evidenced by the memoranda they sign at the beginning of the training class.

3. **Precept Training:** After completing the training portion, new employees enter a precept phase of training. During this time, new VCL Responders are paired with an experienced individual to provide coaching, training and mentoring. On average, VCL Responders complete over 85 days of training and precepting before being released for independent work.

Question 5: How many total text messages have been sent to the VCL? And how many unique individuals have reached out to the VCL?

VA Response: From February 2011 to October 1, 2023, VCL received a total of 342,607 text messages. VCL received 70,361 texts during Fiscal Year (FY) 2023, which is a 53% increase compared to FY 2022. From February 2009 to October 1, 2023, 2,646,975 unique individuals have reached out to VCL by phone, chat and text.

Question 6: How many Suicide Prevention Coordinators (SPC) are employed by the VA? Is there a SPC located at every VA clinic location? Do all SPCs have an office space suitable to conduct meetings with individuals if requested?

VA Response: As of October 1, 2023, VHA employed 447 SPCs at local health care systems as part of suicide prevention teams. SPCs support suicide prevention programming across the VA enterprise.

Staffing for SPCs is directed by VHA Memorandum 2023-08-12, For Action: Guidance for Reporting and Monitoring of Suicide Prevention Program (SPP) Staffing (VIEWS 10685516), published on August 8, 2023. This memo establishes monthly SPC reporting requirements and dictates that each VA Medical Center (VAMC) and Community-Based Outpatient Clinic (CBOC) large enough to serve more than 10,000 unique Veterans per year must appoint and maintain at least one SPC with a full-time commitment to suicide prevention programming activities. As of October 1, 2023, in reviewing all sites of care required to assign an SPC, 24 VAMCs or very large CBOC were reported to not have 1 FTE Suicide Prevention Coordinator. Health care systems staff full suicide prevention teams who support the effort across the enterprise and include the following: SPCs, Suicide Prevention Case Managers and other support staff. Additionally, health care systems staff Community Engagement and Partnership Coordinators, Peer Support Specialists, Program Support Assistants and Education/Outreach Specialists.

Regarding SPC resources and office space, each Veterans Integrated Service Network is responsible to ensure adequate resources, including office space, to support all the responsibilities for local suicide prevention teams and suicide prevention programing (VHA Directive 1160.07 *Suicide Prevention Program*, dated May 24, 2021).

Question 7: What is the average wait time for a veteran to be seen at a VA clinic by a mental health professional? What is the average wait time for a rural veteran to be seen at a VA clinic by a mental health professional?

VA Response: In FY 2023, the average wait time for a new patient for MH services within the VA was 21.2 days. For established patients, the average wait time was 5.8 days. Similarly, for rural Veterans, the wait times were 21.6 days for new patients and 5.5 days for established patients.

Question 8: How many community care appointments for behavioral health have been scheduled for veterans in FY23? How many appointments have been scheduled to veterans living in highly rural areas in FY23?

VA Response: In FY 2023, there were approximately 1.62 million behavioral health appointments provided through community care. Of this total, approximately 34,500 appointments were for patients residing in highly rural areas. These totals are expected to increase slightly over the coming months as additional claims for FY 2023 services are submitted by community providers for processing.

Question 9: Did you receive an incentive pay award as part of the Critical Skill Incentive (CSI)?

VA Response: The Executive Director for Suicide Prevention received a CSI payment; however, this CSI award was cancelled along with that of other senior executives.

Questions for the Record from Senator John Boozman

Question 1: Dr. Miller, on March 23, 2023, Sec McDonough said he was proud of the seven privately funded VA clinical research studies related to MDMA-Assisted Therapy addressing veteran PTSD and suicide. There appears to be clear bipartisan support for the Secretary to continue and expand these efforts at the VA. How long will it take the VA to set up a program so that it's prepared to administer this therapy upon final Food and Drug Administration (FDA) approval, which is expected in 2024?

VA Response: VA is committed to ensuring access to safe and effective treatments that promote the health of the Nation's Veterans. In line with this goal, VA conducts studies under stringent protocols at various facilities nationwide to identify effective treatments for Veterans experiencing PTSD and suicide risk. VA researchers are currently engaged in studies that are examining if compounds such as 3,4-methylenedioxy-methamphetamine (MDMA) and psilocybin can treat Veterans with PTSD, treatment resistant depressive disorder, major depressive disorder and potentially other mental health conditions. VA monitors ongoing psychedelic research outside VA, and based on the scientific evidence, we will continue to evaluate expanding future studies.

VHA's Office of Research and Development (ORD) and OMHSP continually work together on proactive, planful approaches to determine potential benefits of treatments for Veterans. ORD and OMHSP co-hosted a State-of-the-Art (SOTA) Conference: Psychedelic Treatments for Mental Health Conditions in September 2023 with two aims: 1) to better understand the current state of scientific evidence and to identify a strategic framework to conduct future psychedelic treatment research for select mental health conditions and 2) for agents where U.S. Food and Drug Administration (FDA) approval may be anticipated, to determine the necessary steps for potential VA system-wide clinical implementation. Lessons learned from this conference will be applied to inform consideration of research strategy and policy and practice changes for mental health conditions. VA is actively working on the information generated from the SOTA Conference to consider additional research opportunities.

Questions for the Record from Senator Bill Cassidy

Question 1: What is the current employment status of the VCL responder referenced in the 9/14 VAOIG Report? Has this staffer been required to complete additional training? A reprimand? Since this person clearly made serious errors in the course of performing their core work, partially causing the suicide of a veteran in the VA's care, don't you think some kind of personnel response is in order for this employee?

VA Response: The VCL Responder, noted in VA Office of Inspector General (OIG) Report 22-00507-211, is a current VCL employee; however, this employee no longer performs VCL Crisis Responder duties. The employee was removed from regular silent monitoring duties for approximately 10 weeks while an investigation was completed. The employee received additional coaching and training from April 4, 2022, through April 12, 2022.

A VCL organization-wide change went into effect on March 23, 2022, which stipulated that title 5 (non-clinical) employees may no longer perform VCL Crisis Responder duties. VCL is making meaningful progress on all recommendations outlined in the VA OIG Report 22-00507-211, published on September 14, 2023. This includes actions regarding recommendation 1, which directs the VCL Director to conduct a full review of the VCL Crisis Responders management of the Veteran and third-party contacts, in consultation with Workforce Management Consultants (WMC) and Office of General Counsel (OGC). VCL will take actions as warranted.

Question 2: What is the current employment status of the VCL Director for Quality and Training referenced in the 9/14 VAOIG Report? Coaching an employee in how to "appropriately" respond to questions from the OIG is an egregious action for a senior federal employee. If this employee is still an employee of the VA, why? What personnel actions have been taken in regard to this employee?

VA Response: The VCL Director for Quality and Training referenced VA OIG Report 22-00507-211 remains a VCL employee as the Division Director for Quality and Risk Management. VCL is collaborating with the WMC and OGC to complete a review of case details as recommended by the VA OIG report, and VCL will take actions as warranted.

Question 3: What is the current employment status of the Executive Director of the VCL referenced in the 9/14 VA OIG Report? Is it true that this employee has been "promoted" to the position of Senior Advisor for Health to the VA Secretary at headquarters? If this person is a member of the Senior Executive Service, and thereby can be removed from federal service without cause, why is this employee still in federal service?

VA Response: The prior Executive Director of VCL, Dr. Lisa Kearney, was permanently appointed as a Chief Consultant to the Deputy Under Secretary for Health. This was a lateral move in November 2022 within the Senior Executive Service for Dr.

Kearney, who was asked to take the role after the departure of the prior Chief Consultant. While this role is housed within VHA, Dr. Kearney currently serves as the Senior Advisor on Health in the Office of the Secretary.

Question 4: According to information provided in the 9/14 VA OIG Report, the VCL advises its responders to terminate a text session if a customer is silent for 15 minutes. Why is this the case, when an individual veteran who is suffering could do something drastic in less than 15 minutes?

VA Response: In cases where assessed risk for suicide or violent behavior has been mitigated, the VCL Crisis Responder will prompt the customer to re-engage if a customer stops engaging in the ongoing text conversation. If, after 15 minutes, a customer has not replied to the prompt, the VCL Crisis Responder will encourage the customer to reach back out, provide all VCL contact information and conclude the interaction. It is important to note that if there are still risks for suicide or violence that have not been mitigated, the VCL Crisis Responder will not end the interaction after 15 minutes of non-responsiveness. Instead, they will continue their efforts to engage and consult with a supervisor to explore the possibility of attempting outreach through a phone call. This process is outlined in VCL SOP for Digital Services Interaction Flow, dated July 27, 2023, which provides guidance on handling non-responsive text interactions.

Questions for the Record from Senator Kevin Cramer

Question 1: Dr. Miller, I was encouraged to hear your testimony at our September 20 hearing in which you reiterated the need to address veteran suicide as a top priority for the VA. Supporting the mental health needs of our service members is of critical importance. It is crucial veterans have access to proven therapies as they seek treatment for major depressive disorder and difficult-to-treat depression, including non-drug treatment options. Can veterans, under the guidance of their physicians at the VHA, access all FDA-approved therapies for treatment-resistant depression, including vagus nerve stimulation (VNS)? What is inhibiting therapies like VNS or other non-drug treatment options from being available and accessible to veterans who are struggling with depression proven difficult to treat?

VA Response: VA agrees that treatment resistant depression (TRD) is an impactful health condition among Veterans. It is crucial for Veterans to have access to evidence-based treatments for depression. VNS is one of several evidence-based treatments for patients with TRD. With guidance from their health care providers at VA facilities, Veterans utilizing VA services have access to FDA-approved treatments for TRD, both at VA facilities and through referrals to community care. VA data from FY 2022 indicate that 16 VA facilities treated 116 Veterans with VNS either at the facility or through a community care referral. Veteran access to non-pharmacological treatments for TRD such as VNS may be limited by the complexity of the intervention. The availability of trained providers with adequate expertise to place and manage such devices is often limited. Such interventions are complex, requiring coordination between multiple service lines such as psychiatry, surgery, anesthesia and neurology in order to ensure safety and efficacy. In addition, there are other pharmacological interventions for TRD such as ketamine or esketamine that Veterans may choose prior to invasive surgical procedures.

<u>Questions for the Record from Senator Joe Manchin</u>

<u>Question 1</u>: Mental Telehealth Appointments: As I've now learned, many VAMCs offer telehealth appointments as a way to provide mental health care to veterans but from what I'm hearing from veterans in my state is that they prefer in person appointments which is why the veteran who recently reached out to us, sought care in the community. Additionally, a majority of the veterans who reside in West Virginia tend to have limited access to internet due to the rural nature of our state and may even experience challenges using technology to attend a telehealth appointment because half of our veteran population is above the age of 65. I'd like to know how the VA working to ensure that veterans who are seeking mental health care are able to access in person treatment at a VA facility if they so choose?

<u>VA Response</u>: Telehealth is one of many modalities the offers to provide the soonest and best care to Veterans. Veterans always have the option to utilize a face-to-face appointment instead of telehealth for their care needs if they prefer.

<u>Question 2</u>: Suicide Rates Among Rural Veterans: West Virginia is the third most rural state in the nation, with over 51% of the state's population living in rural areas. Ensuring Veterans in rural America have access to the mental health treatment they need is a top priority of mine. Based on the 2022 National Veteran Suicide Prevention Report, rural and highly rural veterans are at a higher risk for suicide. Can you tell me what demographic differences in rural or highly rural veteran populations you believe would contribute to these high rates of suicide? How is the VA's suicide prevention office addressing these specific characteristics that drive rural veteran suicide?

<u>VA Response</u>: The 2022 National Veteran Suicide Prevention Report provides information on suicide rates by rurality, as defined by patient zip codes, among Veteran VHA Users only. Information on suicide rates by rurality among all Veterans is currently not available. The analysis finds elevated suicide rates among Veteran VHA users with rural (including highly rural) residence for all years in the period 2001-2020. The report notes that this disparity is partly attributed to demographic differences among Veteran VHA users by rurality status and cites, in a footnote, with work by <u>Peltzman et. al (2022)</u>, which explores the role of race in explaining rural-urban suicide differences among VHA users. This study, which looked at all VHA users between 2003 and 2017, concluded that differences in the racial composition of rural and urban VHA users were the primary driver of the observed rural-urban suicide disparity, as rural users were significantly more likely to be White, and White VHA users were the group with the highest suicide rate. This conclusion was derived from analyses, which found that when race was added to models comparing rural and urban suicide rates, differences in rural and urban rates overall were not significant. Although this does not change the fact of an observed higher rate among rural VHA users from 2001-2020, it does suggest that this finding is primarily reflective of a persistently higher concentration of White Veteran VHA users in rural settings.

Given this important finding, a supplemental analysis was conducted for the 2022 National Veteran Suicide Prevention Report (results are presented in the aforementioned footnote) comparing rural and urban suicide rates, stratified by race and Hispanic ethnicity. This analysis found that between 2016 and 2020, suicide rates were lower for some groups of rural Veteran VHA users (14.6% lower for American Indian or Alaska Native Veterans, 16.5% lower for Black Veterans) and higher for others (2.7% higher for White Veterans, 3.8% higher for Native Hawaiian or Pacific Islander Veterans, 26.2% higher for Hispanic Veterans and 8.8% higher for Veterans with multiple race categories). Although these rates were not compared in statistical analysis for the report, they support findings from Peltzman (2022), which found that Hispanic VHA users had rates that were significantly higher in rural settings, while differences between rural and urban populations were not significant among White or Black VHA users. Work by Shiner et. al (2023) explored what factors might be driving this disparity and did not find stark demographic, clinical, or community differences in suicide risk between rural and urban Hispanic patients, but did note that mental health diagnoses and particularly substance use disorders were important drivers in both groups.

Questions for the Record from Senator Kyrsten Sinema

Question 1: As you know, the transition from active duty to civilian life or retired status can be an exceptionally challenging period, particularly for servicemembers grappling with substance use disorders. Reliable, ongoing support is vital during this sensitive time, both for the servicemembers themselves and for their families. Within the Department of the Navy, there has been a critically important program aimed at this vulnerable population: NavyMORE (My Ongoing Recovery Experience). This program has offered digitally accessible treatment for substance use disorders, benefiting not only active-duty servicemembers but also their families and veterans. Unfortunately, this program has recently had to suspend its operations due to a lapse in funding, leaving a glaring gap in the continuum of care. Could you provide information on any community-based programs to support Veteran recovery from mental health and substance use disorders, including data on their efficacy over time, similar to the Navy's utilization of and supporting data on outcomes for participants in the Navy My Ongoing Recovery Experience program?

VA Response: VA has a suite of award-winning mobile apps to support Veterans and their families with tools to help them manage emotional and behavioral concerns. Available mobile apps include those for use by Veterans (self-help) to support their ability to cope with personal issues (e.g., PTSD symptoms, PTSD and alcohol use, or smoking cessation) as well as mobile apps designed as an adjunct to psychotherapy and used with a mental health provider to support Veterans' engagement in care and their use of skills learned in therapy. VA's Mobile Apps enable Veterans to engage in self-help before their problems reach a level of needing professional assistance and aim to promote active engagement when they are in care. The goal is to empower Veterans and their families and potentially support VA's efforts to improve access to care. Please see: https://mobile.va.gov/appstore/mental-health.

Step Away is a mobile app for the self-management of drinking behaviors. It is one of the few mobile apps in which there are data from a randomized controlled trial demonstrating its effectiveness in improving drinking outcomes for adults. Stand Down is the Veteran version of the Step Away app. Stand Down is not a VA App and is not located on the VA App Store; however, it was developed with input from VA staff and is currently under study in VA. In an open trial, Veterans who screened positive for hazardous drinking during a primary care visit and were not receiving treatment for their drinking were asked to use the Stand Down app for 4 weeks and to concurrently receive weekly phone support from a Peer Specialist to facilitate engagement with the app. Acceptability of the intervention was high, and patients reported significant reductions in total standard drinks, drinks per drinking day and heavy drinking days over 4 weeks. Similar results were reported in an open trial study of Veterans using the Step Away app as a standalone intervention (without Peer Specialist facilitation). A large randomized controlled trial of the Stand Down app (with and without Peer Specialist facilitation) is currently underway at two VAMCs. If found to be effective in that trial, the Stand Down app can address the VA's goal of offering harm reduction techniques and expanding outreach to Veterans with a substance use problem who are not currently engaged in treatment for these problems at a VA facility.

VetChange is a free online self-management program for active-duty military and Veterans who are concerned about their drinking following military deployment. VetChange was created in 2011 with support from the National Institute on Alcohol Abuse and Alcoholism. The results from a randomized controlled trial (https://psycnet.apa.org/doilanding?doi=10.1037/a0033697) of this early version produced evidence that the intervention helped many Veterans reduce their drinking and PTSD symptoms. The current version was developed by Boston University and VA Boston Healthcare System with support from the National Center for PTSD and the Bristol-Myers Squibb Foundation.

Question 2: Could you speak to the challenges and repercussions of phasing out specialized programs like NavyMORE, especially at a time when our nation is striving to improve mental health and suicide prevention measures for our veterans? How can we ensure that effective programs are not just created but also maintained for the long-term benefit of our servicemembers and veterans?

VA Response: VA did not use or implement the NavyMORE program.VA defers to the Department of Defense (DoD) on sustainment of DoD programs.

Questions for the Record from Senator Thom Tillis

Question 1: Regarding the VA OIG concerning access to care in the Outpatient Mental Health Clinic at the Charles George VA Medical Center in Asheville, NC, the OIG learned that a patient had psychotherapy consults due to misconstrued information from prescribers believing that "permission" from the Behavioral Health Interdisciplinary Program (BHIP) team was required before placing a psychotherapy consult in a patient's health record. Was the VA able to conclude that the patient's death was indeed an accidental death or is it possible that the delayed care resulted in the patient committing suicide by motorcycle?

VA Response: VA concluded the Veteran's death was not a suicide based on the report of the Veteran's spouse and the State Highway Patrol. The Veteran's death certificate was requested and does not indicate suicide.

The OIG report describes their review of a Veteran's VA MH care from 2014-2021 and, specifically, focuses on the 28 days of care in 2021 the Veteran received at the Asheville VAMC for MH treatment. The Veteran did not experience a delay in care. From the first day of engagement with care at the Asheville VAMC on August 10, 2021, until his death 28 days later on September 6, 2021, the Veteran was provided 19 encounters from services across the continuum of care including Same Day MH Service, outpatient MH, Homeless program, Suicide Prevention, Inpatient Medicine with MH consulting, Post 9/11 Case Management and the VCL. He had seven encounters with outpatient MH staff that included medication management and supportive psychotherapy. A Behavioral Health Interdisciplinary Program (BHIP) consult was placed for this Veteran on day one of his outpatient care, and he was scheduled for 2 weeks later, which is not considered delayed per VA access guidelines. The Veteran did not appear for this BHIP consult appointment. In the 7 days following the missed appointment, four attempts were made to reach the Veteran to reschedule the BHIP consult appointment.

On day seven, after the missed appointment, the Veteran's provider was able to contact him and encouraged him to present to the Emergency Department for admission to inpatient psychiatry. The Veteran was admitted to a medical unit due to testing positive for Coronavirus Disease 2019. He was assessed by MH consult and medical staff and released the next day at the Veteran's request. The Veteran was assessed by the MH consult team prior to his release, and it was determined he did not meet the criteria for involuntary commitment. The Veteran received timely follow-up from his outpatient provider 1 day after his discharge from the inpatient medical unit. The Veteran's provider was providing medication management and supportive psychotherapy, including Motivational Interviewing, at each encounter. The Veteran was assessed for suicide risk in three settings (outpatient mental health, emergency department, inpatient medicine) by three different providers over the course of his treatment. While he endorsed vague suicidal ideation in these assessments, he credibly denied intent, plan or means to harm himself.

<u>Question 2</u>: **I know VA was working with nonprofits on suicide prevention well before the Hannon Act and the Fox grants came to be. In one case, VHA's Office or Mental Health and Suicide Prevention teamed up with The Independence Fund based in my state to support their Operation Resiliency combat unit reunions and mental health retreats with peer-to-peer support as the core objective. Does VA collect any data on those earlier and now still ongoing nonprofit engagements that do not require Federal funding, or do you derive any "lessons learned" from those collaborations where VA staff come in direct contact with nonprofits aiding Veterans needing mental health support?**

<u>VA Response</u>: Currently, neither the Office of Mental Health nor the Office of Suicide Prevention have any existing formalized partnerships with The Independence Fund. The Office of Mental Health and Suicide Prevention (OMHSP) and The Independence Fund had a Memorandum of Agreement (MOA) from January 11, 2021, through January 11, 2022. The primary objective of the MOA was to collaborate to expand the reach and awareness of suicide prevention, create awareness and/or educational opportunities and explore opportunities to identify Veterans not enrolled in VHA. While VA did not collect any data on that earlier engagement provided under the 2021 MOA, the Office of Suicide Prevention did assist The Independence Fund with the creation and initial implementation of a program evaluation plan and survey applied to Operation Resiliency. More broadly regarding partnerships and data collection, VA and VHA policy and guidance pertaining to the establishment, maintenance and evaluation of partnership effectiveness do require formalized and agreed-upon key performance indicators consistent with and valid indicators of defined goals and objectives specific to the partnership.

<u>Question 3</u>: **I have heard that in some cases a Veteran may call the Crisis Line and first responders, including police, are sometimes dispatched to check on that Veteran. What is VA doing to connect with law enforcement agencies nationally on a state-by-state basis to help them understand the critical role they play in preventing or de-escalating violence by Veterans in crisis and appropriately diverting them for appropriate mental health care versus arrest and incarceration? I know some of this work is being done by The Independence Fund, a nonprofit in my state, to bridge that gap, but I would think VA has a role to play here as well.**

<u>VA Response</u>: VA Suicide Prevention has developed a strong relationship with the Office of Operations, Security and Preparedness and the VA Law Enforcement Training Center who are leaders in Veteran de-escalation and violence prevention. Our teams work closely to build connections with and present for outside law enforcement agencies at conferences and trainings. The goal is to create understanding of Veteran-specific issues and the importance of prevention, de-escalation and diversion of Veterans from criminal justice and into healthcare. In FY 2023, our VA Suicide Prevention collaborated with the VA Police Service and Veterans Justice Programs to foster the growth of community police interventions designed to deflect Veterans into needed services and out of contact with the criminal justice system. To foster this growth, VAMCs were required to select three-person community partnership teams

consisting of one Veterans Justice Outreach Specialist, one VA Police Officer and one mental health provider to attend a one-time training. The aim of this training is to prepare these local VAMC teams to engage their communities around Veteran deflection efforts, creating pathways into care.

Additionally, in FY 2023 VA Suicide Prevention presented at the National Tactical Officers Association Conference and VA Police Chiefs conference to train community and VA police agencies on specific Veteran drivers of risk, as well as prevention, intervention and educational resources specially designed for police. VA Suicide Prevention also works with Substance Abuse and Mental Health Services Administration though their Crisis Intercept Mapping (https://www.samhsa.gov/smvf-ta-center/crisis-intercept-mapping) program and our Community-Based Interventions for Suicide Prevention program to support communities seeking to increase coordinated crisis care services.

Questions for the Record from Senator Tommy Tuberville

Question 1: What type of predictive analytics does the VA use to determine whether an individual is at a higher risk of self-harm or suicide?

VA Response: VA employs a suicide risk prediction algorithm in a program called Recovery Engagement and Coordination for Health – Veterans Enhanced Treatment (REACH VET) to alert facilities of Veterans at the top 0.1% increased statistical risk for those Veterans in VHA care at those facilities. This algorithm is based on data from the past 2 years of the VA health record to help streamline clinical reviews and provide an additional clinical data point for conceptualization and treatment enhancement by the treatment team. Although identified Veterans are at high statistical risk for adverse outcomes, including suicide, this does not necessarily indicate current acute clinical risk for suicide. REACH VET is intended to supplement, rather than replace, current clinical strategies. REACH-VET has been associated with increased attendance at outpatient appointments, a greater proportion of individuals with new safety plans and reductions in mental health admissions and emergency department visits and reduction in suicide attempts. Please see McCarthy et al. 2021, Evaluation of the Recovery Engagement and Coordination for Health–Veterans Enhanced Treatment Suicide Risk Modeling Clinical Program in the Veterans Health Administration. JAMA Network Open. 4(10):e2129900. doi:10.1001/jamanetworkopen.2021.29900 below.

McCarthy JAMA Net Open - Eval of REAC

Question 2: Has the model flagged veterans who have died by suicide? Have there been any veterans who have died by suicide but were not flagged as high risk of self-harm using the REACH Vet model?

VA Response: Yes, the REACH VET algorithm identifies high-risk Veterans and of those who are identified, some have died from suicide. This is documented in a published evaluation of the effectiveness of the REACH VET algorithm. Please see McCarthy et al. 2021, Evaluation of the Recovery Engagement and Coordination for Health–Veterans Enhanced Treatment Suicide Risk Modeling Clinical Program in the Veterans Health Administration. JAMA Network Open. 4(10):e2129900. doi:10.1001/jamanetworkopen.2021.29900.

Sen. Tuberville Statement: Dr. Miller, last week, the Office of Inspector General published a troubling report regarding a veteran who died by suicide after texting with a Veterans Crisis Line responder for 75 minutes. Of the many issues the report identified, the VCL appears to not have text retention capability, resulting in a family member having to screen shot the text chain back to the VCL to review whether situation was handled appropriately by the responder.

Question 3: There are numerous issues recognized in the report, but at a minimum, has the VCL instituted text message retention since this investigation concluded?

VA Response: As the VA OIG Report 22-00507-211 notes, VCL examined available options for the retention of interaction transcripts in the VCL Medora information system after current and prior text service vendors could not supply this feature. A method of retaining text transcripts was identified through copying and pasting the interaction transcript from the text service to Medora. This method was reviewed and approved by the Privacy/Freedom of Information Act Officer. This method has been in place since May 2022. In addition, VCL enhanced procedures for Silent Monitors to verify the text interaction is pasted into Medora during their review process through a modification of the Policy for Crisis Responder Interaction Standards and Silent Monitoring SOP, dated July 10, 2023. Additionally, the SOP (dated July 28, 2023) for Social Science Specialist (Crisis Responder) Documentation Guidelines now requires VCL Crisis Responders to paste transcripts for chat and text interactions into Medora.

Senator Tuberville Statement: Months after the veteran died by suicide, their family continued to receive information from the VA regarding appointments they had been scheduled for, because their health record had not been updated to reflect their death.

Question 4: Will the VA be reviewing all case files of veterans who have contacted the VCL regarding suicide or self-harm ideations to determine if their health records have been updated accordingly?

VA Response: VA has established guidance to ensure coordination between VCL and facility electronic health record documentation. Specifically, VHA Memorandum 2023-03-21 Enhancing Management and Oversight of Veterans Crisis Line (VCL) Requests (VIEWS 9623904), dated March 15, 2023, established that facility managers must complete regular, ongoing performance reviews of facility SPCs' management of VCL Requests pursuant to VHA Directive 1503(2), Operations of Veterans Crisis Line Center, May 26, 2020, sections 5.n. and 5.o and the minimum requirements described in this memorandum.

The memorandum required facilities to conduct performance reviews within 120 days of publication of the memorandum and to develop an ongoing quality assurance process that established the following requirements:

1. A time-based cadence for VCL Request periods of review;
2. The number or percentage of records to be reviewed within the period;
3. A clinical case review of VCL Request management electronic health record documentation for all required clinical documentation; and
4. Confirmation of SPC compliance with completing VCL outreach attempts that are interspersed over a consecutive 3-day period when outreach efforts to the customer have been unsuccessful.

Department of Veterans Affairs
November 2023

Supplemental Online Content

McCarthy JF, Cooper SA, Dent KR, et al. Evaluation of the Recovery Engagement and Coordination for Health–Veterans Enhanced Treatment suicide risk modeling clinical program in the Veterans Health Administration. *JAMA Netw Open*. 2021;4(10):e2129900. doi:10.1001/jamanetworkopen.2021.29900

eAppendix. Parallel-Trend Assumption Tests for REACH VET Evaluation Outcomes Prior to and After Identification

eTable 1. Mean Continuous Outcomes per Cohort and Time Period

eTable 2. Proportion Outcomes per Cohort and Time Period

This supplemental material has been provided by the authors to give readers additional information about their work.

eAppendix. Parallel-Trend Assumption Tests for REACH VET Evaluation Outcomes Prior to and After Identification

Background

Difference in differences analyses assume that in the absence of an intervention the differences between treatment and control groups would remain constant over time.[1] In cases where parallel trends are not observed in a pre-intervention period, it is appropriate to employ a triple differences (TD) study design, in order to adjust for non-parallel trends. In this study, the parallel trend assumption was assessed for each measure, for two possible differences-in-differences approaches: 1) differences across REACH VET and pre-REACH VET time periods among patients identified in the top 0.1% risk tier, and 2) differences across risk tiers (top 0.1% versus subthreshold) among those in the REACH VET era. Panel a and b in the illustrative figure below show violations of the parallel trend assumption, thus requiring a TD approach, and panel c demonstrates parallel trends, which would be consistent with use of the difference-in-differences approach.

Appendix Figure: Parallel Trends Assumption and Implications for Design: Illustrative Examples

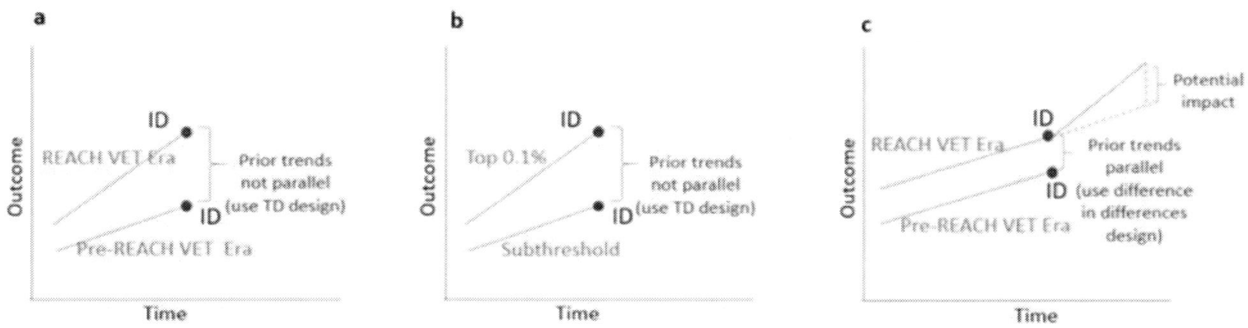

Methods

To assess for parallel trends, outcomes were collected across four 6-month periods prior to each patient's cohort entry (prior 0-6 months, prior 6-12 months, prior 12-18 months, prior 18-24 months). The parallel trend assumption across REACH VET eras among individuals in the top 0.1% risk tier was assessed using an interaction term between time period and REACH VET era (Model 1). The parallel trend assumption across REACH VET risk tiers among those in the REACH VET era was assessed using an interaction between time period and REACH VET risk tier (Model 2). The estimate and 95% confidence intervals for the difference in the associations with time across groups are presented in Appendix Table 1, below. A 95% confidence interval excluding zero indicates a statically significant difference in the pre-identification trends across groups during the 24 months prior to identification into the REACH VET cohort. In these cases, the parallel trend assumption is violated.

Model 1: Parallel Trend Assumption Test for Differences in Differences across REACH VET Eras among the Top 0.1% Risk Tier

$$\text{Outcome}=\beta_0+\beta_1*\text{REACH\_VET\_Era}+\beta_2*\text{Time}+\beta_3*\text{REACH\_VET\_Era}*\text{Time}+\varepsilon_i$$

Population was limited to those in the top 0.1% risk tier.

Time was a continuous indicator for the four 6-month periods prior to the patient's REACH VET identification date.

Model 2: Parallel Trend Assumption Test for Differences in Differences across REACH VET Risk Tiers in the REACH VET Era

$$\text{Outcome}=\beta_0+\beta_1*\text{Top0.1\%Tier}+\beta_2*\text{Time}+\beta_3*\text{Top0.1\%Tier}*\text{Time}+\varepsilon_i$$

Population was limited to those in the REACH VET era.

Time was a continuous indicator for the 4, 6-month periods prior to the patients REACH VET identification date.

While the triple differences estimation adjusts for non-parallel trends across groups, there may be residual differences in trends across comparison groups.[1] To assess any differences in trends within the pre-identification period, we used an interaction between time period, REACH VET risk tier, and REACH VET era (Model 3). Estimates with a 95% confidence interval that did not include zero indicated that adjustment for period and risk-tier was insufficient to eliminate all pre-REACH VET identification trends. There may be unobservable factors contributing to trends in these outcomes even in the absence of the REACH VET program and consequently results for outcomes that violate the triple differences parallel trend assumption should be interpreted with caution.

Model 3: Parallel Trend Assumption for Triple Differences

$$Outcome=\beta_0+\beta_1*Time+\beta_2*REACH\_VET\_Era+\beta_3*Top0.1\% +\beta_4*Time*REACH\_VET\_Era+\beta_5*Time*Top0.1\%$$

$$+\beta_6*REACH\_VET\_Era*Top0.1\%+\beta_7*Time*REACH\_VET\_Era*Top0.1\%+\varepsilon_i$$

Time was a continuous indicator for the four 6-month periods prior to the patients REACH VET identification date.

Results

eAppendix Table. Parallel Trend Assumption Tests[a]

Outcome	Differences in Differences across REACH VET Eras within Top 0.1% Risk Tier Estimate (95% Confidence Interval)	Differences in Differences across Threshold Groups within the REACH VET Era Estimate (95% Confidence Interval)	Triple Differences Estimate (95% Confidence Interval)
Average Scheduled Outpatient Appointments	-0.023 (-0.082, 0.037)	**0.136 (0.075, 0.197)**	0.005 (-0.075, 0.086)
Average Completed Outpatient Appointments	-0.031 (-0.080, 0.018)	0.015 (-0.034, 0.065)	-0.028 (-0.095, 0.037)
Proportion of Scheduled Outpatient Appointments Missed	-0.002 (-0.004, 0.001)	**0.013 (0.011, 0.016)**	0.003 (-0.001, 0.006)
Average Outpatient Mental Health Visits	**0.610 (0.528, 0.691)**	**1.478 (1.381, 1.575)**	**0.531 (0.409, 0.652)**
Average Inpatient Mental Health Admissions	**0.016 (0.014, 0.019)**	**0.040 (0.039, 0.042)**	**0.019 (0.017, 0.022)**
Average Emergency Department Visit Days	**0.020 (0.016, 0.025)**	**0.064 (0.059, 0.069)**	**0.016 (0.010, 0.022)**
Proportion with Any Documented Suicide Attempt	**0.002 (0.002, 0.003)**	**0.005 (0.004, 0.005)**	**0.002 (0.001, 0.003)**
Proportion with Any Safety Plan Documentation	**0.017 (0.016, 0.018)**	**0.015 (0.014, 0.016)**	**0.007 (0.006, 0.009)**

[a] bold indicates significance and violation of parallel trends assumption.

The parallel trend assumption was violated for all differences-in-differences analyses except for average number of scheduled outpatient appointments, average number of completed outpatient appointments, and proportion of scheduled outpatient appointments missed across REACH VET eras, among the top 0.1% risk tier, and for number of completed outpatient appointments across risk tiers, in the REACH VET era. In these instances, a differences-in-differences approach may have been sufficient, yet since all other outcomes indicated that a TD analysis was warranted, that more conservative approach was employed for all outcomes.

The TD parallel trend assumption was violated for all outcomes except the number of scheduled and completed outpatient appointments and the proportion of scheduled outpatient appointments that were missed. The violation of the TD parallel trend assumption does not prevent one from drawing conclusions, yet requires a more nuanced interpretation of the results.[1,2,3,4] Trends for inpatient mental health admissions, emergency department visit days, prevalence of any documented suicide attempt, and prevalence of any safety plan documentation prior to identification into REACH VET were in the opposite direction of the observed associations of the REACH VET program. This suggests that the true magnitude of the REACH VET association may be larger than what was documented, given the presence of non-parallel trends. Meanwhile, the pre-identification trend for outpatient mental health visits was in the same direction as the REACH VET association. However, since the TD assessment of the REACH VET association with outpatient mental health visits was non-significant, the pre-identification trend does not change our conclusions. Overall, pre-identification trends were close to zero and frequently were in the opposite direction from the observed REACH VET TD associations. The latter case suggests that there may be greater REACH VET associations than were ascertained in the TD analysis, because the TD design insufficiently controlled for pre-existing trends in the outcome. We note that significant TD parallel trend assumption tests may reflect the high statistical power of these tests rather than substantive differences in trends.

[1]Olden A, Moen J. The Triple Difference Estimator. NHH Dept. of Business and Management Science Discussion Paper No. 2020/1. 2020. Retrieve from https://ssrn.com/abstract=3582447

[2]Chen Q, Chu X, Wang S, Zhang B. A Triple-Difference Approach to Re-Evaluating the Impact of China's New Cooperative Medical Scheme on Incidences of Chronic Diseases Among Older Adults in Rural Communities. Risk Manag Healthc Policy. 2020;13:643-659. Published 2020 Jun 24. doi:10.2147/RMHP.S244021

[3]Keng SH, Sheu SJ. The effect of national health insurance on mortality and the SES-health gradient: evidence from the elderly in Taiwan. Health Econ. 2013;22(1):52-72. doi:10.1002/hec.1815

[4]Kim S, Kwon S. The effect of extension of benefit coverage for cancer patients on health care utilization across different income groups in South Korea. Int J Health Care Finance Econ. 2014;14(2):161-177. doi:10.1007/s10754-014-9144-y

eTable 1. Mean Continuous Outcomes per Cohort and Time Period

	Pre-REACH Vet Top 0.1%				Pre-REACH Vet 0.3%-0.1%				REACH Vet Top 0.1%				REACH Vet 0.3%-0.1%			
	Prior 6-Months		Subsequent 6-Months		Prior 6-Months		Subsequent 6-Months		Prior 6-Months		Subsequent 6-Months		Prior 6-Months		Subsequent 6-Months	
Outcome	Average	Std Dev	Average	Std Dev	Average	Std Dev	Average	Std Dev	Average	Std Dev	Average	Std Dev	Average	Std Dev	Average	Std Dev
Scheduled Outpatient Appointments	10.70	13.1	16.85	21.6	10.69	12.9	13.82	17.7	11.82	14.8	17.12	22.3	11.62	14.5	13.58	18.0
Completed Outpatient Appointments	6.93	9.9	11.31	17.6	7.33	10.0	9.69	14.4	7.56	11.3	11.50	17.8	8.00	11.2	9.54	14.2
Outpatient Mental Health Visits	30.23	32.2	37.66	52.6	23.51	31.9	23.66	41.6	36.01	37.8	40.74	56.8	26.15	36.1	23.06	43.1
Inpatient Mental Health Admissions	1.22	0.8	0.49	1.0	0.78	0.8	0.21	0.6	1.27	0.9	0.50	1.0	0.74	0.8	0.19	0.6
Emergency Department Visit Days	2.08	2.3	1.30	2.4	1.70	2.0	0.90	1.8	2.21	2.6	1.32	2.6	1.72	2.1	0.87	1.8

eTable 2. Proportion Outcomes per Cohort and Time Period

	Pre-REACH Vet Top 0.1%		Pre-REACH Vet 0.3%-0.1%		REACH Vet Top 0.1%		REACH Vet 0.3%-0.1%	
	Prior 6-Months	Subsequent 6-Months	Prior 6-Months	Subsequent 6-Months	Prior 6-Months	Subsequent 6-Months	Prior 6-Months	Subsequent 6-Months
Outcome	N(%)	N(%)	N(%)	N(%)	N(%)	N(%)	N(%)	N(%)
Scheduled Outpatient Appointments Missed[a]	135,803 (35.0)	194,896 (32.7)	154,785 (31.2)	188,312 (29.7)	170,886 (35.9)	224,649 (32.8)	170,924 (30.8)	193,795 (29.7)
Any Documented Suicide Attempt	3,778 (10.3)	1,040 (2.8)	2,049 (4.3)	468 (1.0)	5,251 (12.9)	1,188 (2.9)	2,214 (4.5)	405 (0.8)
Any Safety Plan Documentation	19,508 (53.3)	7,992 (21.8)	15,774 (33.5)	4,982 (10.6)	28,021 (68.7)	11,778 (28.9)	20,430 (41.9)	6,196 (12.7)
New Safety Plan[b]	---	1,982 (12.8)	---	1,439 (5.2)	---	1,812 (16.8)	---	1,332 (5.6)
All-Cause Mortality[c]	---	712 (1.9)	---	1,349 (2.9)	---	884 (2.2)	---	1,546 (3.2)

[a]Total appointments missed. Cohorts were limited to those with at least one appointment in the prior and subsequent six months (Total N = 158,346).

[b]Cohorts were limited to those with no safety plan in the prior two years (Total N = 77,625)

[c]Mortality ascertained from the Vital Status File. Cohorts were limited to those for which vital status could be ascertained (Total N = 173,305)

Submission for the Record

Drug and Alcohol Dependence 233 (2022) 109296

Contents lists available at ScienceDirect

Drug and Alcohol Dependence

journal homepage: www.elsevier.com/locate/drugalcdep

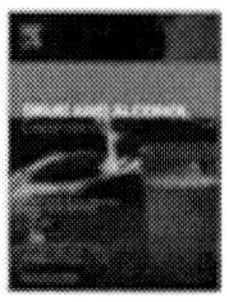

Veteran drug overdose mortality, 2010–2019

Mark R. Begley[a,*], Chandru Ravindran[a], Talya Peltzman[b], Sybil W. Morley[a], Brady M. Stephens[a], Lisham Ashrafioun[a,c], John F. McCarthy[b,d]

[a] Veterans Affairs (VA) Veterans Integrated Service Network 2, Center of Excellence for Suicide Prevention, Canandaigua, NY, USA
[b] VA Serious Mental Illness Treatment Resource and Evaluation Center, Office of Mental Health and Suicide Prevention, Ann Arbor, MI, USA
[c] Department of Psychiatry, University of Rochester, Rochester, NY, USA
[d] Department of Psychiatry, University of Michigan, Ann Arbor, MI, USA

ARTICLE INFO

Keywords:
Drug overdose
Veteran
Veterans Health Administration (VHA)
Mortality trends

ABSTRACT

Background: Prior work documents that Veteran drug overdose mortality increased from 2010 to 2016. The present study assessed trends from 2010 to 2019, by drug type and recent receipt of Veterans Health Administration (VHA) services, and compared rates for Veteran and non-Veteran US adults.

Methods: This retrospective cross-sectional study used data from Veterans Affairs (VA) medical records, the VA/Department of Defense Mortality Data Repository, and CDC WONDER. Trends were compared using Joinpoint regression.

Results: From 2010–2019, age-adjusted overdose mortality rates increased 53.2% among Veterans and 79.0% among non-Veterans. Age-adjusted rates of overdose mortality among Veterans rose from 19.8/100,000 in 2010 to 32.6/100,000 in 2017, before falling to 30.3/100,000 in 2019. Despite the decrease from 2017 to 2019 in overall overdose mortality, rates of overdose deaths involving synthetic opioids other than methadone and involving psychostimulants continued to increase through 2019. In 2019, overdose mortality was lower for male Veterans than male non-Veterans (standardized rate ratio (SRR) = 0.81, 95% confidence interval (CI): 0.77–0.84). Among male Veterans, rates were higher in all years for those with recent VHA use than those without (2019: SRR=1.69, 95% CI: 1.56–1.83). From 2010–2019, overdose mortality rates increased faster among female Veterans without VHA use than those with VHA use.

Conclusions: From 2015 onward, Veteran men experienced lower age-adjusted overdose rates than non-Veteran men. In all years, overdose rates were higher among male Veterans with recent VHA use than those without recent use. While overall rates of Veteran overdose deaths declined from 2017 to 2019, rates involving psychostimulants and synthetic opioids continued to rise.

1. Introduction

From 1999–2019, the United States (US) rate of drug overdose mortality increased by 254.1%. (Hedegaard et al., 2020) The percentage of US overdose deaths that involved opioids rose from 47.8% in 1999 to 70.6% in 2019. Stimulant involvement in overdose deaths rose from 25.9% in 1999 to 45.4% in 2019, with rapid increases in overdose deaths involving cocaine and psychostimulants with abuse potential, such as methamphetamine.

Overdose mortality trends vary by demographic and geographic factors and by the specific drugs involved. The few studies that have examined overdose mortality among US Veterans have primarily focused on patients receiving care in the Department of Veterans Affairs health system, the Veterans Health Administration (VHA). (Ilgen et al., 2016; Lin et al., 2019; Warfield, 2019) For example, research indicates that the fiscal year 2005 rate of opioid overdose mortality in VHA patients was nearly twice that of the general US population. (Bohnert et al., 2011) However, Veterans with recent VHA care comprised only 32.5% of all Veterans in 2018, and VHA findings may not generalize to the overall Veteran population. (U.S. Department of Veterans Affairs Office of Mental Health and Suicide Prevention, 2020a). Indeed, Veterans in VHA care have a higher prevalence of chronic pain, medical, and mental health conditions than other Veterans. (Meffert et al., 2019) Opioid overdose prevention efforts in VHA include reducing opioid prescribing, increasing naloxone distribution, and substance use screening, treatment, and education. (Gellad et al., 2017; U.S. Department of Veterans

* Correspondence to: Center of Excellence for Suicide Prevention, VA Medical Center, 400 Fort Hill Avenue, Canandaigua, NY 14424, USA.
E-mail address: Mark.R.Begley14@gmail.com (M.R. Begley).

https://doi.org/10.1016/j.drugalcdep.2022.109296
Received 4 November 2021; Received in revised form 16 December 2021; Accepted 18 December 2021
Available online 12 January 2022

Table 1
Veteran Overdose Mortality Rates,[a] 2010-2019, Overall and by Drug Type[b].

	All drug overdose			Opioid overdose			Stimulant overdose		
	2010 Rate	2019 Rate	Change from 2010 to 2019	2010 Rate	2019 Rate	Change from 2010 to 2019	2010 Rate	2019 Rate	Change from 2010 to 2019
All Veterans	19.8	30.3	53.2%*	11.1	21.5	93.4%*	3.0	12.9	333.4%*
Sex									
Female	17.9	18.0	0.4%	8.9	11.3	26.3%*	1.9	5.2	168.0%*
Male	20.3	32.8	61.2%*	11.7	23.6	102.5%*	3.1	14.3	361.1%*
Age group (years at death)									
18-24	16.8	16.0	-4.7%	12.1	12.2	1.0%	–[c]	5.7	–
25-34	22.3	38.7	73.4%*	13.8	31.4	127.9%*	2.7	13.7	402.4%*
35-44	21.3	41.8	96.2%*	11.7	29.9	156.6%*	3.2	17.9	454.0%*
45-54	32.2	31.1	-3.4%	17.0	21.0	23.3%*	5.9	14.6	148.8%*
55-64	20.9	41.0	96.7%*	10.2	25.3	147.8%*	4.3	20.5	374.4%*
65+	3.5	9.3	167.2%*	1.1	5.0	337.8%*	0.2	3.9	1490.2%*
Geographic region[d]									
Midwest	20.0	33.6	67.8%*	10.7	24.3	125.6%*	2.9	12.5	334.8%*
Northeast	22.4	52.8	136.1%*	11.9	43.9	267.9%*	3.6	20.8	483.5%*
South	17.7	24.9	40.6%*	10.1	17.7	74.9%*	2.5	10.8	336.3%*
West	22.5	27.3	21.5%*	13.0	15.4	17.7%	3.8	13.5	255.2%*
Race[e]									
American Indian, Alaskan Native	23.3	22.7	-2.6%	11.7	10.4	-10.5%	–	11.0	–
Asian, Hawaiian, or Pacific Islander	15.6	17.4	11.4%	7.8	9.6	22.7%	4.6	8.1	77.2%
Black	16.5	34.5	109.4%*	6.6	22.1	236.3%*	7.8	20.6	164.7%*
Multiple Races	17.2	69.5	304.1%*	7.9	48.0	510.1%*	–	34.6	–
White	15.6	21.5	37.4%*	8.3	14.2	70.2%*	1.9	8.7	358.2%*
Ethnicity[f]									
Hispanic	17.4	20.5	18.1%	10.0	13.1	31.2%*	3.6	9.4	165.3%*
Not Hispanic	15.4	24.0	55.4%*	7.9	15.7	99.6%*	2.5	10.8	322.3%*
Recent Use of VHA Services[g]									
Yes	37.0	41.7	12.8%*	21.0	29.7	41.2%*	5.3	18.0	242.3%*
No	15.6	25.7	65.1%*	8.7	18.3	108.9%*	2.4	10.7	356.0%*

* Statistically significant difference (for rates based on <100 deaths, no overlap of gamma confidence intervals; for rates based on >100 deaths, z-tests with $p < .05$).
[a] Crude rates are presented for age, race, and ethnicity groups. Historic Veteran population estimates were not available stratified by both age and race or ethnicity. Therefore, crude rates are presented for race and ethnicity groups. All other rates presented are age-adjusted.
[b] An overdose death identified as involving both an opioid and a stimulant contributed to rates for each group.
[c] Rates based on fewer than 10 deaths have been suppressed in accordance with privacy standards
[d] US Census Regions, determined by state of death
[e] Race was missing for 2.8% of decedents. Race groups presented reflect individuals identified as exclusively belonging to that category.
[f] Ethnicity was missing for 3.3% of decedents
[g] Recent use defined as a VHA encounter during year of death or year prior

Affairs Opioid Overdose Education & Naloxone Distribution (OEND) Program - Pharmacy Benefits Management Services, 2021) Recent VHA efforts to treat stimulant use disorders include contingency management approaches and evidence-based medication therapies. (DePhilippis et al., 2018; Gordon et al., 2020).

A recent analysis of the entire Veteran population for 2010–2016 suggests that trends in opioid-involved Veteran overdose deaths align with those for the overall US adult population. (Peltzman et al., 2020).

The present analysis builds on this work by examining Veteran overdose mortality in the period of 2010–2019, considering additional drug types, demographic factors, and recent use of VHA services. Finally, the present analysis provides statistical comparisons of rates for Veterans and non-Veteran US adults.

2. Methods

This analysis examined 536,478 drug overdose deaths within the 50 US states and Washington, D.C., from 2010 to 2019. (Hedegaard et al., 2020) Of these, 42,627 were deaths of Veterans. Veterans were defined as "persons who served on federal active duty and were not currently serving at the time of their death", using methodology consistent with the National Veteran Suicide Prevention Annual Report. (U.S. Department of Veterans Affairs Office of Mental Health and Suicide Prevention, 2021a). Veteran deaths were identified using National Death Index search results included in the Department of Veterans Affairs/Department of Defense Mortality Data Repository. (U.S. Department of Veterans Affairs Office of Mental Health and Suicide Prevention, 2021b). Veteran overdose rates were calculated using linearly interpolated estimates of the Veteran Population Projection Model 2018 (VetPop2018) population, calculated to provide a point estimate as of July 1 of each year. (National Center for Veterans Analysis and Statistics, 2021; VA Office of Mental Health and Suicide Prevention, 2021a) Counts of overdose deaths among the general US adult population (ages 18 and older) and corresponding population estimates were obtained from Centers for Disease Control (CDC) Wide-ranging ONline Data for Epidemiologic Research (WONDER). (Centers for Disease Control and Prevention, 2021) Non-Veteran numbers were estimated by subtracting known Veteran counts from general US adult population numbers. Age-adjusted rates were calculated based on the 2000 Projected US population and displayed per 100,000 population. (Klein and Schoenborn, 2001) Standardized rate ratios (SRR) were calculated to compare age-adjusted rates among the Veteran and non-Veteran US adult population, stratified by sex. Use of VHA services was obtained from the Veterans Affairs Corporate Data Warehouse database of patient health records, and recent Veteran VHA users were defined for each calendar year as Veterans who had a VHA encounter in either that calendar year or the prior year. (U.S. Department of Veterans Affairs Office of Mental Health and Suicide Prevention, 2020b). Veteran VHA user populations were determined by tallying the number of recent Veteran VHA users as of July 1 of each year. Numbers of Veterans without recent

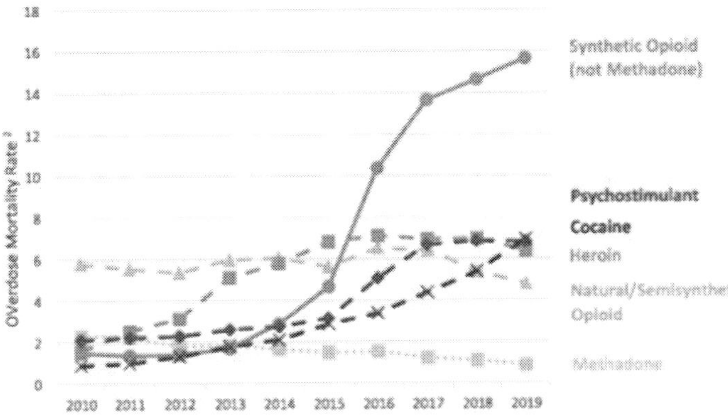

Fig. 1. Age-Adjusted Veteran Overdose Mortality Rate, by Drug Type [1], 2010–2019. [1] *Rates presented are not mutually exclusive, an overdose death involving multiple drugs would contribute to each relevant trend line.* [2] *Age-adjusted mortality rate per 100,000 population.*

VHA use were estimated by subtracting known counts of Veterans with recent VHA use from overall Veteran population numbers. Race and ethnicity were identified for Veterans using VHA administrative data and the United States Veterans Eligibility Trends and Statistics (USVETS) database. Calculations according to geography utilized US Census Regions, determined by state of death. (U.S. Census, 2021).

Overdose deaths were identified according to International Classification of Disease (ICD-10) underlying cause-of-death codes X40–44 (unintentional), X60–64 (suicide), X85 (homicide), or Y10–Y14 (undetermined intent). Identified overdose deaths were examined according to the specific drug involved using multiple cause-of-death codes as follows: heroin (T40.1); natural, semisynthetic, or other opioids (T40.2); methadone (T40.3); synthetic opioids other than methadone (T40.4); cocaine (T40.5); and psychostimulants/methamphetamines (T43.6). Overdose deaths were also examined according to two drug type categories: all opioids (one or more of: T40.0–T40.4, T40.6) and all stimulants (T40.5, T43.6). Overdose deaths having indications of involvement of multiple drug types contributed to the counts and rates for each indicated type. Counts and rates for all listed drug types for the years 2010–2019 are presented in the appendix. Overdose deaths solely involving drugs not listed above (e.g., benzodiazepines) are included within the category "all overdose" but are not presented in drug-specific analyses. This is consistent with CDC Data Brief reporting on drug overdose deaths. (Hedegaard et al., 2020).

For calculations involving rates based on fewer than 100 deaths in any stratum, statistical significance was assessed by comparing gamma confidence intervals for overlap; for rates based on 100 or more deaths, z-tests were used with $p < .05$ determining significance. (Fay and Feuer, 1997) Statistical significance was assessed for SRRs using gamma confidence intervals. Joinpoint 4.8 was used to compare trends across groups, assessing differences in average annual percent change for the best fit Joinpoint regression models selected at alpha = 0.05. (Joinpoint Regression Program, 2020) Pairwise comparisons were used in Joinpoint to test for differences in trends, indicating whether rates of change in overdose mortality were significantly different across groups over the period 2010–2019. (Kim et al., 2004).

This study was conducted as part of VHA operations and program evaluation. Per VA guidance, it was not classified as research and did not require institutional review board review. This work was reviewed and approved by the VA Office of Mental Health and Suicide Prevention.

3. Results

From 2010–2019, there were 42,627 overdose deaths among US Veterans, including 18,573 Veterans with recent VHA care and 24,054 Veterans without recent VHA care. The average Veteran population during this period was 21,367,900 (standard deviation: 1,021,234).

As shown in Table 1, from 2010 to 2019, the age-adjusted rate of drug overdose mortality among Veterans increased by 53.2% overall, by 93.4% for overdoses involving opioids, and by 333.4% for overdoses involving stimulants. The percentage of Veteran overdose deaths that involved opioids increased from 51.5% (n = 1891) in 2010 to 65.7% (n=3,197) in 2019; for stimulants it increased from 16.7% (n = 612) in 2010–44.6% (n = 2172) in 2019.

Male Veterans experienced a 61.2% increase in overall overdose mortality from 2010 to 2019, with age-adjusted rates of opioid-involved deaths doubling from 11.7 to 23.6 per 100,000, and rates of stimulant-involved deaths more than quadrupling from 3.1 to 14.3 per 100,000. Female Veterans did not experience a statistically significant change in overall overdose mortality from 2010 to 2019, despite statistically significant rate increases of 26.3% for opioid-involved deaths and 168.0% for stimulant-involved deaths.

Veterans aged 65+ experienced the largest relative increase in overdose mortality from 2010 to 2019. Veterans aged 25–34, 35–44, and 55–64 experienced comparable increases in overdose mortality, roughly doubling during this time, while Veterans aged 45–54 did not experience a statistically significant change. Among US Census regions, the largest absolute and relative increases in rates of overdose mortality occurred in the Northeast. Among race groups compared, Veterans identified as being of multiple races had the highest crude rate of overdose mortality in 2019, with 69.5 deaths per 100,000. Veterans identified as non-Hispanic experienced a 55.4% increase in overall overdose mortality from 2010 to 2019. In 2019, age-adjusted overdose mortality rates were 41.7 per 100,000 among Veterans with recent use of VHA services, and 25.7 per 100,000 among Veterans without recent VHA use.

Veteran overdose mortality varied substantially by specific drug involved. From 2010–2019, age-adjusted rates of overdose deaths involving synthetic opioids rose from 1.5 to 15.7 per 100,000 and rates involving heroin rose from 1.6 to 6.4 per 100,000. Rates involving methadone fell by more than half, from 2.3 to 0.9 per 100,000. Rates involving natural/semisynthetic opioids decreased from 5.8 to 4.8 per 100,000. Rates involving stimulants grew notably, increasing by 219.3% for cocaine to 6.9 per 100,000 and by 669.2% for psychostimulants to 7.0 per 100,000 as of 2019. Figs. 1–3.

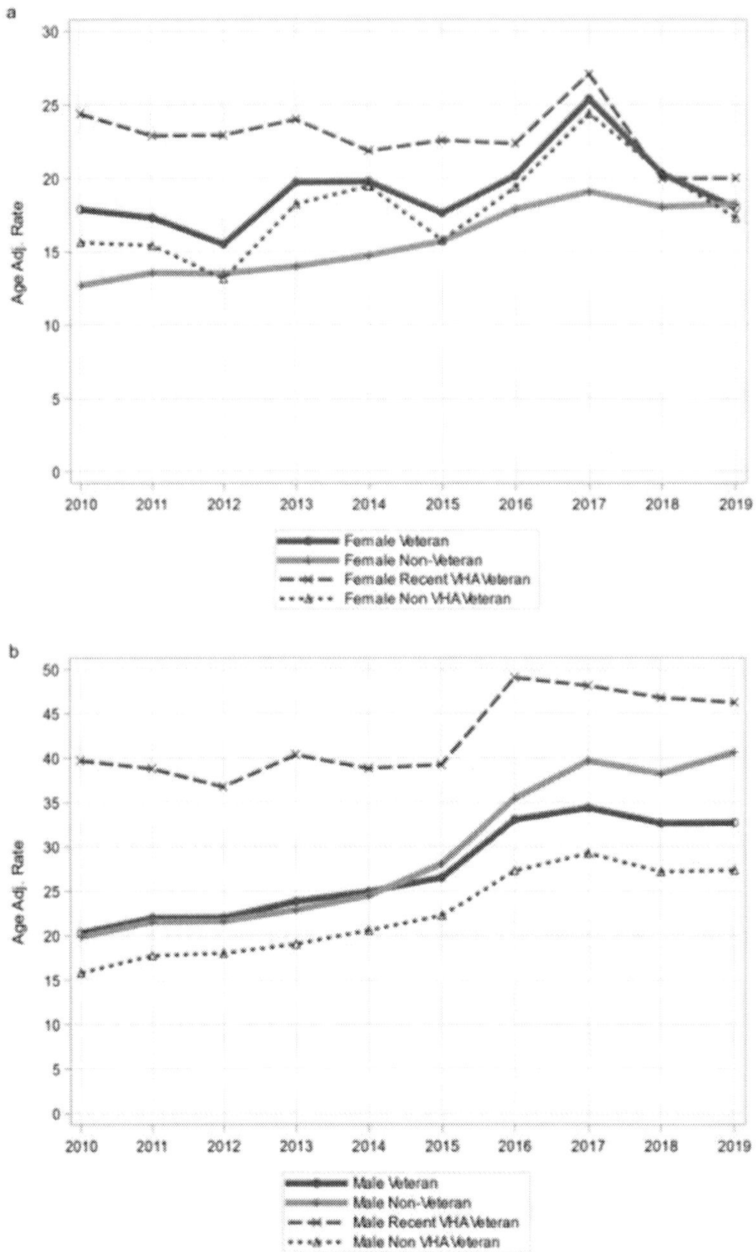

Fig. 2. **a** Among Women: Age-Adjusted Rates of Drug Overdose Deaths, by Veteran Status and VHA Use, 2010–2019. **2 b:** Among Men: Age-Adjusted Rates of Drug Overdose Deaths, by Veteran Status and VHA Use, 2010–2019.

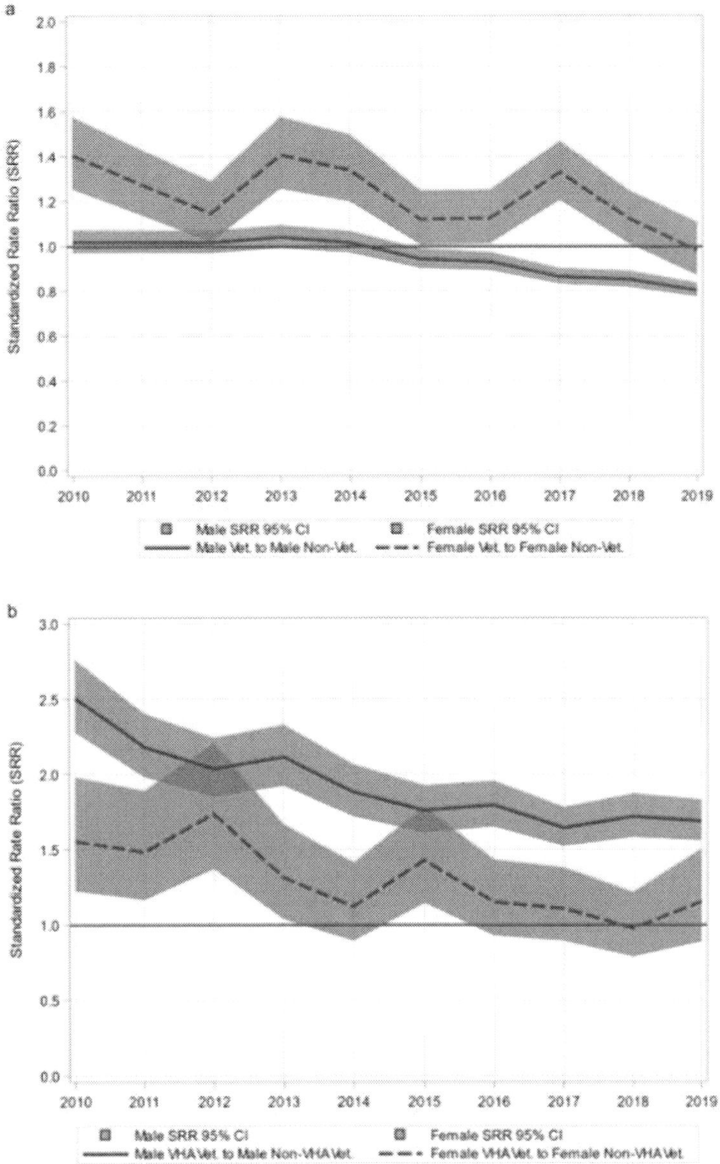

Fig. 3. **a** Age-Adjusted Rate Ratio of Overdose Mortality, Veteran vs. Non-Veteran US Adults, by Sex. **3 b**. Age-Adjusted Rate Ratio of Overdose Mortality, VHA-Using Veteran vs. Non-VHA-Using Veteran, by Sex.

The 2019 age-adjusted rate of overdose mortality was 19% lower for male Veterans than for male non-Veteran US adults (SRR 0.81, 95% CI [0.77, 0.84]). The 2019 age-adjusted rate of overdose mortality was 69% higher among male Veterans with recent VHA use than those without recent VHA use (SRR 1.69, 95% CI [1.56, 1.83]). In 2019, rates among women were not significantly different according to Veteran status or recent VHA use.

From 2010-2019, age-adjusted overdose mortality increased among both male Veterans and male non-Veteran US adults. However, the average annual percent change (AAPC) was significantly lower for male

Table 2
Veteran Overdose Deaths, Crude and Adjusted Rates by Drug.

Year of death	Drug	Deaths	Veteran population estimate	Crude rate per 100,000	Age adjusted rate per 100,000
2010	All Overdose	3669	22,752,000	16.1	19.8
2011	All Overdose	3737	22,521,000	16.6	21.0
2012	All Overdose	3624	22,193,000	16.3	20.8
2013	All Overdose	3866	22,000,000	17.6	23.2
2014	All Overdose	4010	21,666,000	18.5	24.0
2015	All Overdose	4130	21,241,000	19.4	25.0
2016	All Overdose	4820	20,863,000	23.1	30.8
2017	All Overdose	5119	20,480,000	25.0	32.6
2018	All Overdose	4787	20,166,000	23.7	30.4
2019	All Overdose	4865	19,797,000	24.6	30.3
2010	All Opioids	1891	22,752,000	8.3	11.1
2011	All Opioids	1894	22,521,000	8.4	11.6
2012	All Opioids	1854	22,193,000	8.4	11.4
2013	All Opioids	2084	22,000,000	9.5	13.6
2014	All Opioids	2314	21,666,000	10.7	15.0
2015	All Opioids	2441	21,241,000	11.5	16.0
2016	All Opioids	3010	20,863,000	14.4	20.7
2017	All Opioids	3236	20,480,000	15.8	22.4
2018	All Opioids	3080	20,166,000	15.3	21.3
2019	All Opioids	3197	19,797,000	16.1	21.5
2010	All Stimulants	612	22,752,000	2.7	3.0
2011	All Stimulants	605	22,521,000	2.7	3.2
2012	All Stimulants	660	22,193,000	3.0	3.5
2013	All Stimulants	771	22,000,000	3.5	4.3
2014	All Stimulants	861	21,666,000	4.0	4.7
2015	All Stimulants	1031	21,241,000	4.9	5.8
2016	All Stimulants	1395	20,863,000	6.7	8.2
2017	All Stimulants	1719	20,480,000	8.4	10.4
2018	All Stimulants	1955	20,166,000	9.7	11.7
2019	All Stimulants	2172	19,797,000	11.0	12.9
2010	Cocaine	444	22,752,000	2.0	2.1
2011	Cocaine	430	22,521,000	1.9	2.2
2012	Cocaine	439	22,193,000	2.0	2.3
2013	Cocaine	493	22,000,000	2.2	2.6
2014	Cocaine	504	21,666,000	2.3	2.8
2015	Cocaine	571	21,241,000	2.7	3.2
2016	Cocaine	879	20,863,000	4.2	5.1
2017	Cocaine	1087	20,480,000	5.3	6.7
2018	Cocaine	1145	20,166,000	5.7	6.9
2019	Cocaine	1187	19,797,000	6.0	6.9
2010	Heroin	232	22,752,000	1.0	1.6
2011	Heroin	362	22,521,000	1.6	2.5
2012	Heroin	429	22,193,000	1.9	3.2
2013	Heroin	655	22,000,000	3.0	5.1
2014	Heroin	770	21,666,000	3.6	5.8
2015	Heroin	896	21,241,000	4.2	6.8
2016	Heroin	1006	20,863,000	4.8	7.1
2017	Heroin	980	20,480,000	4.8	7.0
2018	Heroin	987	20,166,000	4.9	7.0
2019	Heroin	977	19,797,000	4.9	6.4
2010	Methadone	389	22,752,000	1.7	2.3
2011	Methadone	355	22,521,000	1.6	2.2
2012	Methadone	284	22,193,000	1.3	1.8
2013	Methadone	285	22,000,000	1.3	1.8
2014	Methadone	268	21,666,000	1.2	1.7
2015	Methadone	234	21,241,000	1.1	1.5
2016	Methadone	236	20,863,000	1.1	1.5
2017	Methadone	202	20,480,000	1.0	1.2
2018	Methadone	192	20,166,000	1.0	1.1
2019	Methadone	142	19,797,000	0.7	0.9
2010	Natural and Semi-Synthetic Opioids	1023	22,752,000	4.5	5.8
2011	Natural and Semi-Synthetic Opioids	972	22,521,000	4.3	5.6
2012	Natural and Semi-Synthetic Opioids	948	22,193,000	4.3	5.4
2013	Natural and Semi-Synthetic Opioids	997	22,000,000	4.5	6.0
2014	Natural and Semi-Synthetic Opioids	1078	21,666,000	5.0	6.1
2015	Natural and Semi-Synthetic Opioids	1005	21,241,000	4.7	5.6
2016	Natural and Semi-Synthetic Opioids	1104	20,863,000	5.3	6.5
2017	Natural and Semi-Synthetic Opioids	1076	20,480,000	5.3	6.4
2018	Natural and Semi-Synthetic Opioids	932	20,166,000	4.6	5.4
2019	Natural and Semi-Synthetic Opioids	819	19,797,000	4.1	4.8
2010	Psychostimulants	182	22,752,000	0.8	0.9
2011	Psychostimulants	185	22,521,000	0.8	1.0
2012	Psychostimulants	236	22,193,000	1.1	1.3
2013	Psychostimulants	299	22,000,000	1.4	1.8
2014	Psychostimulants	385	21,666,000	1.8	2.1
2015	Psychostimulants	488	21,241,000	2.3	2.9
2016	Psychostimulants	565	20,863,000	2.7	3.4
2017	Psychostimulants	718	20,480,000	3.5	4.4
2018	Psychostimulants	897	20,166,000	4.4	5.4
2019	Psychostimulants	1106	19,797,000	5.6	7.0
2010	Synthetic Opioid Other than Methadone	280	22,752,000	1.2	1.5
2011	Synthetic Opioid Other than Methadone	247	22,521,000	1.1	1.4
2012	Synthetic Opioid Other than Methadone	239	22,193,000	1.1	1.4
2013	Synthetic Opioid Other than Methadone	288	22,000,000	1.3	1.7
2014	Synthetic Opioid Other than Methadone	417	21,666,000	1.9	2.9
2015	Synthetic Opioid Other than Methadone	662	21,241,000	3.1	4.7
2016	Synthetic Opioid Other than Methadone	1343	20,863,000	6.4	10.4
2017	Synthetic Opioid Other than Methadone	1828	20,480,000	8.9	13.7
2018	Synthetic Opioid Other than Methadone	1971	20,166,000	9.8	14.6
2019	Synthetic Opioid Other than Methadone	2214	19,797,000	11.2	15.7

Veterans (AAPC=6.4) than male non-Veterans (AAPC=9.6) during this period. Among male Veterans, the rate of increase did not significantly differ according to recent VHA use. From 2010-2019, age-adjusted overdose mortality did not significantly increase among female Veterans but did significantly increase among female non-Veterans. The rate of increase was not significantly different between these two groups. Among female Veterans, the rate of change was significantly lower among those with recent VHA use (AAPC = −1.2)[1] than those without recent VHA use (AAPC = 3.9).

Overdose rates among male Veterans decreased relative to male non-Veterans after 2014. The comparison between female Veterans and female non-Veterans fluctuated throughout the study period, but suggests an overall decline with rates higher among female Veterans from 2010

[1] Note: the 2010-2019 AAPC among female Veterans with recent VHA use was not statistically significantly different from 0. All other AAPC values presented were statistically significantly different from 0.

Table 3
Veteran Drug Overdose Mortality Counts 2010–2019, Overall and by Drug Category [a].

	Overall drug overdose		Opioid overdose		Stimulant overdose	
	2010 Deaths	2019 Deaths	2010 Deaths	2019 Deaths	2010 Deaths	2019 Deaths
All Veterans	3669	4865	1891	3197	612	2172
Sex						
Female	356	372	172	229	35	102
Male	3313	4493	1719	2968	577	2070
Age group (years at death)[b]						
18–24	57	42	41	32	< 10	15
25–34	393	619	243	583	48	219
35–44	574	897	314	642	87	384
45–54	1268	912	670	615	231	428
55–64	1064	1530	521	944	220	763
65+	312	853	102	457	22	358
Geographic region[c]						
Midwest	775	1074	376	750	122	420
Northeast	526	989	258	787	87	385
South	1405	1770	734	1168	224	802
West	963	1032	523	492	179	565
Race						
American Indian, Alaskan Native	38	37	19	17	< 10	18
Asian, Hawaiian, or Pacific Islander	48	69	24	38	14	32
Black	414	853	165	546	195	508
Multiple Races	59	317	27	219	< 10	158
White	3011	3460	1604	2282	367	1406
Unknown	99	129	52	95	30	50
Ethnicity						
Hispanic	210	311	121	199	43	143
Not Hispanic	3331	4395	1703	2886	551	1975
Recent Use of VHA Services[d]						
Yes	1575	2158	807	1410	269	1004
No	2094	2707	1084	1787	343	1168

[a] An overdose death identified as involving both an opioid and a stimulant contributed to counts for each group.
[b] Age was missing for one decedent.
[c] US Census Regions, determined by state of death
[d] Recent use defined as a VHA encounter during year of death or year prior

to 2018 then not significantly different in 2019.

4. Discussion

This report presents new information on overdose mortality among US Veterans. The analyses examine the most recent available Veteran mortality data, through 2019. Age-adjusted rates of Veteran drug overdose deaths increased 64.6% from 2010 to 2017, decreased 6.7% from 2017 to 2018, and were not significantly different between 2018 and 2019. This work offers the first comparison of drug overdose mortality among Veterans and non-Veteran US adults. Findings by sex suggest that overdose rates among Veterans diminished relative to non-Veterans during the study period: Adjusting for age, after 2014 Veteran men had lower overdose mortality rates than non-Veteran men, and in 2019 previously elevated rates among Veteran women fell to become not significantly different from those of non-Veteran women. Similar findings were observed for overdose deaths specifically involving opioids and for those involving stimulants.

The study also evaluates differences in overdose mortality within Veteran population subgroups, comparing those with recent use of VHA health care to those without recent use. Among male Veterans, those with recent VHA use had higher rates of overdose mortality than other male Veterans. This may reflect a more complex clinical profile among Veterans with recent VHA care and it highlights the importance of overdose prevention efforts in the context of health care encounters. Among female Veterans, those with recent VHA use experienced higher rates of overdose mortality compared to other female Veterans in 2010–2018, however not in 2019. While female Veterans with recent VHA use did not experience significant average annual increases in overdose mortality from 2010 to 2019, significant increases were documented for female Veterans without recent VHA use.

Findings are consistent with prior reports showing higher opioid overdose mortality among VHA patients compared to the general US population (Bohnert et al., 2011), and they emphasize the importance of overdose prevention efforts for Veteran men who use VHA care, among whom risk concentration is highest. However, prevention efforts should also consider Veterans not in VHA care, who have the greatest number of overdose deaths (2707 in 2019 among Veterans not in VHA care, versus 2158 among Veterans in VHA care). Targeted approaches may be warranted to address the unique needs of Veteran subgroups.

Veteran overdose deaths involving opioids increased from 1891 in 2010 to 3,197 in 2019. Although Veteran overdose deaths involving heroin, methadone, and natural and semi-synthetic opioids have decreased or remained steady since 2016, Veteran overdose deaths involving synthetic opioids have continued to rise substantially. VHA has worked to address Veteran opioid overdose through a multifaceted approach including reducing opioid prescriptions, improving naloxone distribution, and increasing use of evidence-based medications for opioid use disorder. (Gordon et al., 2020; Lin et al., 2017; Rubin, 2019) Stimulants, while still involved in a minority of Veteran overdose deaths (44.6% in 2019), also present cause for concern: age-adjusted rates of Veteran overdose deaths involving stimulants more than quadrupled from 2010 to 2019 (from 3.0 to 12.9 per 100,000). In 2019, one quarter of Veteran overdose deaths involving opioids also involved a stimulant, and further work is needed to understand and address this growing trend.

This analysis had several limitations. Overdose deaths may be mistakenly attributed to other causes such as cardiac arrest, potentially resulting in undercounting of cases. (Tseng et al., 2018) Rates involving non-Veterans were estimated by removing counts of known Veterans from the general population, and are therefore influenced by the availability of Veteran status data. Improvements in toxicology testing during the study period may account for some of the observed increase in cases reported. Availability of overdose mortality reporting varies by state and may impact regional trends presented. (Centers for Disease Control and Prevention, National Center for Health Statistics, 2020). Race and ethnicity were classified for Veteran decedents using medical record and administrative data, and although self-reported data were prioritized where available, may not reflect personal identity or experience.

5. Conclusions

This study provides an improved understanding of trends in overdose deaths among Veterans and offers information that can be used to target prevention efforts to reach those most at risk. In particular, our findings highlight the need to address overdose risk by Veteran subgroup given that results differ by recent VHA use history and by sex. The high rates among recent VHA users underscores the need for ongoing prevention efforts by VA. Despite decreases in overdose rates among Veterans relative to rates among the broader US population, current CDC projections and challenges posed by the COVID-19 pandemic suggest that this topic needs to be an ongoing area of attention for VA. Provisional data from CDC's National Center for Health Statistics indicate a projected 30.8% increase in overdose deaths from 2019 to 2020 among the general US population. (Ahmad et al., 2021) Future analyses will assess whether Veteran trends follow a similar pattern.

Role of funding source

This work was supported by the VA Office of Mental Health and Suicide Prevention.

Credit authorship contribution statement

All listed authors made a substantial contribution. C.R., T.P., S.M., and B.S. provided input on the structure of the analysis and presentation of results. S.M. and T.P. provided guidance on appropriate statistical methodology. J.M. provided editorial review and supervision. M.B. conducted the statistical analysis and drafted the manuscript with input from all authors. L.A. provided subject matter expertise and input on VHA initiatives related to substance use. All authors have approved this manuscript.

Declaration of Competing Interest

The authors declare that they have no known competing financial interests or personal relationships that could have influenced or appeared to influence the work reported in this paper.

Acknowledgments

With thanks to Dr. Joseph Liberto, National Mental Health Director, Substance Abuse Disorders, Office of Mental Health and Suicide Prevention, US Department of Veterans Affairs, for comments on this manuscript.

Appendix

See Tables 2–3.

References

Ahmad FB, Rossen LM, Sutton P., 2021. Provisional drug overdose death counts. National Center for Health Statistics. Designed by LM Rossen, A Lipphardt, FB Ahmad, JM Keralis, and Y Chong. National Center for Health Statistics. 〈https://www.cdc.gov/nchs/nvss/vsrr/drug-overdose-data.htm〉 (Accessed Oct 15, 2021).

Bohnert, A.S.B., Ilgen, M.A., Galea, S., McCarthy, J.F., Blow, F.C., 2011. Accidental poisoning mortality among patients in the department of veterans affairs health system. Med. Care 49, 393–396. https://doi.org/10.1097/MLR.0b013e318202aa27.

U.S. Census. Census Regions and Divisions of the United States. 〈https://www2.census.gov/geo/pdfs/maps-data/maps/reference/us_regdiv.pdf〉 (Accessed Mar 2, 2021).

Centers for Disease Control and Prevention, National Center for Health Statistics, 2021. Multiple Cause of Death 1999–2019 on CDC WONDER Online Database, released in 2020. Data are from the Multiple Cause of Death Files, 1999–2019, as compiled from data provided by the 57 vital statistics jurisdictions through the Vital Statistics Cooperative Program. 〈http://wonder.cdc.gov/mcd-icd10.html〉 (Accessed Aug 12, 2021).

Centers for Disease Control and Prevention, National Center for Health Statistics, 2020. 2018–2019 Heroin Overdose Data: Changes in drug overdose death rates involving heroin by select states, United States, 2018 to 2019. 〈http://wonder.cdc.gov/mcd-icd10.html〉 (Accessed Oct 12, 2021).

DePhilippis, D., Petry, N.M., Bonn-Miller, M.O., Rosenbach, S.B., McKay, J.R., 2018. The national implementation of contingency management (CM) in the department of veterans affairs: attendance at CM sessions and substance use outcomes. Drug Alcohol Depend. 185, 367–373. https://doi.org/10.1016/j.drugalcdep.2017.12.020.

Fay, M.P., Feuer, E.J., 1997. Confidence intervals for directly standardized rates: a method based on the gamma distribution. Stat. Med. 16, 791–801. 〈https://wonder.cdc.gov/wonder/help/cancer/fayfeuerconfidenceintervals.pdf〉.

Gellad, W.F., Good, C.B., Shulkin, D.J., 2017. Addressing the opioid epidemic in the United States: lessons from the department of veterans affairs. JAMA Intern. Med. 177 (5), 611–612. https://doi.org/10.1001/jamainternmed.2017.0147.

Gordon, A.J., Drexler, K., Hawkins, E.J., Burden, J., Codell, N.K., Mhatre-Owens, A., Dungan, M.T., Hagedorn, H., 2020. Stepped care for opioid use disorder train the trainer (SCOUTT) initiative: expanding access to medication treatment for opioid use disorder within veterans health administration facilities. Subst. Abus. 41 (3), 275–282. https://doi.org/10.1080/08897077.2020.1787299.

Hedegaard H., Miniño A.M., Warner M., 2020. Drug overdose deaths in the United States, 1999–2019. NCHS Data Brief, no 394. Hyattsville, MD: National Center for Health Statistics. 〈https://www.cdc.gov/nchs/products/databriefs/db394.htm〉.

Ilgen, M.A., Bohnert, A.S.B., Ganoczy, D., Bair, M.J., McCarthy, J.F., Blow, F.C., 2016. Opioid dose and risk of suicide. Pain 157, 1079–1084. https://doi.org/10.1097/j.pain.0000000000000484.

Joinpoint Regression Program, Version 4.8.0.1 - April 2020; Statistical Methodology and Applications Branch, Surveillance Research Program, National Cancer Institute.

Kim, H.J., Fay, M.P., Yu, B., Barrett, M.J., Feuer, E.J., 2004. Comparability of segmented line regression models. Biometrics 60, 1005–1014. https://doi.org/10.1111/j.0006-341X.2004.00256.x.

Klein, R.J., Schoenborn, C.A., 2001. Age Adjustment Using the 2000 Projected U.S. Population. Healthy People Statistical Notes. National Center for Health Statistics,, Hyattsville, MA. 〈https://www.cdc.gov/nchs/data/statnt/statnt20.pdf〉.

Lin, L.A., Bohnert, A.S.B., Kerns, R.D., Clay, M.A., Ganoczy, D., Ilgen, M.A., 2017. Impact of the opioid safety initiative on opioid-related prescribing in veterans. Pain 158, 833–839. https://doi.org/10.1097/j.pain.0000000000000837.

Lin, L.A., Peltzman, T., McCarthy, J.F., Oliva, E.M., Trafton, J.A., Bohnert, A.S.B., 2019. Changing trends in opioid overdose deaths and prescription opioid receipt among veterans. Am. J. Prev. Med. 57, 106–110. https://doi.org/10.1016/j.amepre.2019.01.016.

Meffert, B.N., Morabito, D.M., Sawicki, D.A., Hausman, C., Southwick, S.M., Pietrzak, R. H., Heinz, A.J., 2019. US veterans who do and do not utilize veterans affairs health care services: demographic, military, medical, and psychosocial characteristics. Prim. Care Companion CNS Disord. 21. https://doi.org/10.4088/PCC.18m02350.

National Center for Veterans Analysis and Statistics. Veteran population (VetPop) models by age and gender. Extracted 2010–2018. 〈https://www.va.gov/vetdata/Veteran_population.asp〉 (Accessed Feb 3, 2021).

Peltzman, T., Ravindran, C., Schoen, P.M., Morley, S.W., Drexler, K., Katz, I.R., McCarthy, J.F., 2020. Brief report: opioid-involved overdose mortality in United States veterans. Am. J. Addict. 29, 340–344. https://doi.org/10.1111/ajad.13027.

Rubin, R., 2019. VA efforts to reduce opioid overdose deaths in at-risk veterans. JAMA 322, 2374. https://doi.org/10.1001/jama.2019.20562.

Tseng, Z.H., Olgin, J.E., Vittinghoff, E., Ursell, P.C., Kim, A.S., Sporer, K., Yeh, C., Colburn, B., Clark, N.M., Khan, R., Hart, A.P., Moffatt, E., 2018. Prospective countywide surveillance and autopsy characterization of sudden cardiac death: POST SCD Study. Circulation 137, 2689–2700. https://doi.org/10.1161/CIRCULATIONAHA.117.033427.

U.S. Department of Veterans Affairs Office of Mental Health and Suicide Prevention. 2021b. Joint Department of Veterans Affairs and Department of Defense Mortality Data Repository. 〈https://www.mirecc.va.gov/suicideprevention/documents/VA_DoD-MDR_Flyer-92421.pdf〉 (Accessed 10/18/2021.).

U.S. Department of Veterans Affairs Office of Mental Health and Suicide Prevention, 2020a. 2005–2018 National Suicide Data Appendix. 〈https://www.mentalhealth.va.gov/docs/data-sheets/2018/2005-2018-National-Data-Appendix-508.xlsx〉 (Accessed Feb 5, 2021).

U.S. Department of Veterans Affairs Office of Mental Health and Suicide Prevention, 2020b. 2020 National Veteran Suicide Prevention Annual Report. 〈https://www.mentalhealth.va.gov/docs/data-sheets/2020/2020-National-Veteran-Suicide-Prevention-Annual-Report-11-2020-508.pdf〉 (Accessed Feb 5, 2021).

U.S. Department of Veterans Affairs Office of Mental Health and Suicide Prevention, 2021a. 2021 National Veteran Suicide Surveillance Methods Summary. 〈https://www.mentalhealth.va.gov/docs/data-sheets/2020/Suicide_Report_Methods_508.pdf〉 (Accessed Oct 12, 2021).

U.S. Department of Veterans Affairs Opioid Overdose Education & Naloxone Distribution (OEND) Program - Pharmacy Benefits Management Services, n.d. 〈https://www.pbm.va.gov/PBM/academicdetailingservice/Opioid_Overdose_Education_and_Naloxone_Distribution.asp〉 (Accessed Mar 2, 2021).

Warfield, S.C., 2019. Characteristics and patterns of opioid-related overdoses among veterans. Graduate Theses, Dissertations, and Problem Reports. 3902. 〈https://researchrepository.wvu.edu/etd/3902〉 (Accessed Mar 3, 2021).

Statements for the Record

Syracuse University
D'Aniello Institute for Veterans & Military Families
JPMorgan Chase & Co., Founding Partner

Statement for the Record

Senate Committee on Veterans' Affairs Hearing:
Invisible Wounds of War: Improving Mental Health and Suicide Prevention Measures for our Nation's Veterans.

Prepared by:
D'Aniello Institute for Veterans and Military Families (IVMF) at Syracuse University

September 20, 2023

Background

Successfully addressing and preventing veteran suicide requires a comprehensive and holistic approach at the individual, community, and policy levels. This collective approach must include addressing the variety of upstream, non-medical drivers of mental health that contribute to a veteran's overall health outcomes and risk of suicide. Examples of non-medical drivers of health include socioeconomic status, financial strain, housing stability, food security, and access to reliable transportation. The complex nature and interactions of these contributing factors present *multiple opportunities to intervene* when a veteran is at risk of suicide. At each of these steps, community-based organizations and government agencies have the chance to prevent further deterioration of the veteran's health by providing resources to meet the veteran's material and non-material needs. Due to their long-standing presence and trusted partnerships, non-profit community-based organizations (CBOs) are particularly well poised to intervene and assist veterans who are at risk of suicide.

Established in 2020 with the passing of the Commander John Scott Hannon Veterans Mental Health Care Improvement Act, the Staff Sergeant Parker Gordon Fox Suicide Prevention Grant Program (SSG Fox SPGP) plays a vital role in addressing the pressing issue of veteran suicide in the United States. By providing funding to CBOs to address underlying causes of veteran suicide in addition to facilitating referrals for clinical care, the SSG Fox SPGP recognizes the complex nature of factors leading to veteran suicide and takes *meaningful action to partner with and support communities in the prevention effort.*

In September, the D'Aniello Institute for Veterans and Military Families (IVMF) at Syracuse University hosted several events in recognition of National Suicide Prevention Month at the National Veterans Resource Center. In addition to local attendees, we invited our community partners that are recipients of the SSG Fox SPGP to join in person. During the gathering, we convened a roundtable where SSG Fox SPGP grantees had the opportunity to share valuable insights on both the program's successes and the challenges it faces. The feedback provided in this document represents the collective viewpoints of eleven grantees from across the country who actively engaged in this discussion.

Eligibility

One topic the roundtable participants discussed related to eligibility was restrictions based around level of risk. Participants noted that these restrictions prevent them from potentially capturing high-risk individuals who don't meet the administrative eligibility, such as the 24-month requirement. the potential expansion of the SSG Fox SPGP to support additional populations.

Participants also recognized instances where individuals scored within an eligible range for some assessment metrics but fell short in others, leading to disqualification from SSG Fox SPGP intervention. For example, grantees noted that individuals who score high on psychosocial assessments but not on the Columbia Suicide Severity Rating Scale (C-SSRS) still present a potential risk and should be eligible. In a few more dire cases, despite exploring other avenues to assist these individuals, communities reported they had witnessed tragic outcomes, including suicide. Our discussion emphasized that understanding the *motivations behind* individuals declining assessments could lead to a more comprehensive approach.

Grantees also highlighted constraints to eligibility regarding covered services. They raised significant concerns about barriers to entry into the SSG Fox SPGP, both in terms of outreach and getting to the point of screening. Many individuals struggle with transportation, as it isn't covered until a client becomes officially enrolled in the program. Others are more responsive to initial outreach efforts that are more social in nature, rather than focused specifically on mental health. Providing veterans with material resources such as food and transportation assistance simultaneously reduces risk factors and builds trust with individuals in their communities.

Additionally, specific barriers were recognized as potentially addressable by non-SSG Fox SPGP funding, such as the Supportive Services for Veteran Families (SSVF) for housing. Still, these programs may have their own entry challenges, and keeping track of different federal funding sources for similar activities can be burdensome.

One other topic that arose was the idea of expanding populations eligible for the program. These populations might include Reservists, National Guard members, and even family members. For example, if a veteran enrolled in SSG Fox SPGP dies by suicide, their spouse may subsequently experience suicidal ideations. However, the program is currently unable to provide the needed support.

Screening

In addition to the eligibility side of screening, a range of crucial issues regarding screening tools and process emerged. While supportive of the selected assessments in general, as noted above, grantees want to eliminated situations where a veteran would be automatically disqualified despite the potential risk still present. This dilemma prompted discussions on how to make the screening process more comfortable and conducive to open conversations, as well as addressing its labor-intensive and formal nature. Suggestions included actively seeking feedback from grantees to enhance comfort, promoting organic and conversational interactions, involving non-clinicians in the screening process, and exploring ways to distill necessary information from more natural conversations.

One of our presenters in another session (Joe Geraci, PhD, Director of the Transitioning Servicemember/Veteran and Suicide Prevention Center at the VISN 2 MIRECC) shared a 17-question screener used by his team, which *includes the C-SSRS questions*. Many participants seemed to believe this screener would be a valuable asset, relative to the host of other screeners currently part of SSG Fox SPGP.

Participants acknowledged that screenings are subjective and contingent on a client's truthfulness, adding to the complexity of the process. There's also a culture clash between current military culture and openly discussing mental health. To overcome this hurdle, grantees stressed the importance of finding effective ways to communicate in the language of the service member and to reshape their perspective on mental health. In light of these challenges, participants and our team underscored the trusted standing that CBOs hold within their communities, and how they play a critical role in engaging with veterans and creating the space they need to obtain support and assistance.

And lastly, while the Fox grantees' programs and interventions differ from one another, the screening tools and eligibility criteria are uniform. Many of the participants expressed interest in collaboration and efforts to share resources more effectively, particularly when a practice was working well in one community but not another.

VA Referrals & Process

The process of referring eligible individuals to the VA has revealed both successful practices and areas necessitating improvement. One success reported was direct collaboration between the VA and the grantee, where they were able to work directly with the Suicide Prevention Coordinator (SPC) to create procedures for enrollment. These actions not only streamlined the referral process, but also enhanced understanding of the VA's capacity to accommodate these referrals.

However, there have been notable challenges in the referral process. Though well-intentioned, the Office of Mental Health and Suicide Prevention has sometimes fallen short in ensuring local VA Medical Centers (VAMCs) follow programmatic guidance and intent. Successful collaboration with SPCs as described above was the exception, and levels of support seem to vary highly from VAMC to VAMC. Even where partnerships were strong, they were not stable in the event of turnover.

Furthermore, VAMCs may not have the readiness to accommodate referrals through this channel. Suicide Prevention teams, often stretched thin, have cited capacity constraints. Another critical issue is the absence of a specific code in the intake to identify SSG Fox SPGP participants, leading to delays in care due to administrative hurdles. There is also a need for improved tracking of clients' treatment history across different systems to streamline the referral process and ensure seamless coordination between the VA and CBOs.

Grantees also noted that the referral process would benefit from being more bidirectional, particularly at the point where patients may be discharged from VA care. Communities faced discrepancies in whether their local VA was willing to take the appropriate steps to authorize releases of information. They noted that the services they are able to provide can often make an enormous difference to veterans' experiences managing their mental health and day-to-day lives.

Overwhelmingly, our partners remained positive about the potential of the SSG Fox SPGP. They believe that by continuing to build upon the partnerships with CBOs through the program, the VA can continue to provide comprehensive care for veterans that aims to address root causes of health and wellness that allow veterans to thrive.

Data Collection & Sharing

While grantees acknowledged ongoing improvements from the VA and MITRE, data collection remains a challenge. One prominent issue revolves around the lack of clarity on how the MITRE dashboard will display important and relevant information. Grantees agreed it feels as if they're sending data off without a clear sense of how it will be shared or utilized. Participants also emphasized the necessity for more immediate feedback and quicker turnaround on screening scoring. Others suggested more flexibility in the required data forms, depending on any changes that may come to screening process requirements.

We also noted other missed opportunities to capture meaningful data. For example, while this program is in its early stages and therefore still improving, it would be beneficial to track individuals who score high on psychosocial assessments but zero on the C-SSRS screening, those who screen positive but face administrative-caused ineligibilities, and those who refuse assessments. There is also a desire for more comprehensive data on those screened but not deemed eligible, including insights into their circumstances. Participants have expressed a perception of limited interest from the SSG Fox SPGP data team regarding information on individuals who do not strictly meet the eligibility criteria. Additionally, they expressed concern over the omission in collecting information about why individuals withdraw from the program. There was a strong willingness to collect and share this type of information with the VA, if more data was available in return.

As a final point on data collection and reporting, grantees conveyed the complexity with managing multiple federal grants that have specific coverage and measurement requirements. There was wide agreement that there is an opportunity to increase efficiency and consider the ways in which data can be standardized and aligned throughout the process of administering different programs.

In response to data challenges, programs have undertaken their own tracking and documentation of program data to understand the broader context better, integrate into their other operations more effectively, and address the pain points described above. We know that robust and accessible data is necessary to effectively address the underlying causes of poor mental health and veteran suicide. Both the IVMF and our partners strongly hope that data from SSG Fox SPGP is collected thoughtfully, incorporated into meaningful analysis, and transparently shared.

Conclusion

We thank the Committee for the opportunity to share these insights and for its continued focus on the target and shared goal of preventing veteran suicide. The SSG Fox SPGP provides the needed support to CBOs to address upstream factors of mental health that contribute to a veteran's risk of suicide. We look forward to seeing how veteran health continues to improve with the incorporation of this feedback to strengthen the SSG Fox SPGP and ensure its long-term viability and sustainability.

Chairman, Ranking Member, and Members of the Committee,

My name is Heath Steel. I serve as the Executive Vice President & Chief Business Officer for Volunteers of America Northern Rockies, and I am here today to testify on behalf of the Staff Sergeant Parker Gordon Fox Suicide Prevention Grant Program.

I want to thank senior United States Senator Jon Tester for inviting us to be here today. Senator Tester has been a longtime ally to Veterans in Montana, and his support is critical to the services we provide.

Volunteers of America Northern Rockies is the largest private provider of Veteran services in Montana, Wyoming, and Western South Dakota. We serve more than 3,300 Veterans annually with homeless prevention, rapid rehousing, employment, and moral injury services. We are honored to be of service to the men and women who sacrificed so much for our great Nation.

The Staff Sergeant Parker Gordon Fox Suicide Prevention Grant Program is having tremendous impact on communities in our region. I want to start by applauding the United States Veterans Affairs Department for welcoming the out of the box thinking that produced this grant. I don't need to lecture you on the devastating reality that is the current Veteran Suicide rate of 31.7 per 100,000. It breaks our heart … and having served Veterans for more than a decade, 31.7 isn't just a number to Volunteers of America - it is clients, staff, and friends.

Moral injury is the internal pain we feel when life's experiences violate our own understanding of right and wrong. This wounding of the soul may leave us feeling emotionally broken, distrustful of others, or of ourselves. Such a burden on our soul limits our capacity to live fully and to live in peace.

Volunteers of America is incredibly proud of our staff and the work they do through our Mending Moral Injury program. In this non-clinical peer-led program, Veterans begin the healing process by sharing their stories, processing grief and trauma, and walking through forgiveness. Then, our staff are able to reconnect them with purpose, hope, faith and the community.

Volunteers of America was awarded a Staff Sergeant Fox Grant in 2022, and while the application process was straightforward, the implementation process was burdensome and delayed the start of our program, as well as many other awardees, by three months.

In the nine months since we began operation, we've served 59 veterans, including 16 of their family members through the Mending Moral Injury Program. We currently have five paid staff and 35 volunteer facilitators. These individuals have organized seven groups in six communities and continue to expand the footprint of this program daily.

By using Veteran volunteer facilitators, we are able to empower those who have found healing from their own morally injurious experiences to provide healing for others, resulting in tremendous impact on the rural communities we serve.

Immediately after participating in our 8 to 12 week Mending Moral Injury Program, the Patient Health Questionnaire (PHQ9) surveys show that Veterans are less depressed and have less suicidal ideation. We are currently collecting and analyzing six-month follow-up data. These results are inspiring and can be realized firsthand through this Veteran testimony...

I want to share one quick story from Mac LaVerne McDonald. Mac wanted to be sure each and every one of you heard that "not all veterans have physical wounds that you can see and easily get healing from" - She came to the VOA Mending Moral Injury Program with deep military sexual trauma. She proudly shared "The experience I had within the group was supportive and encouraging, and I would not be alive today if it was not for Volunteers of America and their Mending Moral Injury Program supported by the Staff Sergeant Parker Gordon Fox Suicide Prevention Grant. Thank you for providing this supportive program, it saved my life."

Again, I want to thank Senator Tester for this opportunity to share the impact of the Staff Sergeant Parker Gordon Fox Suicide Prevention Grant. This program is saving the lives of America's Veterans like Mac and transforming their ability to engage with their families and their communities. I urge you to protect these funds in advocacy for our Nation's heroes.

God bless you all, and God bless our Nation.

WESTERN GOVERNORS' ASSOCIATION

MARK GORDON
GOVERNOR OF WYOMING
CHAIR

MICHELLE LUJAN GRISHAM
GOVERNOR OF NEW MEXICO
VICE CHAIR

JACK WALDORF
EXECUTIVE DIRECTOR

September 25, 2023

The Honorable Jon Tester
Chairman
Committee on Veterans' Affairs
United States Senate
412 Russell Senate Office Building
Washington, DC 20510

The Honorable Jerry Moran
Ranking Member
Committee on Veterans' Affairs
United States Senate
412 Russell Senate Office Building
Washington, DC 20510

Dear Chairman Tester and Ranking Member Moran:

In light of the Committee's September 20, 2023 hearing, Invisible Wounds of War: Improving Mental Health and Suicide Prevention Measures for our Nation's Veterans, attached please find Western Governors' Association (WGA) Policy Resolutions 2023-08, Veterans, and 2022-07, Physical and Behavioral Health Care in Western States.

In the veterans resolution, Western Governors urge the Department of Veterans Affairs to improve mental health care for veterans by: prioritizing the integration of peer support and behavioral health services for traumatic brain injury into mental health care models; providing training and support for peer specialists; focusing on workforce development and retention; supporting suicide prevention programs; ensuring equitable access to essential health care services in rural areas; and conducting ongoing evaluations for the effective implementation of these practices. The health care resolution outlines Western Governors' behavioral health policies and highlights the need to improve the quality and quantity of behavioral health services available to all western residents.

I request that you include these documents in the permanent record of the hearing, as they articulate Western Governors' policy positions and recommendations related to this urgent issue.

Thank you for your attention to this matter and your consideration of this request. Please contact me if you have any questions or require further information.

Sincerely,

Jack Waldorf
Executive Director

Attachments

1700 Broadway, Suite 500, Denver, CO 80290 | (303) 623-9378 | WESTGOV.ORG

WESTERN GOVERNORS' ASSOCIATION

Policy Resolution 2023-08
Veterans

A. BACKGROUND

American military personnel often return home to a hero's welcome after completing their service, but they face a series of complex challenges. Veterans, whether they volunteered or were drafted, commonly confront a range of issues such as food insecurity, homelessness, unemployment, physical and psychological wounds, and bureaucratic barriers when seeking support services. Western Governors recognize the need to support veterans and address the challenges they face. With one-third of the known veteran population residing in western states, Governors recommend federal regulatory and statutory changes to foster an environment that facilitates access to support services for veterans and encourages further investment in initiatives tailored to assist them.

B. GOVERNORS' POLICY STATEMENT

1. Western Governors urge the Department of Veterans Affairs (VA) to prioritize the integration of peer support services and behavioral health services for Traumatic Brain Injury (TBI) into mental health care models. Additionally, Western Governors urge the VA to address staffing models to support the increasing health concerns for memory care (Dementia, Alzheimer's) and other neurological disorders. VA should also provide continuous training and support for peer specialists and focus on developing and retaining the behavioral health care workforce. Western Governors have highlighted substantive health care workforce recommendations in our health care policy resolution. Ongoing evaluations should be conducted to ensure effective implementation of these practices, which should be disseminated across all VA health care settings to ensure broad access to peer support services for all veterans.

2. Western Governors acknowledge the importance of the VA Governor's Challenge and urge VA to continue its provision of support for programs aimed at effectively addressing the issue of veterans' suicide.

3. Recognizing the need to improve health program services for women veterans, Western Governors urge VA to take urgent action to address gaps in the VA health care system. Improving the promotion of, access to, and the quality of health care for women veterans is essential and requires timely and effective measures to be implemented across VA. Western Governors recommend that VA initiate research programs to study health issues specific to women veterans.

4. Western Governors recognize the significance of expanding access to health care services for veterans, especially those residing in remote areas. VA should take action to increase the accessibility of:

    a. VA Community Care for veterans residing in areas that do not have access to VA health care facilities. It is imperative that VA consult with Governors to ensure that veterans living in rural areas are not disadvantaged in accessing health care;

b. Vet Centers for veterans living in rural areas, to ensure that they have access to necessary health services and support;

c. Health care professionals in rural areas, to provide flexibility for veterans and allow them to access the health care provider of their choosing; and

d. Telemedicine services, which are a vital tool that can help bridge the gap in accessing health care services.

5. Western Governors recommend that VA seek consultation and input from tribal leaders and communities to inform the development and administration of its programs and services for American Indian, Alaska Native, and Native Hawaiian veterans.

6. To ensure that veterans have timely access to high-quality health care, Western Governors recommend that Congress prioritize providing VA with the necessary resources, authority, and ability to recruit, hire, train, and retain health care professionals. This includes physicians, nurses, mental and behavioral health providers, long-term care professionals, and administrative staff. In addition, Western Governors believe VA should streamline the hiring process, offer competitive salaries and benefits, and provide ongoing training and professional development opportunities for health care professionals.

7. Western Governors believe VA should collaborate with states and territories to improve and expand the Highly Rural Transportation Grants program. This includes identifying counties that require assistance, simplifying the application and implementation process, and consulting early with Governors for valuable input on their state's needs. Additionally, VA should reevaluate and expand the current eligibility criteria to ensure that more veterans can benefit from the program.

8. Western Governors urge VA to conduct a comprehensive evaluation of the Veteran Transportation Services (VTS) exam and implement necessary revisions to reduce its complexity, facilitating the process for individuals to obtain a license to transport veterans to VA health care facilities and authorized non-VA health care appointments.

9. Western Governors call on VA to improve community care for veterans by enforcing timely referrals and appointments, particularly for programs like VA Community Care. VA should also streamline reimbursement processes to third-party health care providers in line with industry standards and ensure prompt access to services and increased provider participation.

10. To ensure that our nation's veterans receive the benefits and services they are entitled to in a timely and efficient manner, Western Governors urge VA to continue to improve and streamline the claims process, especially with the new Sergeant First Class (SFC) Heath Robinson Honoring our Promise to Address Comprehensive Toxics (PACT) Act (Pub. L. 117-168) claims.

11. Western Governors recommend that VA implement a policy allowing veterans to select their own care providers, including those who are not affiliated with VA health care

facilities. By doing so, veterans would have greater flexibility and choice when seeking health care services.

12. Western Governors recognize the necessity of conducting a comprehensive review of VA regulations regarding payments for State Veterans Homes and urge VA to consult with states to identify the unique needs of each state. Additionally, Western Governors recommend expanding coverage to include all specialty care services, and prioritize funding for specialized cognitive care.

13. Western Governors recommend that VA authorize and prioritize the expansion of VA programs to provide comprehensive financial support for third-party assisted living and nursing facilities, which offer varying levels of care for long-term care services to our nation's veterans.

14. Western Governors urge Congress to pass legislation that requires VA and the Department of Defense (DOD) to modernize their electronic health record-keeping systems and mandate VA to upgrade its overall technology infrastructure. These upgrades are necessary to streamline access to critical health information, enhance coordination between the two departments, and improve the claims process for veterans, which is a priority for the Governors.

15. Western Governors recommend that the federal government provide funding for state and congressionally chartered Veterans Service Organizations (VSOs) to offset the costs of training and to enhance the workforce capacity of VSOs. This would help to improve the level of support and care provided to veterans and their families by such VSOs, ensuring that they have access to the resources and services they need to thrive.

16. Western Governors emphasize the need for VA to provide Veteran Services Officers with access to vital information, enabling them to better assist veterans in navigating VA's programs and services. This will ensure that veterans receive the support and resources necessary to thrive.

17. Western Governors recommend that VA expand its dental services to all veterans enrolled in the VA health care system, regardless of their service-connected dental issues or other narrow criteria.

18. Western Governors urge Congress to authorize and appropriate funds for VA to provide grants to state, territorial, and tribal governments. The purpose of these grants is to increase outreach and assistance to veterans and their families by raising awareness of benefits and aiding them in applying for VA benefits. Priority should be given to areas with high rates of veteran suicide and a shortage of Veteran Services Officers.

19. Western Governors support the idea that service members should be given the opportunity to receive credit or professional credentials for the training they undergo in the military, which can then be transferred to the private sector or educational institutions. This initiative will help veterans transition into civilian careers by providing them with the necessary credentials and recognition for the skills developed through their military service.

20. Western Governors urge Congress to provide diligent oversight over VA and DOD to ensure that transitioning service members receive comprehensive information on VA benefits at least twelve months prior to their transition to civilian life. This includes ensuring that service members are aware of the full range of programs and support services available to them.

21. Western Governors recommend that VA conduct a comprehensive study on their efforts to reduce homelessness and identify those programs that have provided the highest return on investment.

C. GOVERNORS' MANAGEMENT DIRECTIVE

1. The Governors direct WGA staff to work with congressional committees of jurisdiction, the Executive Branch, and other entities, where appropriate, to achieve the objectives of this resolution.

2. Furthermore, the Governors direct WGA staff to consult with the Staff Advisory Council regarding its efforts to realize the objectives of this resolution and to keep the Governors apprised of its progress in this regard.

This resolution will expire in June 2026. Western Governors enact new policy resolutions and amend existing resolutions on a semiannual basis. Please consult http://www.westgov.org/resolutions for the most current copy of a resolution and a list of all current WGA policy resolutions.

Policy Resolution 2022-07

Physical and Behavioral Health Care in Western States

A. BACKGROUND

1. Ensuring access to high-quality, affordable health care is critical to enhancing the quality of life in western states for our growing populations and is the foundation of building and maintaining healthy and vibrant communities and economies.

2. The COVID-19 pandemic illustrated the importance of our health care and public health systems and the urgency with which we must improve health inequities and disparities. Despite warnings of an impending global pandemic, federal, state, local and Tribal governments encountered significant issues containing and responding to the virus, resulting in economic turmoil, supply chain shortages, and a devastating loss of life. In addition, inequities and disparities fueled the spread of COVID-19, affecting many racial and ethnic minority groups who are more likely to live and work in suboptimal conditions.

3. Western states face unique challenges in health care that have been compounded by the pandemic, including growing rates of behavioral health conditions, which encompass mental health and substance use disorders; provider shortages in underserved and rural areas; and limited access to broadband, which has limited the availability of telehealth services. Low population densities and the vast distances between population centers also make it difficult for providers to establish economically sustainable health care practices in rural areas.

4. In addition, distance and density inhibit construction of the technology infrastructure that would provide or improve broadband connectivity in underserved and rural areas. Expanding broadband access provides numerous quality-of-life benefits for rural Americans, including economic development, social connectivity, education, public safety, and access to telehealth and telemedicine.

5. Telehealth utilization has skyrocketed due to the loosening of federal and private insurance restrictions to meet emergency needs during the pandemic. Telehealth is an essential tool to advance health care access, especially in rural areas and among underserved populations, but its use has been limited over the years by federal regulations and licensing barriers.

6. The health care sector faces severe workforce shortages in western states despite efforts of Western Governors, such as the foundation of Western Governors University and other medical training programs in western states, to ensure adequate numbers of qualified medical personnel. This issue has been further exacerbated by COVID-19 and is particularly acute in the West's underserved and rural areas. Ensuring access to health care services requires an adequate number and distribution of physicians, nurses, mental and behavioral health counselors, and other trained health care professionals. Population growth, aging residents, and challenges involving Tribal health care and services for veterans require a renewed focus on developing our nation's health care workforce.

7. Social and economic factors distinct from medical care are powerful predictors of health outcomes and disease burden throughout a person's life. The U.S. Department of Health and Human Services (HHS) defines these social determinants of health (SDOH) as conditions in the environments in which people live, learn, work, play, worship, and age that affect a wide range of health, functioning, and quality-of-life outcomes and risks. It has also identified five key areas of SDOH: economic stability; education; social and community context; health and health care; and neighborhood and built environment.

8. In many cases, SDOH disproportionately affect communities of color and other minority populations in the West and drive disease, worsen health disparities, and present barriers to accessing health care. As such, the integration of health and human services is important to promote a whole person orientation to care that is focused on prevention and is delivered in a culturally and linguistically appropriate manner. Understanding the effect of SDOH on health and health care can inform the development of effective policy to increase access and improve health outcomes for these populations.

9. Western states have a unique body of experience, knowledge, and perspective with respect to health care. The Western Governors' Association (WGA) is ideally situated to collect and disseminate information, including best practices, case studies and policy options, that states can use to improve the foundation for health care services and advocate for shared policy priorities on behalf of their citizens.

Behavioral Health Integration

10. Behavioral health needs are often associated with negative stigma and harmful misperceptions, which can have many detrimental effects, including: a lack of understanding by family members, friends, coworkers, and others; reduced professional, educational, and personal opportunities; various forms of discrimination; and bullying, physical violence, or harassment. Stigma can result in a reluctance to seek help or treatment and contribute to self-doubt and shame associated with behavioral health conditions, including mental health and substance use disorders.

11. Two-thirds of all diagnosable mental illness onset before adulthood, yet the vast majority of adolescents do not receive any treatment. Access to prevention and early intervention services and support for children and youth helps treat behavioral health conditions before they become debilitating and lead to negative outcomes in adulthood.

12. Western states experience higher than average suicide rates. Suicide is the second leading cause of death among youth, and the ten states with the highest suicide rates in the nation are all located in the West.

13. Integrating behavioral and physical health care services and supports can have many positive effects on health outcomes and health care spending. Behavioral health integration presents a more holistic approach to patient care and offers increased access for consumers. Integration can also be an effective tool to de-stigmatize treatment for behavioral health.

14. Substance use disorders (SUDs), including alcohol and drug misuse, are a major public health and safety crisis affecting nearly 21 million Americans. They are particularly prevalent in western states, where individuals are more likely to experience SUDs or have a family member who has. SUDs cross all social and economic lines and tragically take the

lives of tens of thousands of Americans every year. Much attention has been focused on opioid use, and recent federal investment has prioritized opioid prevention and treatment. In western states, however, methamphetamine overdose deaths outpace those resulting from opioid use. It is important to recognize that SUDs encompass all drug classes and polysubstance misuse, and to balance federal SUD investments accordingly. While state and federal progress has been made to address SUDs, additional efforts are necessary to help bridge prevention, treatment, and recovery gaps in western states.

15. Jails and prisons have become de facto behavioral health treatment facilities, which are unequipped to provide needed care. This reality results in inefficient use of public resources and poor outcomes for patients. Youth experiencing a first episode of psychosis are too often sent to juvenile halls, and adults with mental illness and SUD become incarcerated without proper treatment for their underlying chronic behavioral health conditions.

16. Many people experiencing homelessness also struggle with a behavioral health condition, which contributes to the risk of being unhoused. Both supportive housing and adequate, coordinated health and social services must be available to prevent and reduce homelessness for people with mental health and SUDs.

17. The quality and completeness of patient records is an important element of care coordination and patient safety. Ensuring the protection and privacy of these records is a critical aspect of maintaining patient confidence in the health care system and ensuring that patients are forthcoming about their behavioral health needs.

18. Currently, federal privacy rules prohibit SUD treatment providers from fully participating in health information exchanges. This may leave health care providers without a full understanding of a patient's medical history and use of medications, which can reduce the quality of care and lead to negative patient outcomes, including potentially deadly medication interactions.

19. Electronic health records (EHR), state Prescription Drug Monitoring Programs (PDMP), and Health Information Exchange (HIE) are important tools in improving care coordination and addressing the opioid crisis, allowing prescribers and pharmacies to help prevent opioid misuse. At present, there are instances of limited interoperability between EHRs and PDMPs that reduce the potential positive effect of these tools on patient safety. Robust systems for HIE can help to address these shortfalls.

20. Current federal statute limits the ability of state Medicaid programs to cover inpatient and residential treatment and recovery services at facilities with more than 16 beds, also known as the Institutions for Mental Diseases (IMD) exclusion. This antiquated limitation prevents many adults with behavioral health needs from receiving adequate treatment in a licensed health care facility. Waivers for this exclusion offered by the U.S. Department of Health and Human Services (HHS) have provided states with important flexibility and improved access to treatment for patients with SUD, but barriers still remain.

21. Medication-assisted treatment (MAT), including opioid treatment programs, combines behavioral treatment and recovery services with medications to treat SUDs. While MAT has been proven to improve health outcomes and reduce mortality among opioid addiction patients, stigma and myths surrounding the use of MAT limit its potential use in SUD treatment and recovery.

22. The passage of the SUPPORT for Patients and Communities Act in 2018 was a significant step forward for MAT, including by promoting greater flexibility in its use and expanding access to and coverage for MAT. However, significant limits remain on MAT use and providers' ability to take full advantage of these treatment methods.

23. Support from individuals with lived experience, peer support groups, and community-based organizations, including faith-based and cultural organizations, are important components of effective treatment and recovery for SUD and other behavioral health conditions.

B. GOVERNORS' POLICY STATEMENT

1. Federal efforts to address health care workforce and access needs should reflect early, meaningful, and substantive input from Governors, who are best positioned to assess the needs of their states and help develop solutions to meet these needs. State-federal collaboration and coordination are integral to addressing these health care challenges. Wherever possible, and where appropriate, the federal government should respect state authority and maximize flexibility granted to states and Governors.

2. The federal government should work with states to facilitate the deployment of broadband to underserved and rural areas, recognizing that adequate broadband access has a direct correlation to rural populations' ability to access telehealth and telemedicine.

3. Western Governors urge the federal government to make permanent regulatory changes based on waivers and authorizations granted during the COVID-19 public health crisis to provide flexibility and increase access to telehealth and telementoring. We propose actions to create an environment conducive to the expansion of telehealth beyond the pandemic, including but not limited to permanently changing provisions of 42 CFR and Section 1834(m) of the Social Security Act (SSA) such as:

   a. Eliminating the requirement for physicians and non-physician practitioners to perform in-person visits for nursing home residents and allowing visits to be conducted, as appropriate, via telehealth options (42 CFR 483.30);

   b. Waiving interactive telecommunications systems requirements and permitting audio-only visits for certain services (Section 1834(m)(1) of the SSA);

   c. Removing requirements specifying the types of practitioners that may bill for their services when furnished as Medicare telehealth services from the distant site, which expands the type of practitioner that can provide services through telehealth and allows all practitioners eligible to bill Medicare for services to deliver those services via telehealth (Section 1834(m)(4)(E) of the SSA);

   d. Making Federally Qualified Health Centers and Rural Health Clinics qualified distant site providers of telehealth services (1834(m) of the SSA);

   e. Granting clinicians the ability to provide remote patient monitoring services to new and established patients for both acute and chronic disease management and for patients with only one disease condition (1834(m) of the SSA);

f. Eliminating originating site requirements to allow patients to take visits from their homes (42 CFR 409.46(e)); and

g. Expanding geographies to include all counties, not just those located outside metropolitan statistical areas or in health professional shortage areas (1834(m) of the SSA).

Any changes to federal telehealth policy should ensure that patient needs are at the center of those changes. Any changes should also ensure that patient choice to receive in-person services is preserved and only clinically appropriate services are provided via telehealth.

4. Despite efforts by Western Governors to address the shortage of qualified health care workers, significant challenges remain. Governors urge the federal government to examine and implement programs to ensure states have an adequate health care workforce – including in primary care, behavioral and oral health as well as other in-demand specialties – that is prepared to serve diverse populations in urban, suburban, and rural communities. Additionally, the federal government should consider funding new types of personnel, such as community health workers or promotores, in order to further extend the health care team and ensure that patients are connected to resources. Understanding that there remain significant disparities in access and treatment for many populations, Governors also support efforts to increase diversity and representation in the health care workforce to improve health outcomes for all.

5. Western Governors recognize the role that social determinants of health (SDOH) have on the health outcomes and well-being of our citizens, and the effect that social determinants – including economic stability, education, social and community context, and neighborhood and built environment – have on an individual's health status. Western Governors support efforts to identify risks facing high utilizers of health care services, including food insecurity, domestic violence risk, unmet transportation needs, lack of housing and housing instability, utility, and other essential supports and services, and to develop innovative models designed to improve coordination of medical and non-medical services and use of evidence-based interventions. These models can provide valuable information on how meeting non-health needs and addressing other social determinants can improve overall health status and decrease health spending.

6. Western Governors encourage Congress to adopt legislation that would empower states and local governments to address persistent economic and social conditions – like limited access to health care providers, stable housing, reliable transportation, healthy foods, and high-quality education – that often hinder health outcomes. Such legislation would assist states in developing plans to target social determinants that negatively affect health outcomes for western populations.

7. Western Governors acknowledge the importance of improving our nation's public health preparedness and response systems. The federal government must examine the lessons learned from COVID-19 in collaboration with states and ensure that we have the capability and necessary public health infrastructure investment to effectively confront future public health challenges. We recommend that the federal government clarify pandemic response roles and build operational capacity within the appropriate health-related agencies. The federal government should also consider how to expand our international health surveillance and public health threat detection mechanisms.

Behavioral Health Policy

8. Western Governors believe patients should have the same access to behavioral health care as they have for physical health care, including prevention and early intervention services and supports for chronic conditions like mental illness.

9. Western Governors support efforts to improve the quality and quantity of behavioral health services and supports available to our residents, as these services and supports are essential to reducing suicide rates and treating a range of behavioral health conditions, including mental illness and SUDs.

10. Western Governors recognize and support efforts at the federal, state, and local levels to promote the integration of physical and behavioral health services. The Governors encourage Congress to adopt legislation and the Administration to implement policies that support states' integration efforts and that encourage health care providers to better integrate behavioral and physical health into their practice of care.

11. Western Governors also support innovation within the behavioral health workforce to create new classifications and address gaps in the continuum of care professionals.

12. Western Governors believe the federal government should work toward treating addiction as a chronic illness and work with Western Governors to develop strategies for addressing SUD that work in concert with state efforts and recognize regional variations in SUD patterns.

13. Western Governors believe that the federal government should take steps to increase opportunities for early intervention and law enforcement diversion to prevent entry into the justice system for individuals with behavioral health conditions. That includes providing law enforcement and emergency service providers with the resources and training they need to divert when appropriate and expanding the availability of community reentry programs that provide appropriate treatment for underlying behavioral health conditions that contribute to involvement in the justice system.

14. Western Governors support efforts to increase the availability of transitional and permanent supportive housing with coordinated health and social services to more fully support and sustain recovery for people with behavioral health conditions.

15. Western Governors encourage Congress to pass legislation that aligns federal privacy requirements for SUDs (42 CFR Part 2) with the requirements for all other types of medical conditions under the Health Insurance Portability and Accountability Act (HIPAA) to improve care coordination and reduce stigma for patients with SUD.

16. The exchange of health information is fragmented and often does not occur, limiting the ability of a provider or team of providers to understand the complete needs of a patient and provide whole-of-person care. Western Governors believe the federal government should take steps to support and help sustain states' administration of PDMPs and ensure that EHRs and PDMPs are fully interoperable between states and the federal government, accessible to relevant health care providers, including opioid treatment providers, and include adequate protections for patients from stigmatization and discrimination.

17. Western Governors support legislation to address the so-called Institutions for Mental Diseases (IMD) exclusion to improve access to SUD treatment and recovery services at residential and inpatient facilities with more than 16 beds, as well as to the full continuum of community-based behavioral health care. This policy solution must also improve access to both inpatient and ongoing, recovery-focused treatment in community settings. Until a legislative solution is enacted, the federal government should continue working with states to provide IMD waivers that offer important flexibility and improve access to treatment for patients with SUD. Implementation of these waivers must also occur in connection with expansions of the full community-based continuum of behavioral health care so that consumers receive services in the lowest level of clinically appropriate care in the community whenever possible.

18. Western Governors support legislative action to increase access to MAT for patients with SUD. This includes eliminating the unnecessary and burdensome registration requirements for physicians, physician assistants, and nurse practitioners to obtain a waiver from the Drug Enforcement Administration to treat opioid use disorder with buprenorphine, which would provide health care professionals with additional flexibility to use MAT to treat opioid-related SUD.

19. Western Governors urge the federal government to develop an evidence-based, culturally competent national education and awareness campaign to reduce the stigma associated with mental health and SUDs and encourage individuals to seek help for these health conditions.

C. GOVERNORS' MANAGEMENT DIRECTIVE

1. The Governors direct WGA staff to work with congressional committees of jurisdiction, the Executive Branch, and other entities, where appropriate, to achieve the objectives of this resolution.

2. Furthermore, the Governors direct WGA staff to consult with the Staff Advisory Council regarding its efforts to realize the objectives of this resolution and to keep the Governors apprised of its progress in this regard.

This resolution will expire in December 2024. Western Governors enact new policy resolutions and amend existing resolutions on a semiannual basis. Please consult http://www.westgov.org/resolutions for the most current copy of a resolution and a list of all current WGA policy resolutions.

Chapter 4

Mission Transition: Evaluating Mental Health Support Programs for Separating Servicemembers*

Committee on Veterans' Affairs

Statement of Melissa Cohen, Executive Director, Outreach, Transition, and Economic Development (OTED) Service Veterans Benefits Administration (VBA) Department of Veterans Affairs (VA) Before the House Committee on Veterans' Affairs Subcommittee on Economic Opportunity, U.S. House of Representatives September 10, 2024

Chairman Van Orden, Ranking Member Levin, and distinguished members of the Subcommittee, I appreciate the opportunity to appear before you today to discuss access to mental health care programs and services during the transition from military to civilian life. Accompanying me today from the Veterans Health Administration (VHA) is Ms. Jill DeBord, LCSW, Executive Director, Care Management and Social Work. I appreciate your continued support of the Nation's Veterans, their families, caregivers, and survivors. Within VA, our focus is on increasing transparency, improving collaboration, and keeping Veterans at the center of everything we do.

The transition period can present many challenges for Service members, including increased risk for suicide, homelessness, post-traumatic stress, and substance use disorders, to name just a few. In the 2023 National Veteran Suicide Prevention Annual Report[1] 48,100 adult Americans died by suicide. Of those, 6,392 (13.3%) were Veterans. This report also shows that rates of suicide in the 12 months following separations ranged from 34.8 per 100,000, for Veterans who separated in 2010, to 48.9 per 100,000, for Veterans who separated in 2019. These numbers reflect individual lives prematurely ended and grieved by family members, loved ones, and the Nation as a whole.

---

* This is an edited, reformatted and augmented version of Oversight Hearing, before the Committee on Veterans' Affairs Subcommittee on Economic Opportunity Publication, dated September 10, 2024.

1 https://www.mentalhealth.va.gov/docs/data-sheets/2023/2023-National-Veteran-Suicide-Prevention-Annual-Report-FINAL-508.pdf.

In: Supporting Our Veterans
Editor: Gina P. Sharpe
ISBN: 979-8-89530-504-1

VA must always do everything we can to drive that number to zero – especially during transition, which arguably is one of the most vulnerable periods in a Service member's life.

Transition Support

TAP is an interagency effort designed to help the nearly 200,000 transitioning Service members annually. Together with Department of Defense (DoD), Department of Labor (DOL), the Small Business Administration, the Department of Homeland Security, the Department of Education, the Office of Personnel Management and the military services, we equip Service members with the tools they need to succeed in civilian life and we connect them with the benefits and services they have earned and deserve. VA works closely with our interagency federal partners at the Department of Labor (DOL) and Department of Defense (DoD), and our collective efforts are aimed at ensuring transitioning Service members receive comprehensive, standardized, and non-clinical individualized self-assessments across VA and DoD; are informed and educated about all post-separation VA, DOL, and DoD benefits and services for which they are eligible, and are equipped with the tools they need to succeed and reintegrate into their communities.

The VA Benefits and Services course delivered as part of the week -long TAP course provides an overview of the wide array of benefits and services, available to transitioning Service members and Veterans, and addresses topics specific to health care, mental health care, suicide risk factors, and available mental health programs and resources. For example, included in the curriculum is information about the VA Liaison Program which utilizes VA social workers and nurses either onsite at DoD installations or providing virtual support to coordinate a clinical transition of health and mental health care to VHA, customized to the needs of the individual transitioning Service member.

Through this process, a transitioning Service member is registered for VA health care and connected to the Post-9/11 Military2VA (M2VA) Case Management Program at their home VA medical facility and over 80% of the time, have initial VA health care appointments scheduled prior to separation from the military. In fiscal year (FY) 2023, over 14,240 Service members received a coordinated transition of health and mental health care from DoD to VA through the VA Liaison Program.

In addition to the VA Benefits and Services course, Service members and their families have access to Military Life Cycle (MLC) modules. MLC modules are 45- to 60- minute information sessions that may be taken at any time and address a specific in- depth topic such as benefits; education; home loans or life insurance; social and emotional health resources; integration into a civilian community; or survivor and casualty assistance.

VA TAP also provides one-on-one sessions with a Benefits Advisor, offering Service members individualized assistance. One-on-one assistance sessions are based on the individual's needs and are driven by the information covered during the VA Benefits and Services course. The most requested discussion topics include VA home loans, education benefits, and disability compensation.

Warm Handovers

VA strives to ensure Service members are connected with the specific resources they need at the time they need them. Our interagency partners share that commitment. DoD TAP Counselors and VA Benefits Advisors utilize a combination of local, state and National resources and contacts on a myriad of topics spanning mental health, disability compensation, health care resources, education, and housing, to name a few.

Concurrently, VA and interagency partners continue to pursue more seamless connections to transitioning servicemembers. In May 2022, VA launched a pilot across 30 DoD military installations to test a single point of entry, where DoD TAP Managers initiate a warm handover during Capstone (90 days before separation) to VA in areas of education, disability compensation, health care, housing, mental health resources and other VA services. This single point of entry allowed for tracking and validation of the warm handover from DoD to VA. During the pilot (May 2022 – June 2024), VA confirmed 100% of transitioning Service members identified as needing a warm handover (288 individuals), were connected to VA by a DoD TAP manager. VA is currently analyzing the findings to develop a way forward to ensure Service members and Veterans receive timely warm handover to benefits and services they need.

M2VA Case Management Program

Additionally, recently separated Veterans who are receiving coaching services through DoD's inTransitionTransition Program and who request assistance with accessing VA mental health care are referred via a referral to the Post-9/11 M2VA Case Management Program at their local VA medical facility.

Embedded within each VA health care system, Post-9/11 M2VA teams are led by a social work or nurse program manager and comprised of clinical case managers and a non-clinical transition patient advocate. Post-9/11 M2VA teams serve as the point of entry into VA health care systems for tens of thousands of transitioning Service members and Post-9/11 era Veterans annually. Moreover, these teams provide personalized, proactive screenings to over 200,000 transitioning Service members and Post-9/11 era Veterans newly establishing their care at VA medical facilities annually.

The purpose of these screenings is to identify at risk Veterans (such as those with suicidal ideations or housing instability), and when a risk factor is identified, further assessment is completed to determine ongoing clinical case management needs in collaboration with the Veteran. Case management services include care coordination and monitoring, and linkage to VA care, benefits and services as well as community resources that will support a Veteran's health and wellness. Ongoing case management is provided to approximately 38,000 Post-9/11 era Veterans annually by these Post-9/11 M2VA teams.

VA Solid Start (VASS)

The VASS Program launched on December 2, 2019, as part of the Military to Civilian Readiness Pathway to make early, consistent, and caring contact with newly separated Veterans. On October 17, 2022, VASS was signed into law (P.L. 117-205), permanently authorizing VA to expand VASS with DoD coordination. VASS calls all eligible Veterans, regardless of their character of discharge, at 3 key stages (90-, 180-, and 365-days post-separation) during their first year after separation from active duty. Using data provided by DoD, VASS provides priority contact to Veterans meeting certain mental health risk factors, supporting continuity of care and lowering any barriers to access to mental health care treatment and support through VA. These representatives receive special training to recognize the signs of crisis and, when needed, can provide a direct transfer to the Veterans and Military Crisis Line for additional support. Veterans, Service members, and their loved ones can call 988 and Press 1, chat online, or send a text message to 838255 to receive confidential support 24 hours a day, 7 days a week, 365 days a year.

VASS representatives address challenges the Veteran may be facing at the time of the call by connecting the Veteran with the appropriate benefits or resources for assistance. VASS calls are not scripted. Representatives ask open-ended questions that seek to establish the current status and potential needs of the Veteran. Each call is different and is driven by the needs of each Veteran at the time of the call. There are no talk time limitations for the calls. By establishing this relationship with Veterans in the first critical year post-separation from active duty, VASS aims to increase the likelihood that they will get connected to VA earlier and utilize VA benefits and services, to include mental health resources, when needed.

From the program launch in December 2019 through August 2024, VASS has successfully connected with 511,460 (73.9%) recently separated Veterans, helping them connect with the benefits and services they have earned. For example, in calendar year 2023, of Veterans who had a successful VASS connection, 67.19% applied for or are receiving compensation benefits and 69.52% applied for, or are enrolled in, VHA services. Veterans who did not have a successful connection with VASS had utilization rates of 22.94% and 41.74%, respectively.

To further assist Veterans with access to VHA care, including mental health services, VASS representatives can make referrals to the Post-9/11 M2VA Case Management Program at their local VA medical facility. VASS successfully connected 3,644 Veterans to their local Post-9/11 M2VA team from October 2020 to August 2024.

VASS provides priority contact to Veterans meeting certain risk factors (such as having a mental health appointment) during their last year of active duty. From December 2019 through August 2024, VASS successfully connected with 90,948 Priority Veterans (representing 83.0% of the eligible population). Additionally, since the program launch in December 2019, through August 2024, VASS has successfully connected with 9,046, or 55.8%, of recently separated Veterans with an other than honorable (OTH) discharge.

Furthermore, in July 2023, VASS launched a VSignals survey to assess Veteran satisfaction with the VASS program. Since its launch through August 2024, VASS- eligible Veterans rated their satisfaction with the VASS program as 4.5 on a 5-point Likert scale.

Economic Factors During the Transition Period

Some Veterans report difficulty in transitioning to civilian positions and translating military-related skills to higher-paying civilian jobs. Unemployment and poverty are correlated with homelessness among Veterans. Financial hardship and economic stressors are major predictors of mental health crisis and Veteran suicide. VBA provides a variety of benefits and services that can help reduce or eliminate risk factors associated with suicide and promote protective factors for some Veterans. Benefits such as disability compensation, pension, Veteran Readiness and Employment services and education/GI Bill benefits assist Veterans with transitioning to civilian life, connecting with benefits, establishing, and achieving educational, vocational, and career goals, and supporting financial well-being. Below are some examples of programs used to support transitioning Service members pre- and post-service that can impact their financial stability and lessen economic stressors.

Personalized Career Planning and Guidance (PCPG)

PCPG, also known as Chapter 36 services, fulfills 38 U.S.C. § 3697A requirements by supporting transitioning Service members, Veterans, and qualified dependents. PCPG services provide participants with personalized counseling and support to help guide career paths, ensure the most effective use of VA benefits, and achieve educational and career goals. Services are available to transitioning Service members within 6 months of leaving the military, to Veterans who have left the military within the past 12 months, or (at any time) to individuals who are eligible to use a VA education benefit. PCPG career and education counseling services include résumé support; education and employment planning; detailed skills assessment; a personalized action plan to achieve education and career goals; adjustment counseling to successfully transition to civilian employment; and a direct connection to VA benefits and services. From October through July of FY 2024, PCPG received 7,308 applications requesting services.

Separation Health Assessment (SHA)

Executive Order 13822 of January 9, 2018, established requirements for the Secretary of Defense, the Secretary of Veterans Affairs, and the Secretary of Homeland Security to submit a Joint Action Plan describing actions to provide seamless access to mental health care and suicide prevention resources for transitioning uniformed Service members during the year following discharge, separation, or retirement. Since the order, VA and DoD have partnered in including mental health screening questions in the SHA questionnaire.

The SHA establishes a consistent opportunity for separating Service members to discuss illnesses, injuries, and psychological harm incurred or aggravated during military service, including but not limited to, those arising from or related to occupational exposures, physical hazards, or sexual trauma. The SHA promotes efficient, effective, standardized electronic processes for obtaining and documenting information to support continuity of health care, development of transition support plans, understanding of potential health effects of military service, and contemporaneous or future determinations of eligibility for disability benefits and services from VA.

The mental health assessment elements of the SHA require a person-to-person discussion between the examining clinician and the Service member. DD Form 3146/SHA Part A includes a general self-assessment of the Service member's mental health at separation. The SHA includes screening questionnaires on post-traumatic stress disorder (PTSD), depression, and alcohol use. The examining clinician reviews these screening results along with the results of a clinical assessment to provide a suicide risk assessment and violence risk assessment and, if indicated, refer the Service member for mental health transition assistance.

When a Service member applies for disability compensation through VA's Benefits Delivery at Discharge (BDD) Program, VA conducts the SHA examination. When SHA mental health screening indicates a risk or mental health condition, the VA examining provider refers the Service member to DoD's inTransition Program for mental health assistance. The inTransition program is a free, confidential program that offers specialized coaching and assistance for active-duty service members, National Guard members, Reservists, Veterans, and retirees who need access to mental health care.

In consultation with VA, DoD assists Service members' by providing information and referrals, if necessary, for care, treatment, and other services that VA may provide. Information provided includes available clinical services resources (counseling and treatment for PTSD and other mental health conditions), other care and treatment services, information on private sector sources of treatments available in the member's community and assistance to enroll in VA for health care benefits.

Outreach

Transition can be a time of great stress for Service members, increasing risks of homelessness, substance use, and economic hardships, all of which are high-risk factors for suicide and more likely to occur in underserved communities. That is why VBA maintains a robust outreach program to frequently share and connect Veterans to the resources and benefits available to them. For special emphasis populations, VBA maintains policies to ensure these vulnerable populations are regularly connected. VA believes that no Veteran should be without a place to call home and is committed to assisting in ending homelessness among Veterans. Our focus is threefold.

- Outreach: Conducting coordinated outreach to proactively seek out Veterans and transitioning Service members in need of assistance.
- Claims: Expediting claims for benefits for those who are homeless or at risk of homelessness.
- Stakeholders: Collaborating with Federal and state agencies, community nonprofits, and others to ensure Veterans are connected with services they need to attain and remain in permanent, stable housing.

VBA has Homeless Veterans Outreach Coordinators (HVOC) at 25 regional offices (RO). These individuals are dedicated full-time employees, who provide access to VA benefits and information through outreach efforts to homeless Veterans and to Veterans at risk of being homeless. As of October 2023, five new locations (Denver, Honolulu, Portland, Reno, and San Diego) received full-time HVOCs.

Table 1. Regional offices with full-time homeless veteran outreach coordinators

Atlanta	Detroit	Nashville	Phoenix	Saint Petersburg
Boston	Honolulu	New York	Portland	San Diego
Chicago	Houston	Newark	Reno	Seattle
Cleveland	Indianapolis	Oakland	Roanoke	Waco
Denver	Los Angeles	Philadelphia	Saint Louis	Winston-Salem

VBA has Homeless Veterans Claims Coordinators (HVCC) in the remainder of ROs to expedite processing of claims from Veterans who are homeless or in imminent risk of homelessness and to report on prioritization of homeless claims activities. VBA provides homeless program updates to the homeless coordinators via the quarterly National Outreach Call and hosts an annual Homeless Veterans Outreach Training Symposium. As of July 31,

2024, VBA Outreach held 1,965 homeless Veteran events in FY 2024, totaling 6,575 hours of outreach to homeless Veterans.

To ensure VA meets the needs of the rural Veteran population, ROs designate one regional outreach coordinator (ROC) to provide VA benefits information to Veterans, dependents, and survivors residing in rural areas. As of July 31, 2024, VBA Outreach has held 1,412 rural Veteran events in FY 2024, totaling 2,230 hours of outreach to rural Veterans.

VA is committed to providing outreach to LGBTQ+ Service members and Veterans. VA recognizes the need for direct outreach to ensure awareness of the VA benefits and services to which they may be entitled. Each RO must host at least one event per quarter for this special emphasis group. As of July 31, 2024, VBA Outreach has held 631 LGBTQ+ Veteran events in FY 2024, totaling 913 hours of outreach to LGBTQ+ Veterans.

Military Sexual Trauma (MST) Survivors Coordinators at ROs assist Veterans who have experienced MST. VBA established the MST Outreach Program to educate, empower, and spread awareness about increased benefits and special services that may be available to this Veteran population. MST Coordinators assist by:

- conducting outreach and disseminating MST-related information,
- navigating the process of filing a claim related to MST,
- providing trauma-sensitive customer service, and
- initiating telephone contact with Veterans.

Each of VA's 56 ROs must provide 12 hours of outreach per quarter related to MST. VBA exceeded the fiscal year requirement of 2,688 hours by hosting 2,264 MST Veteran events, totaling 3,983 hours of outreach to MST Veterans.

Additional programs embedded in VBA's outreach program to assist in spreading information about benefits and getting transitioning Service Members and Veterans connected to their benefits. For example, transitioning Service members, Veterans, and their families are educated about employment opportunities, special hiring authorities, and career support resources, through VBA-hosted Economic Development Initiative (EDI) events. EDIs are 2 or 3 -day, no-cost events, which connect Veterans with resources promoting financial stability, career opportunities, mental health, and wellness initiatives. Veterans can obtain information on benefits from VA and other organizations, get help filing disability compensation claims, receive private, on-site disability medical examinations, learn about education and home loan guaranty benefits, and find resources for mental health support.

VA also partners with the Off-Base Transition Training (OBTT) pilot. OBTT workshops are currently scheduled as virtual 1-hour sessions with 45 minutes of material and 15 minutes for questions and answers. OBTT is a supplemental briefing for Veterans, beneficiaries, and caregivers who fall outside of the TAP eligibility window as well as any National Guard and Reserve members.

VHA's Readjustment Counseling Service (RCS) consists of more than 300 Vet Centers located in all 50 states, the District of Columbia, Puerto Rico, the U.S. Virgin Islands, Guam, and American Samoa. Vet Centers are community-based counseling centers that provide a wide range of social and psychological services, including professional readjustment counseling to eligible Veterans, active-duty service members, including National Guard and Reserve components, and their families. Readjustment counseling is offered to make a successful transition from military to civilian life or after a traumatic event experienced in the military. Individual, group, marriage and family counseling is offered in addition to referral and connection to other VA or community benefits and services. Vet Center counselors and outreach staff, many of whom are Veterans themselves, are experienced and prepared to discuss the tragedies of war, loss, grief, and transition after trauma.

Character of Discharge Final Rule

Eligibility for VA benefits depends upon type of military service performed, duration of service, and character of discharge (COD) or separation. Former service members (FSMs) must receive a COD under other than dishonorable conditions (honorable, under honorable conditions, general) to be eligible for most VA benefits. Veterans with a dishonorable discharge or statutory bar pertaining to a period of service are prohibited from receiving most VA benefits based on that period of service. Other types of discharges, such as OTH, Undesirable, or Bad Conduct discharges, require VA to make a COD determination for eligibility for VA health care and/or compensation and other monetary benefits.

In September 2022, the Veterans Experience Office published the report "Veteran Journeys: Other than Honorable (OTH) Discharge," which summarized customer research to better understand current and desired experiences over the lifetime of OTH Veterans. This research found that Veterans with an OTH discharge often do not receive adequate information or support to connect with the VA benefits and services they are eligible for, which may have detrimental downstream effects on a population already prone to crisis situations such as mental health emergencies, suicidality, and homelessness. The report findings also noted that because the OTH discharge process typically does not provide support or services for those who have experienced trauma, OTH Veterans often struggle to adjust to life after the military - making crises, such as mental health emergencies, suicidality, homelessness, and/or drug/alcohol addiction, common. The report identified opportunities to simplify eligibility pathways to mental health, addiction, and housing support for OTH Veterans.

VA addressed this opportunity in the final rule (AQ95), "Update and Clarify Regulatory Bars to Benefits Based on Character of Discharge," (https://www.federalregister.gov/documents/2024/04/26/2024-09012/update-and-clarify-regulatory-bars-to-benefits-based-on-character-of-discharge), which became effective on June 25, 2024. VA recognizes there are some Service members, even those with an OTH discharge, who may have earned the status of "Veteran" and the benefits to which Veterans are entitled. VA also recognizes the extraordinary situations and circumstances involved in service, which could lead to injuries or other circumstances that increase risk for behaviors or conduct that military commanders deem inappropriate.

To ensure VA considers all facts and circumstances in each case, VA included a compelling circumstances exception in this final rule which is applicable to the willful and persistent misconduct and moral turpitude regulatory bars and the "absent without leave" statutory bar to VA benefits. This ensures VA considers the length and character of service exclusive of a period of misconduct and potential mitigating reasons for the misconduct such as mental and physical health, hardship, sexual abuse/assault, duress, obligations to others, age, education, cultural background, and judgmental maturity. Although not specifically included in the regulatory text, VA will consider discrimination, including based on race or sex, in the compelling circumstances analysis.

The compelling circumstances exception, coupled with more specific criteria defined for the willful and persistent misconduct regulatory bar, will serve to expand eligibility to additional Veterans. These modifications will help distinguish those who committed serious misconduct that renders their service dishonorable from those whose misconduct comes with a mitigating circumstance or is outweighed by otherwise meritorious service.

While relaxing the bars to eligibility, this final rule does not extend VA benefits eligibility to all FSMs. FSMs who do not meet the criteria for benefits eligibility may still be entitled to certain critical benefits to address the harms caused by their military service, such as mental health and substance use care, emergent suicide care, and medical care in emergency situations.

Too often, FSMs are either incorrectly told or self-select away from VA, based on the belief that the OTH discharge makes them ineligible for VA benefits and services. However, in many instances, FSMs may be found eligible to receive health care and/or disability compensation. VA encourages FSMs to file a claim and let VA determine their eligibility to benefits. In addition, any FSM with a previous unfavorable character of discharge determination from VA may request a new determination under the new final. VA, in all its efforts, is always looking to ensure that benefits and services are provided to all who are entitled to them.

Updated VA Form 21-0781

With the enactment of P.L. 117-271, VA Peer Support Enhancement for MST Survivors Act and P.L. 117-303 MST Claims Coordination Act, VA combined two previous forms related to PTSD[2] and personal assault[3] into a single form titled Statement in Support of Claimed Mental Health Disorder(s) Due to an In-Service Traumatic Event(s), released June 29, 2024. By combining the forms, VA reduced the respondent burden, which is the estimated number of minutes it takes for a respondent to fill out a form, by 50%.

This reduction in the respondent burden also decreases the potential for respondents to provide information that is not needed and allowing for other mental health conditions (other than PTSD) to be submitted on the form. When developing the new form, VA utilized a workgroup of subject matter experts including clinicians from the VHA, to balance the need for collection of pertinent information and trauma sensitivity. The new VA Form 21-0781 includes new sections that help the Veteran complete the form for their type of in-service traumatic event(s), guidance with examples for describing the traumatic event(s), and expansion of the behavioral changes question, among other changes.

Although the previous VA Form 21-0781a was discontinued when the new form was released, VA recognizes that requesting the new VA Form 21-0781 when a completed VA Form 21-0781a is received has the potential to retraumatize the Veteran. As such, on or after June 29, 2024, when a completed VA Form 21-0781a is received, claims processors will review outdated and discontinued versions of the forms to determine their evidentiary value and ensure that requests for an examination or claim development are not unnecessarily delayed. This will

[2] VA Form 21-0781, Statement in Support of Claim for Service Connection for PTSD.
[3] VA Form 21-0781a, Statement in Support of Claim for Service Connection for PTSD Secondary to Personal Assault.

help ensure a more streamlined and trauma-informed experience for Veterans who submit claims for mental health conditions related to in-service traumatic events.

Employee Training

VA follows the tenets of the S.A.V.E. model (Signs of suicide, Ask about suicide, Validate feelings, Encourage help/Expedite treatment) when training employees to identify Veterans at risk and provide assistance. VA S.A.V.E. training is a yearly mandatory requirement for all employees. For VBA positions that involve direct contact with Veterans, such as RO public contact teams and National Contact Center call agents, training is comprehensive and aimed at providing care and support when talking with individuals in crisis. Veteran-facing employees complete mandatory training as new hires and subsequently receive at least two refresher training hours each calendar year focused on crisis management and suicide prevention.

Additional Initiatives

VA understands that news of a reduction, severance, or adverse action regarding VA benefits can increase strain on Veterans. This is especially concerning for Veterans already identified as high-risk. Economic and financial uncertainty can increase the risk of suicide. In March 2024, VA launched a new website to help Veterans manage financial stressors that can affect their mental health and wellbeing.[4] Developed by the National Veterans Financial Resource Center (FINVET), the website aims to boost protective factors that promote mental health and reduce suicide risk by helping Veterans learn about and manage their finances. Economic and financial uncertainty can increase the risk of suicide. FINVET helps mitigate that risk by connecting Veterans to trustworthy financial tools, information, videos, calculators, and worksheets – serving as a one-stop website for Veterans to learn a variety of essential information to help meet their financial goals. Using simple navigation, FINVET empowers Veterans to learn about financial goals such as meeting basic needs, saving or earning more money, lowering bills and debt, and protecting their assets.

VBA is increasing suicide prevention awareness for employees by providing training in lethal means safety, and trauma-informed communications, especially with Veterans who experienced MST. VBA has conducted extensive efforts to improve trauma-informed communications and interactions for MST survivors by updating forms, written communication, and providing staff training in trauma-informed best practices.

Conclusion

We appreciate the Committee's continued support and collaboration in this shared mission. Mr. Chairman, this concludes my statement. My colleague and I are ready to answer any questions you and the Committee may have.

---

[4] https://news.va.gov/press-room/va-financial-website-reduce-suicide/.

DOD and VA Transition Programs
Recommendations for Improving Mental Health Support
United States Government Accountability Office Testimony Before the Subcommittee on Economic Opportunity, Committee on Veterans' Affairs, House of Representatives
September 10, 2024

Why GAO Did This Study

Thousands of service members transition from military service to civilian life each year—about 175,000 in calendar year 2022. Research has shown that during this transition period service members are especially vulnerable. One study found that the suicide rate within the first year of separation was about 2.5 times higher than for the active duty population.

To help address this concern, DOD and VA have various programs and processes available to support transitioning service members and veterans who may need mental health assistance. GAO's past work has identified areas for improvement to these programs and processes.

This statement summarizes GAO's recent work examining DOD's and VA's efforts to support service members and veterans with mental health needs during the transition from military to civilian life. This includes recommendations GAO made regarding (1) DOD's inTransition program; (2) DOD's warm handover process; (3) VA's Solid Start program; and (4) the DOD-VA Joint Executive Committee's assessment of mental health services across the transition continuum.

This statement is primarily based on three GAO reports issued between January 2023 and July 2024 (GAO-23- 105699, GAO-24-106248, and GAO-24-106189). GAO also reviewed documents from DOD and VA related to steps the agencies have taken to address GAO's recommendations.

What GAO Found

The Departments of Defense (DOD) and Veterans Affairs (VA) administer a number of transition programs to support separating service members and veterans, including those with mental health needs. GAO has recently reported on some of these programs and on DOD's and VA's efforts to assess their effectiveness in facilitating access to mental health services during the transition period. Since January 2023, GAO has made 11 recommendations to DOD and three to VA to improve their support for the transitioning population. As of August 2024, the departments had taken steps to implement some of these recommendations. Fully addressing them would help ensure that transitioning service members and veterans have the support they need and deserve.

- *DOD's inTransition program.* This program is intended to help facilitate connections to mental health services for service members and veterans during times of transition to ensure the continuity of their care. In July 2024, GAO reported that inTransition did not successfully connect with over 70 percent of the eligible service members it identified in 2022. This was due, in part, to its reliance on telephone calls and not other forms of outreach, such as email. GAO recommended that inTransition expand its outreach methods. DOD did not provide a formal response to this recommendation.

- *DOD's warm handovers.* To assist service members who may be at risk for a difficult transition—including those with mental health needs—DOD has a process to provide a person-to-person connection, known as a "warm handover," to other agencies. In March 2024, GAO reported that DOD does not reliably verify that warm handovers occur and has not assessed their helpfulness. GAO made multiple recommendations, including that DOD develop a plan to assess the helpfulness of warm handovers. DOD concurred with the recommendations and is working to implement them.
- *VA's Solid Start program.* This program proactively connects new veterans with resources and benefits and designates transitioning service members as "priority veterans" for outreach if they received mental health care in the year prior to separation. In January 2023, GAO reported that VA had not collaborated with veterans organizations to address outreach challenges, such as using cold calls to contact veterans or connecting with hard-to-reach veterans. GAO recommended that VA collaborate with veterans organizations to identify and address any outreach gaps and assess outreach strategies for hard-to-reach veterans. VA concurred and has implemented the recommendation.
- *DOD-VA Joint Executive Committee's assessment of programs.* This committee serves as an interagency body for coordinating the resources and benefits of the departments, including military transition assistance activities. In July 2024, GAO reported that the Committee had not assessed the overall effectiveness of the departments' various efforts to facilitate access to mental health services for transitioning service members and veterans and made a recommendation that it do so. VA concurred with this recommendation, but DOD did not provide a formal response.

Chairman Van Orden, Ranking Member Levin, and Members of the Subcommittee:

Thank you for the opportunity to discuss our work on the Department of Defense's (DOD) and the Department of Veterans Affairs' (VA) efforts to provide mental health support for service members and veterans during their transition from military to civilian life. Thousands of service members separate from the military every year—about 175,000 in calendar year 2022. This transition period can be an especially vulnerable time, bringing challenges such as the loss of a sense of purpose, familial and financial strain, and difficulty readjusting to social and civilian life. Recent research and a 2018 Executive Order found that the suicide rate for veterans in the first year of separation was about 2.5 times higher than for the active-duty population and about twice the overall rate for all veterans.[5]

DOD and VA have a number of programs to support separating service members and veterans during the transition period. For example, DOD has a voluntary program, called inTransition, intended to help facilitate connections to mental health services for service members and veterans during their transitions. Additionally, to assist service members who

[5] Chandru Ravindran, et al., "Association of Suicide Risk with Transition to Civilian Life among U.S. Military Service Members," *JAMA Network Open*, vol. 3, no. 9 (2020), and Exec. Order No. 13,822, 3 C.F.R. 320 (2019), reprinted in 38 U.S.C. § 1712A note at 349-50 (2020).

may be at risk for a difficult transition—including those with mental health needs—DOD, through its Transition Assistance Program (TAP), facilitates a person-to-person connection, known as a "warm handover," to other agencies. Within VA, the Solid Start program connects new veterans with resources and benefits, and it prioritizes outreach to those who received mental health care in the year prior to separation.

DOD and VA's Joint Executive Committee is an interagency body established by law to oversee the departments' coordination with health care and benefits, including the various programs and processes that may assist service members and veterans across the transition continuum, which it defines as 1 year before and 1 year after separation.[6] Given the Committee's ability to look collectively across DOD's and VA's programs and various efforts, it is uniquely positioned to assess the departments' overall efforts to assist and support the transitioning population.

We have recently reported on these programs and on DOD's and VA's efforts to assess their effectiveness in facilitating access to mental health services during the transition period.[7] Our work identified a number of issues, and, since January 2023, we have made eleven recommendations to DOD and three recommendations to VA to improve the departments' support for transitioning service members and veterans. The departments have taken initial steps to implement some of these recommendations, and we will continue to monitor their actions to fully address them.[8]

My remarks today summarize key findings from our recent work examining DOD's and VA's efforts to provide mental health and other support for transitioning service members and veterans, including recommendations we have made to DOD and VA related to

1. DOD's processes for enrollment, outreach, and performance assessment for its inTransition program;
2. DOD's approach for tracking and verifying who receives a warm handover and assessing its helpfulness;
3. VA's outreach for its Solid Start program; and
4. The DOD-VA Joint Executive Committee's assessment of mental health services across the transition continuum.

This statement is based on our recent work issued between January 2023 and July 2024 reviewing DOD's and VA's efforts to support transitioning service members and veterans who may need mental health resources or other types of assistance. Detailed information on the objectives, scope, and methodology of this work can be found in each issued report. For this

---

[6] National Defense Authorization Act for Fiscal Year 2004, Pub. L. No. 108-136, div A, tit. V, § 583(a)(1), 117 Stat. 1392, 1490 (2003) (codified, as amended, at 38 U.S.C. § 320).

[7] GAO, DOD and VA Health Care: Actions Needed to Better Facilitate Access to Mental Health Services During Military to Civilian Transitions, GAO-24-106189 (Washington, D.C.: July 15, 2024); Service Members Transitioning to Civilian Life: Agencies Can Improve Warm Handovers for Additional Assistance, GAO-24-106248 (Washington, D.C.: Mar. 21, 2024), and Veterans Benefits: VA Could Enhance Outreach for Its Solid Start Program by Increasing Collaboration with Veterans Organizations, GAO-23-105699 (Washington, D.C.: Jan. 5, 2023).

[8] As of September 10, 2024, all 11 of the DOD recommendations remain open and 2 of the 3 VA recommendations remain open. We also made one recommendation to the Department of Labor in GAO-24-106248, which remains open.

statement, we reviewed DOD and VA documentation related to the status of efforts to implement our recommendations since the reports were issued.

We conducted the work on which this statement is based in accordance with generally accepted government auditing standards. Those standards require that we plan and perform the audit to obtain sufficient, appropriate evidence to provide a reasonable basis for our findings and conclusions based on our audit objectives. We believe that the evidence obtained provides a reasonable basis for our findings and conclusions based on our audit objectives.

Background: DOD's in Transition Program

Established in 2010, DOD's inTransition program is intended to help facilitate connections to mental health services for individuals at various transition points, including transitioning between duty stations or out of the military, to ensure continuity of care.[9] It is a voluntary and confidential program with licensed psychological health clinicians, called coaches, who provide support services by telephone to the program's enrollees during times of transition. DOD's Defense Health Agency is responsible for managing inTransition, which is implemented by a contractor.[10]

Individuals may enroll in the program one of two ways—through a referral or through the program's automatic enrollment process for eligible transitioning service members. Individuals may be referred to inTransition by a provider or they may self-refer. Under automatic enrollment, inTransition identifies eligible service members using data on military separations and medical histories. Specifically, the program automatically enrolls service members who had received mental health or moderate-to- severe traumatic brain injury (TBI) care in the year prior to their separation.[11]

Once auto-enrollees are identified, the program is to conduct outreach to determine whether these individuals want to "accept" their enrollment and participate in the program, or if they wish to opt out. The inTransition contractor is to conduct up to 3 outreach phone calls to each automatically enrolled service member within specific time frames.[12] The program's coaches may refer service members to mental health providers, as well as provide information on community resources and support groups, among other services. Coaches do not provide telephonic mental health care or other health care services.

---

9 Transitioning service members include those relocating to another assignment, returning from deployment, transitioning from active duty to reserve, transitioning from reserve to active duty, preparing to leave military service or recently separated from service. The program is available to active-duty service members, U.S. Coast Guard personnel, National Guard members, reservists, veterans, and retirees, regardless of time in service, time from service, or characterization of discharge.

10 Officials from the current inTransition contractor told us they started work in October 2021. The contract has an initial base year plus 4 option years, with a total value of approximately $29 million over the 5-year period.

11 More specifically, the program automatically enrolls service members who have had a mental health or moderate-to-severe TBI encounter in the 30 days prior to separation, at least two outpatient mental health or moderate-to-severe TBI encounters in the year before separation, or at least one inpatient mental health or moderate-to-severe TBI encounter in the year before separation.

12 The contract active during the time of our review provided that while the number of calls made to each name on the monthly list is three, monthly requirements for the number of calls may be reduced to two or even one based on monthly consultation of government assessment and need.

DOD Warm Handovers

When eligible service members prepare to separate from the military, they are required to participate in TAP, which provides individualized counseling sessions, tailored classes, and a final review of compliance with program requirements, also known as a capstone. The goal of TAP is to help service members achieve career readiness standards, such as developing a financial plan or completing an individual transition plan, prior to re-entering civilian life. According to DOD's policy, service members are generally expected to begin TAP at least 1 year before they anticipate leaving military service, but not later than 90 days before separation.[13]

When a service member does not meet career readiness standards, a TAP counselor, commander, or commander designee may determine that a service member needs a warm handover. The warm handover is a person-to-person connection of service members to services from an interagency partner, such as VA or the Department of Labor (DOL), with follow-up resources as needed. For example, warm handovers could assist service members in connecting to mental health care available through the VA. According to DOD policy, a commander or commander's designee is supposed to confirm a warm handover for service members who do not meet career readiness standards or who are anticipated to face other transition challenges, such as a lack of peer support or major readjustment, health care, or employment challenges.[14] According to the policy, the warm handover "provides a confirmed introduction and assurance that the appropriate interagency partner acknowledge(s) that an eligible service member requires post-military assistance." Further, the policy states that "the interagency partner follows through on providing assistance to meet the needs of service members, mitigate risk, and assist them in attaining their post-transition goals and a successful transition." In doing so, the warm handover is designed to help vulnerable service members achieve a successful transition into civilian life. See figure 1.

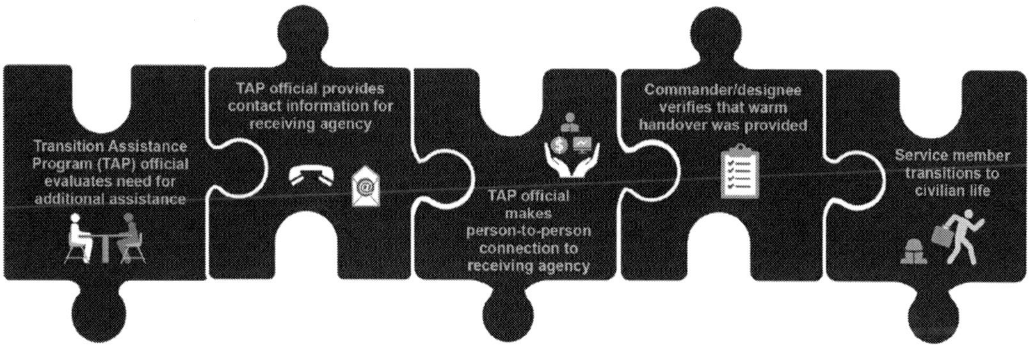

Source: GAO analysis of Department of Defense policy.

Figure 1. General Overview of the Warm Handover Process. | GAO-24-107752.

---

[13] We have previously found that 70 percent of service members did not start TAP more than 1 year in advance, as generally required. For more information, see GAO, *Servicemembers Transitioning to Civilian Life: DOD Can Better Leverage Performance Information to Improve Participation in Counseling Pathways*, GAO-23-104538 (Washington, D.C.: Dec. 12, 2022).

[14] Department of Defense Instruction 1332.35, *Transition Assistance Program (TAP) For Military Personnel* (Washington, D.C.: Sept. 26, 2019).

VA's Solid Start Program

VA launched the Solid Start program in 2019 to proactively connect new veterans with resources and benefits, including mental health and other medical care, employment assistance, and education assistance.[15] Under the program, Solid Start representatives call veterans to determine their needs and proactively connect them to VA benefits. Representatives are to call and email new veterans at three intervals: 90, 180, and 365 days after separation. Once representatives speak with the veteran, they are to follow up with a personalized email with more information. See figure 2.

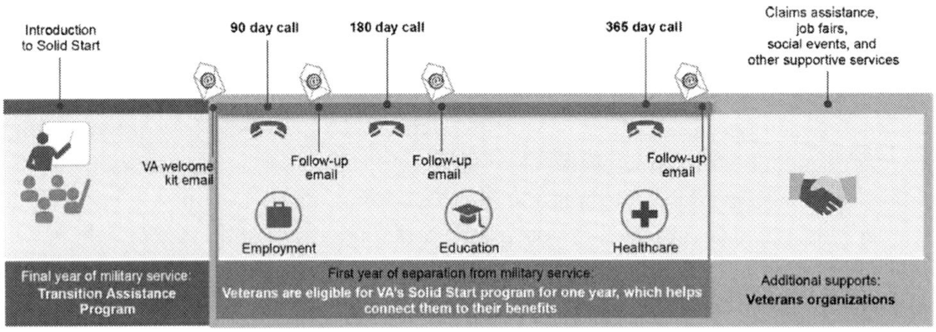

Source: GAO analysis of documentation and interviews with the Department of Veterans Affairs (VA). | GAO-24-107752.

Note: The Transition Assistance Program, with limited exceptions, is a mandatory program that helps separating service members prepare for their transition to civilian life. For the Solid Start program, if the Department of Veterans Affairs (VA) Solid Start representatives speak with a veteran, they send a personalized follow-up email. General informational emails are also sent throughout the year of eligibility. VA continues to offer benefits and resources to veterans after the first year of separation. Veterans organizations are non-governmental organizations that assist veterans with a range of services.

Figure 2. Examples of Supports for New Veterans, Including Solid Start Communication Milestones.

VA designates transitioning service members as priority veterans if they had an appointment with a mental health care professional in the year prior to separation. Priority veterans receive earlier outreach than other veterans.[16] During phone calls, Solid Start representatives share information on specific benefits, as well as offer personalized guidance based on the veteran's needs and interests. In 2021, Solid Start successfully contacted 75 percent of priority veterans.

According to VA officials, the program's telephone outreach strategy was informed by private industry consultants with expertise on the number of calls needed to successfully connect with people.[17] VA defines a successful contact as a phone conversation with an

[15] A law codifying Solid Start was enacted on October 17, 2022. Pub. L. No. 117-205, 136 Stat. 2232 (codified at 38 U.S.C. § 6320).

[16] According to VA officials, representatives must discuss VA mental health benefits during every answered call. If the veteran is experiencing a mental health crisis, the representative is to transfer them to the Veterans Crisis Line—a confidential service for veterans at immediate risk of self-harm provided at no cost to the veteran.

[17] At each time interval, representatives are to make seven attempts to phone the veteran and leave voicemails on the first, third, and seventh attempts. Even if a veteran has answered the 90-day call and spoken to a representative, Solid Start representatives continue to phone them at the 180-day and 365-day call intervals.

individual veteran that covers all required and requested benefits information at least once during the 365-day period of eligibility for Solid Start. VA's goals for successful contacts with eligible veterans in fiscal years 2020 and 2021 were 40 and 50 percent, respectively, which it exceeded both years.[18]

The DOD-VA Joint Executive Committee

The DOD-VA Joint Executive Committee was established to oversee DOD's and VA's coordination with providing health care and benefits and to provide annual reports to Congress on its efforts.[19] In this capacity, the Committee serves as the primary federal interagency body for overseeing military transition assistance activities. In September 2019, the Joint Executive Committee approved the "Military to Civilian Readiness" framework. This framework is a timeline that lays out the various independent processes and programs that may assist service members and veterans across the transition continuum. See figure 3.

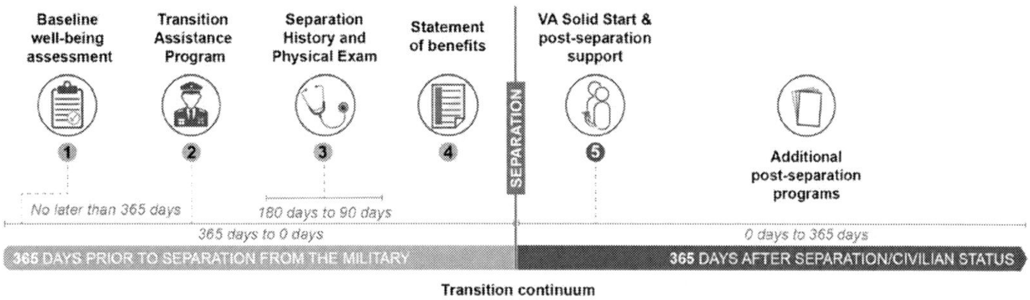

Source: GAO analysis of DOD-VA Joint Exclusive Committee information (information): GAO (icons); barks/stock. Adobe.com (soldier icon). |GAO-24-107752.

Figure 3. Department of Defense (DOD)-Department of Veterans Affairs (VA) Joint Executive Committee's Military to Civilian Readiness Framework.

Implementing GAO's Recommendations Could Improve inTransition's Processes for Enrollment, Outreach, and Performance Assessment

In our July 2024 report, we found several issues with the inTransition program that impeded its ability to successfully assist eligible transitioning service members and veterans who may have mental health needs.[2016] We made four recommendations to the Defense Healthy Agency to address these issues, including recommendations related to the timing of the inTransition's automatic enrollment process, its outreach strategy, and its assessment of program performance. DOD did not provide a formal response to these recommendations.

inTransition's automatic enrollment occurs 2 to 3 months after separation. We found that the program identified most of its enrollees— about 85 percent (91,224 of 107,649

[18] According to VA officials, they established annual successful contact goals for Solid Start based on the contact rates of other VA outreach programs.
[19] See 38 U.S.C. § 320(c).
[20] GAO-24-106189.

enrollees) in calendar year 2022—2 to 3 months after their separation from the military through its automatic enrollment process. This timing coincides with the last 9 months of the 24-month transition continuum, which may result in a post-separation gap in assistance for some service members during a vulnerable period. As we noted in our July report, this timing also affects the program's ability to accomplish its primary objective of ensuring continuity of mental health services during times of transition.

Per inTransition's policy, the program automatically enrolls any service member who meets its criteria of having received care for mental health or moderate-to-severe traumatic brain injury in the year prior to their separation. Agency officials said that accurate execution of the policy's automatic enrollment criteria requires them to conduct this process after service members have separated. According to the contractor who identifies these enrollees, the timing of this process is also impacted by when the military services report their separations data, which generally accounts for a 2- to 3-month time lag.

Identifying eligible service members for automatic enrollment prior to their separation would help inTransition better ensure the continuity of any needed mental health services during the critical transition period. For example, under revised criteria, service members with mental health needs could be identified prior to separation through their participation in mandatory transition processes like TAP. We recommended that the Defense Health Agency revise the program's criteria to identify and enroll these eligible service members prior to their separation from the military.

inTransition's outreach strategy contributed to difficulties in contacting enrollees. We also found the inTransition program was unable to successfully connect with over 70 percent of the service members it identified through its automatic enrollment process (65,545 of 91,224), based on our analysis of inTransition data for 2022.[21] As a result, these service members may not have known that they were identified through inTransition's automatic enrollment process and may not have been aware of the program and the assistance it could provide. See figure 4.

The inTransition program was unable to reach some automatically enrolled service members because DOD did not have up-to-date or accurate contact information to provide to the program. Our analysis of 2022 data showed that the program could not contact about 6 percent (5,710) of the total automatically enrolled service members because of incorrect or missing contact information.

We also found that the number of outreach attempts may have affected the program's overall rate of successful connections. inTransition program officials told us for certain months in 2022 they did not require the contractor to make the up to three outreach telephone calls to each automatically enrolled service member, as provided for in the contract. For example, from July through December, only one phone call was made to each auto enrollee. Officials told us this was becauseinTransition experienced larger-than-expected enrollment lists and a shortage of contract funds. According to inTransition officials, the program received additional funding

[21] This is generally consistent with the rate reported by the DOD's Office of the Inspector General in November 2021. Specifically, that report found an approximately 28 percent successful contact rate for the inTransition program's automatically enrolled service members from fiscal year 2017 through 2020. See Department of Defense Office of the Inspector General, *Evaluation of the Department of Defense's Implementation of Suicide Prevention Resources for Transitioning Uniformed Service Members*, Report No. DODIG- 2022-030 (Nov. 9, 2021). We defined a successful contact as inTransition speaking or connecting with an automatically enrolled service member to inform them of inTransition's services. We defined an unsuccessful contact as inTransition not speaking or connecting with an automatically enrolled service member.

in April 2023, which allowed the contractor to return to making up to three outreach calls for each automatically enrolled service member.

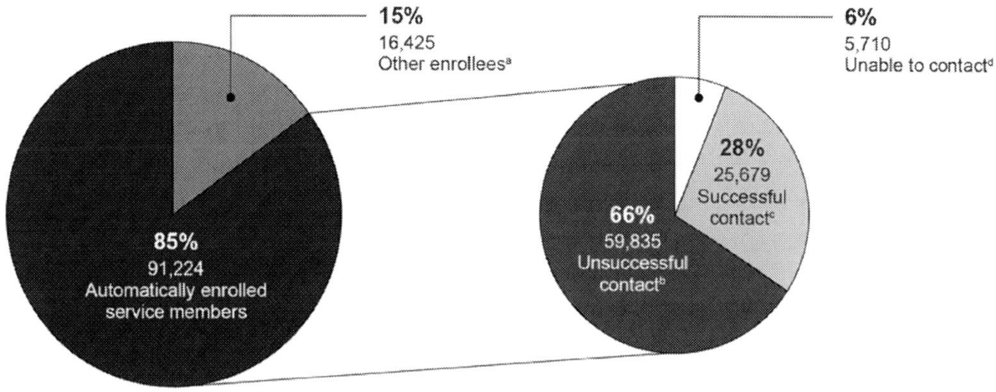

Source : GAO analysis of DOD data. | GAO-24-107752.

[a]Enrollees who were referred or who self-referred to the program.

[b]Enrollees who did not answer or return inTransition's phone calls offering assistance. [c]Enrollees who answered or returned inTransition's phone calls offering assistance. [d]Enrollees who could not be contacted due to missing or incorrect phone numbers.

Note: During this period, the inTransition program was unable to make the up to three calls, provided for in the contract, from April through December, according to officials. inTransition program officials said that was due to larger-than-expected enrollment lists and a shortage of contract funds. Nonetheless, the contact rate we calculated for 2022 was generally consistent with the contact rate reported by the DOD Office of Inspector General in November 2021. Specifically, that report found an approximately 28 percent successful contact rate for the inTransition program's automatically enrolled service members from fiscal years 2017 through 2020.

Figure 4. Department of Defense's inTransition Enrollees and Telephone Call Response Rates to Automatically Enrolled Service Members, 2022.

Program officials explained that the program's method of outreach— telephone calls— may help explain the program's difficulty in successfully connecting with its automatically enrolled service members, because cold calls are an outdated form of communication. When asked about using alternative methods of outreach, program officials said that the program's policy requires phone calls as the primary contact method.[22]

Expanding the program's outreach methods could potentially improve its ability to successfully connect with eligible service members, and in turn, increase participation. Additionally, when coupled with identifying automatically enrolled service members before they separate, the program would likely have more accurate contact information for these individuals. We recommended that the Defense Health Agency revise inTransition's policy to expand its outreach methods for contacting automatically enrolled service members, such as with text messages, email, or the use of services that help locate individuals with outdated or incorrect contact information.

inTransition lacks performance goals. Finally, our July 2024 report found that the inTransition program regularly monitors a number of measures on program performance, but it has not defined the level of performance it aims to achieve. inTransition program officials

[22] Defense Health Agency-Procedural Instruction 6490.01, *inTransition Program* (July 12, 2019).

said that they review the contractor's reported data, such as data on enrollees' military service branch and enrollees' decisions on whether to stay enrolled or opt out, on a monthly, quarterly, and yearly basis. However, despite the difficulties the contractor has faced in successfully connecting with automatically enrolled service members, program officials said they have no changes planned to improve the program, and that the program is working as intended.

Establishing measurable performance goals that have quantitative targets and time frames would help inTransition program officials assess program performance by comparing planned and actual results. For instance, the inTransition contractor tracks and reports how many automatically enrolled service members it contacts, but the program does not have related goals for how many automatically enrolled service members it aims to successfully connect with each month (e.g., such as a targeted percentage of the monthly automatically enrolled service members).

We recommended the program establish performance goals as well as implement a process to use the performance information to assess its effectiveness and make any needed improvements. Taking these steps would give decision-makers baseline information and longitudinal data to determine whether changes to the program are needed. This, in turn, could result in more enrollees participating in the program and more transitioning service members obtaining needed assistance.

DOD Is Taking Steps to Improve Warm Handovers and Assess Their Helpfulness to Service Members Transitioning to Civilian Life

In our March 2024 report, we found several issues with DOD's warm handover process that could prevent the agency from providing transition support to service members.[23] We made eight recommendations to address these issues, including that DOD 1) develop plans to analyze warm handover data, 2) develop additional guidance to commanders and their designees on verifying warm handovers, and 3) develop a plan to assess the helpfulness of warm handovers. DOD concurred with these recommendations and is taking steps to implement them.

DOD is not tracking why some service members do not receive warm handovers. We found that DOD does not know why some service members who do not meet career readiness standards are not receiving a warm handover because DOD has not analyzed available data to determine the reasons why they did not receive them. According to our analysis of DOD's available TAP data and policy, at least 4,300 service members who separated from the military from April 1, 2021, to March 31, 2023, should have received a warm handover but did not.[24]

DOD collects and maintains information on the activities that each service member completes, including whether they complete a financial plan or other requirements for the career readiness standards. However, our report found DOD does not analyze data on the

[23] GAO-24-106248.

[24] According to DOD's available TAP data, 267,745 service members separated from the military during this period. Of this group of service members, 40,998 (15 percent) received at least one warm handover. These data do not include the Reserves, National Guard, Coast Guard, or the Space Force. Army data from November 2022 to June 2023 were unavailable due to data migration and not included in our analysis. These data reflect warm handovers as recorded in DOD data; we did not independently verify whether all steps in the warm handover process were completed. Service members may receive more than one warm handover.

characteristics or circumstances of service members who did not meet these requirements and who did not receive a warm handover. Moreover, in some cases, available data on why a warm handover is not provided may be limited.

According to DOD officials, TAP counselors and commanders make individualized decisions on whether transitioning service members should receive a warm handover. TAP officials may decide not to provide a warm handover even when the service members did not meet career readiness standards. However, TAP officials are not required to record a reason why the warm handover is not provided.

Analyzing data to determine why service members did not receive warm handovers would help DOD ensure that it refers service members who need additional assistance to the relevant resources. We recommended that DOD develop a written plan to analyze its available TAP data to identify reasons why transitioning service members who should receive a warm handover are not receiving one and take action to collect additional warm handover data. In May 2024, DOD indicated that it plans to update its TAP Evaluation Plan with a written analysis regarding warm handovers, modify its TAP data collection form to require reasons why transitioning service members who should receive warm handovers are not receiving one, and provide support for officials involved in data collection. DOD estimated that it will complete these efforts by September 2026.

DOD does not reliably verify who receives a warm handover. We also found that DOD is not reliably verifying whether warm handovers occur. In some cases, warm handovers were provided but not verified in the database, and in other cases warm handovers were not provided but were verified.[25] For instance, according to available DOD data for a 2- year period (April 1, 2021, to March 31, 2023), commanders or their designees verified that a warm handover was provided to 77,711 transitioning service members who were not recorded as receiving one, calling into question the reliability of commander and designee verifications.[26] TAP officials we interviewed during our site visits said that many commanders and designees are not sure about their responsibility to verify with service members that warm handovers occur.

Having a reliable mechanism for verifying that a warm handover has occurred would help DOD ensure that it is assisting service members in finding employment, accessing benefits, and becoming aware of mental health and other resources available to them. We recommended that DOD develop additional guidance to commanders and their designees on verifying warm handovers and on recording the verifications in the TAP database. In May 2024, DOD said that the TAP Interagency Governance Structure is developing a course and written commander's guide to better educate commanders and their designees on the importance of verifying warm handovers and recording the verifications in the TAP database.

DOD plans to develop the commander guidance by March 2025 and incorporate it into the course by June 2025.

DOD has not assessed the helpfulness of warm handovers. Our March 2024 report also found that DOD generally does not know whether service members who were identified as needing a warm handover received services or achieved positive post-transition outcomes.

Stakeholders, such as TAP officials, said that warm handovers could be especially beneficial to younger and lower-ranked service members and to service members facing

---

[25] We considered a warm handover to have been provided when DOD's data included a warm handover reason and an agency type. If either of these data elements were missing, we considered no warm handover to have occurred.

[26] These data do not include the Reserves, National Guard, Coast Guard, or the Space Force. Army data from November 2022 to June 2023 were unavailable due to data migration and not included in our analysis.

unanticipated separations for short-notice, administrative, or medical separations. However, DOD does not have a plan to assess whether service members received services from other agencies or organizations they were referred to or achieved positive post- transition outcomes after a warm handover is provided.

Developing an assessment plan to examine program outcomes would help DOD better understand the helpfulness of the warm handover process and inform future improvement efforts. We recommended that DOD, in coordination with interagency partners, such as DOL and VA, develop a plan to assess the helpfulness of warm handovers as a part of its overall assessment of TAP. In May 2024, DOD said it plans to integrate a written analysis to assess the efficacy of warm handover data into the existing TAP Evaluation Plan. This will be done through the interagency Performance Management Work Group, which includes representatives from DOD, DOL, and VA, among other agencies.

According to DOD, this updated plan will include an assessment of the overall helpfulness of warm handovers. DOD estimates that it will complete this action by March 2025.

VA Implemented GAO's Recommendation to Collaborate with Veterans Organizations to Improve Outreach for Its Solid Start Program

In our January 2023 report, we found that VA had systematically phoned eligible veterans about available benefits and additional resources, and prioritized veterans with prior mental health appointments. However, we also found that VA had not collaborated with veterans organizations to address the outreach challenges they identified with VA's communication tools (e.g., cold calls) and building relationships with veterans.[27] We recommended that VA's Under Secretary for Benefits collaborate with veterans organizations, such as veteran service organizations, in identifying and addressing any outreach gaps, and assessing Solid Start outreach strategies for hard-to-reach groups of veterans. VA concurred with this recommendation and implemented it in May 2023.

Many nongovernmental organizations advocate for and work to support veterans, such as veteran service organizations, which assist veterans with their benefit claims, sponsor a range of programs for veterans, and advocate on behalf of veterans, among other things. Veterans organizations can support veterans throughout their year of Solid Start eligibility, and beyond. Representatives from six of the seven veterans organizations we spoke with told us that using phone calls as Solid Start's primary communication tool may present a challenge because veterans may be reluctant to answer phone calls, especially if the calls are unexpected or labeled as spam. VA officials acknowledged that reaching younger veterans has been a challenge, as shown in lower success rates for contacting veterans under age 23. Other hard-to-reach veterans include those living in remote areas, experiencing homelessness, or who did not receive an honorable discharge.

In addition, representatives from all seven veterans organizations told us there were barriers for Solid Start program representatives in trying to create relationships with the veterans. Such barriers may include Solid Start representatives who lack military experience, or who

[27] GAO-23-105699.

potentially lack cultural competency when interacting with racial and ethnic minorities, and LGBTQ+ veterans.[28] These barriers may result in veterans' hesitancy to speak with or trust VA.

In response to our recommendation, in May 2023, VA implemented an updated veteran service organization engagement plan for more regular collaboration to ensure veteran service organizations have the necessary training, information, and tools to promote Solid Start. VA also implemented additional engagement efforts, such as additional targeted emails promoting the benefits of engaging with Solid Start, and a prominent social media presence, to connect with younger veterans.

DOD-VA Joint Executive Committee Would Benefit from Assessing the Effectiveness of Efforts to Facilitate Access to Mental Health Services

In our July 2024 report, we found that the DOD-VA Joint Executive Committee had not assessed the effectiveness of the departments' efforts overall in facilitating access to mental health services for transitioning service members. We recommended that the Committee assess the effectiveness of DOD and VA programs and processes overall in facilitating access to mental health services across the transition continuum, and recommend any needed changes to DOD and VA, including changes to address any gaps or unnecessary overlap or duplication. VA concurred with the recommendation, but DOD did not formally respond to it.

As described in our report, officials told us that the Committee directed the Transition Executive Committee (its subcommittee focused on transitioning from the military) to identify DOD and VA mental health- related programs and processes across the transition continuum in 2022.[29] The Transition Executive Committee identified a number of DOD and VA programs and processes that may provide mental health touchpoints for service members during this time.

However, officials responsible for the review told us that they limited their review to an inventory of available mental health resources, and they did not assess the effectiveness of these efforts. Specifically, the officials said that they did not evaluate whether or how these programs and processes collectively facilitate continuous access to mental health services across the transition continuum.

Such an assessment—which could build off the inventory of mental health touchpoints—would align with the Committee's strategic goal of enhancing the transition experience. It would also provide the Committee with a more comprehensive understanding of how and when service members and veterans can access mental health services across the transition continuum. As we noted in our report, this would better position the Committee to identify and address issues with any service gaps, overlap, or duplication. For example, we found that approximately 95 percent of the veterans on VA's Solid Start lists of "priority" veterans also

---

[28] LGBTQ+ stands for lesbian, gay, bisexual, transgender, queer or questioning. The "plus" is meant to be inclusive of identities that may not be covered by the acronym LGBTQ, such as asexual, intersex, non-binary, and two-spirit.

[29] The Transition Executive Committee provides oversight and direction related to transition assistance to service members and veterans. The National Defense Authorization Act for Fiscal Year 2024 added the Transition Executive Committee as a statutory committee of the DOD-VA Joint Executive Committee. Prior to this legislation, the Transition Executive Committee operated as a directed committee of the DOD-VA Joint Executive Committee's co-chairs. Pub. L No. 118-31, div. A, tit. XVIII, § 1805, 137 Stat. 136, 687 (2023).

appeared on DOD's inTransition lists of automatically enrolled service members for calendar year 2022. As a result, almost all of these veterans may have received multiple outreach calls from both programs during the same post-separation time period, which could be confusing for them. An assessment would help to determine whether this overlap is problematic and, if so, what steps the Committee could take to help resolve it.

In closing, ensuring that service members and veterans have access to mental health support and other services during the transition continuum is critical, especially in light of the many challenges they may face in readjusting to civilian life. Both DOD and VA have programs geared towards helping this population, but critical improvements are needed to ensure they are effectively reaching and assisting them. Fully addressing our recommendations would help ensure that transitioning service members and veterans have the support they need and deserve. We will continue to monitor their efforts to do so.

Chairman Van Orden, Ranking Member Levin, and Members of the Subcommittee, this concludes my statement. I would be pleased to respond to any questions that you may have at this time.

GAO Contacts and Staff Acknowledgments

If you or your staff members have any questions concerning this testimony, please contact Alyssa M. Hundrup at (202) 512-7114 or HundrupA@gao.gov for questions about DOD's inTransition program or the DOD-VA Joint Executive Committee and John D. Sawyer at (202) 512-7215 or SawyerJ@gao.gov for questions about DOD's warm handover process or VA's Solid Start program. Contact points for our Office of Congressional Relations and Public Affairs may be found on the last page of this statement. Individuals who made key contributions to this testimony statement include Bonnie Anderson (Assistant Director), Amy Andresen (Analyst in Charge), Nick Bartine, Adrienne Bober, Meeta Engle, Kristen Jones, Paul Schearf, and Alexandra Squitieri. Also contributing to this statement were Mimi Nguyen, Aaron Olszewski, Roxanna Sun, Cathy Hamann Whitmore, and Jennifer Whitworth.

Related GAO Reports

Transition to Civilian Life: Better Collection and Analysis of Military Service Data Needed to Improve Oversight of the SkillBridge Program. GAO-24-107352. August 22, 2024.

DOD and VA Health Care: Actions Needed to Better Facilitate Access to Mental Health Services During Military to Civilian Transitions.

GAO-24-106189. Washington, D.C.: July 15, 2024.

Defense Health Care: DOD Should Improve Accuracy of Behavioral Health Provider Information in TRICARE Directories. GAO-24-106588. Washington, D.C.: July 8, 2024.

Veterans Health Care: Opportunities Exist to Improve Assessment of Network Adequacy for Mental Health. GAO-24-106410. Washington, D.C.: June 3, 2024.

Service Members Transitioning to Civilian Life: Agencies Can Improve Warm Handovers for Additional Assistance. GAO-24-106248. Washington, D.C.: March 21, 2024.

VA Health Care: Opportunities Exist to Further Meet Student Veterans' Mental Health Needs. GAO-24-106620. Washington, D.C.: February 15, 2024.

Defense Health Care: DOD Should Monitor Urgent Referrals to Civilian Behavioral Health Providers to Ensure Timely Care. GAO-24-106267. Washington, D.C.: February 6, 2024.

Defense Health Care: DOD Assessment Needed to Ensure TRICARE Behavioral Health Coverage Goals Are Being Met. GAO-24-106597. Washington, D.C.: December 20, 2023.

Veterans Benefits: VA Could Enhance Outreach for Its Solid Start Program by Increasing Collaboration with Veterans Organizations. GAO-23-105699. Washington, D.C.: January 5, 2023.

Servicemembers Transitioning to Civilian Life: DOD Can Better Leverage Performance Information to Improve Participation in Counseling Pathways. GAO-23-104538. Washington, D.C.: December 12, 2022.

VA Vet Centers: Opportunities Exist to Help Better Ensure Veterans' and Servicemembers' Readjustment Counseling Needs Are Met. GAO-22-105039. Washington, D.C.: May 17, 2022.

Military and Veteran Support: DOD Has Taken Steps to Help Servicemembers Transfer Skills to Civilian Employment but Has Limited Evidence to Determine Program Effectiveness. GAO-22-105261. Washington, D.C.: February 17, 2022.

Military Personnel: DOD's Transition Assistance Program at Small or Remote Installations. GAO-21-104608. Washington, D.C.: July 21, 2021.

Military and Veteran Support: Performance Goals Could Strengthen Programs that Help Servicemembers Obtain Civilian Employment. GAO-20-416. Washington, D.C.: July 9, 2020.

GAO's Mission

The Government Accountability Office, the audit, evaluation, and investigative arm of Congress, exists to support Congress in meeting its constitutional responsibilities and to help improve the performance and accountability of the federal government for the American people. GAO examines the use of public funds; evaluates federal programs and policies; and provides analyses, recommendations, and other assistance to help Congress make informed oversight, policy, and funding decisions. GAO's commitment to good government is reflected in its core values of accountability, integrity, and reliability.

Connect with GAO

Connect with GAO on Facebook, Flickr, Twitter, and YouTube. Subscribe to our RSS Feeds or Email Updates. Listen to our Podcasts. Visit GAO on the web at https://www.gao.gov.

To Report Fraud, Waste, and Abuse in Federal Programs

Contact FraudNet:
Website: https://www.gao.gov/about/what-gao-does/fraudnet

Automated answering system: (800) 424-5454 or (202) 512-7700

Congressional Relations

A. Nicole Clowers, Managing Director, ClowersA@gao.gov, (202) 512-4400, U.S. Government Accountability Office, 441 G Street NW, Room 7125, Washington, DC 20548.

Public Affairs

Sarah Kaczmarek, Acting Managing Director, KaczmarekS@gao.gov, (202) 512- 4800, U.S. Government Accountability Office, 441 G Street NW, Room 7149 Washington, DC 20548.

Strategic Planning and External Liaison

Stephen J. Sanford, Managing Director, spel@gao.gov, (202) 512-4707.

U.S. Government Accountability Office, 441 G Street NW, Room 7814, Washington, DC 20548.

Not for publication until released by the Committee

Prepared Statement of Susan Orsega, DSc (Hc), MS, NP, Deputy Assistant Secretary of Defense, Health Services Policy & Oversight Health Affairs Regarding

Mission Transition: Evaluating Mental Health Support Programs for Separating Service Members Before the House Veterans' Affairs Committee, Subcommittee on Economic Opportunity, September 10, 2024

Chairman Van Orden, Ranking Member Levin, and distinguished Members of the House Veterans' Affairs Committee, Subcommittee on Economic Opportunity, thank you for the opportunity to testify before you today. I am pleased to represent the Office of the Assistant Secretary of Defense for Health Affairs to discuss the Department of Defense's (DoD's) commitment to mental health support programs for separating Service members.

The DoD is committed to providing the highest level of mental health care to Service members. We ensure that those who serve our nation receive timely and high-quality health care, including care to address their mental health needs. This is particularly important during the transition from military to civilian life, when Service members are most vulnerable to suicide and some experience challenges such as the loss of a sense of purpose, post-traumatic stress disorder, and other mental health symptoms.

In this testimony, we will inform the Subcommittee about the Department's current mental health programs and resources during the transition from military to civilian life – including the inTransition program, the Transition Assistance Program (TAP), and Military OneSource, as well as the Department's implementation of recommendations from the U.S. Government Accountability Office (GAO) report, "DOD AND VA HEALTH CARE: Actions Needed to Better Facilitate Access to Mental Health Services During Military to Civilian Transitions" (GAO-24-106189).

The DoD created the inTransition program in 2010 in response to a 2007 report by the DoD Task Force on Mental Health, which revealed that a number of Service members were disengaging from mental health care treatment as they transitioned from the DoD to the Department of Veterans Affairs (VA) health care system, contributing to their worsened mental health. For 14 years, inTransition has facilitated continuity of care and connection to continued mental health resources for Service members receiving mental health and/or moderate to severe traumatic brain injury (TBI) care as they move into civilian life. The program supports a Service member's efforts to achieve and maintain wellness and enables continuity of needed services, including mental health services.

The inTransition program supports all transitioning Service members and veterans regardless of the duration of their service, time since discharge, or category of discharge. All Service members who are leaving the military service and who have received care for mental health and/or moderate to severe TBI within one year of their separation are automatically enrolled in the inTransition program, and Service members can also get connected to services through self- or provider-referrals.

Automatic enrollment is an "opt out" process, where neither written consent from the patient nor a signed authorization is required to enroll the Service member in the inTransition Program; however, Service members are provided a choice to remain in or opt out of the program. If the Service member does not opt out of the program, health care providers or designated staff can, in collaboration with the Service member, start enrollment by calling the inTransition number at (800) 424-7877. During this process, health care providers or designated staff provide the name, contact information, destination or discharge status, and diagnosis to the inTransition coach. Service members may also be made aware of the inTransition program and self-refer through multiple channels, including the TAP curriculum, provider referrals, and inTransition program marketing and outreach activities. If not self-referred or provider-referred, all eligible service members are automatically enrolled and called by the inTransition program to discuss the program and provide services.

The inTransition program includes a call center that operates 24/7, 365 days a year, where program staff are available to respond to Service member questions concerning their mental health, and to inform Service members of local resources to meet their mental health needs. The program also provides Service members with specialized one-on-one motivational coaching, information, support, and education to encourage Service members to continue to engage with any needed mental health services. Coaches maintain regular telephonic contact (weekly, or at the preference of the Service member) until the Service member has been transitioned to the new provider and/or opts out of the program.[30] Coaches work with Service

[30] Defense Health Agency Administrative Instruction (DHA-AI) 6490.02, "inTransition Program," March 7, 2024.

members to identify eligible referral destinations, support connecting them with a new mental health provider, and facilitate "warm handoff" referrals to VA personnel who guide Service members through the VA healthcare system to a VA mental health provider.[31,32] Through DoD's inTransition program, the program staff, coaches, and separating Service members work together to help continue Service member engagement with mental health care services in accordance with the individual needs, preferences, and circumstances of each Service member.

Since 2019 the DoD has leveraged an Interactive Customer Evaluation (ICE) tool, which collects feedback on services provided within the DoD. All Service members and Veterans who participate in inTransition coaching services are requested to evaluate the program through the completion of an ICE survey. Since its inception, ICE data demonstrates that Service members who have participated in the inTransition program have indicated their satisfaction with the program and its ability to help connect them with necessary mental health supports and resources during their transition. The inTransition program regularly receives positive feedback from the field, including from military medical treatment facility staff, the VA, Vet Centers, and the Veterans Crisis Line—reflecting the program's significant and successful role within the DoD and VA community.

In addition to inTransition, the DoD implements TAP, which is the result of an interagency partnership among the DoD, VA, the Departments of Labor, Education, and Homeland Security, the Small Business Administration, and the Office of Personnel Management.[33] TAP addresses the many facets of a Service member's transition while providing information, resources, and tools to Service members to help them prepare for the move from military to civilian life. TAP includes counseling from DoD, VA, and DOL on various benefits, programs, services, tools, and other important resource entitlements for which Service members may be eligible, as well as curriculums that educate Service members on VA mental health resources that they can engage with during their transition and when they have reintegrated into civilian life.[34] Through TAP, if it is determined that a Service member is not prepared for transition, there is a warm handover between TAP counselors and the appropriate partner or agency to connect Service members with the needed resources to further assist them post- transition.

Service members participate in TAP up to one year prior to separation or two years prior to retiring to help prepare for their transition and to proactively inform them of available resources to maintain their mental health during their journey back to civilian life.[35] Service members who have participated in TAP have indicated that the program is valuable and that they are satisfied with its ability to educate them on accessing resources, with 91% of respondents confirming that they know how to access transition-related resources, according to 2023 survey results.

Military OneSource is a 24/7 resource available to all Service members and families regardless of whether they are transitioning to civilian life. One element of Military OneSource offers transitioning Service members consultations on navigating their transition and provides information on the resources and programs available to help Service members have a successful transition.[36] Through Military OneSource, Service members have access to confidential non-

---

[31] DHA-AI 6490.02.
[32] Health.mil; "inTransition."
[33] DoDTAP.mil; "Partnering Agencies."
[34] DoDTAP.mil; "TAP Curriculum."
[35] DoD Instruction 1332.35, "Transition Assistance Program (TAP) for Military Personnel," September 26, 2019.
[36] Militaryonesource.mil; "Military OneSource's Transitioning Veterans Consultation."

medical counseling up to a year after their separation or retirement.[37] These resources, along with programs like inTransition and TAP, offer transitioning Service members with a comprehensive set of tools to promote continuity of mental health care.

The mental health of Service members remains a priority for the DoD, and we are continuously identifying opportunities to improve the delivery of mental health support for those who serve our nation. The recently published GAO report, "DOD AND VA HEALTH CARE: Actions Needed to Better Facilitate Access to Mental Health Services During Military to Civilian Transition" (July 15, 2024), reviewed access to mental health services for transitioning Service members, which included examining elements of the DoD's inTransition program and the DoD- VA Joint Executive Committee's (JEC) assessment of the effectiveness of efforts to facilitate access to mental health services for transitioning Service members.

The GAO's review identified challenges for inTransition to conduct outreach to Service members and to connect with Service members that are automatically enrolled in the program. Consequently, GAO provided the following five recommendations, which included a revision of inTransition's enrollment criteria and outreach policy, establishment of inTransition performance goals, and an assessment by the DoD-VA JEC of the departments' efforts to facilitate access to mental health services:

- Recommendation 1: The Defense Health Agency (DHA) should revise the inTransition program's criteria for auto-enrollment as outlined in its policy to identify and enroll eligible Service members prior to their separation from the military.
- Recommendation 2: DHA should revise the inTransition program's policy to expand the outreach methods used by the program to contact automatically enrolled Service members, such as by adding requirements for outreach through email, text, or the use of location services.
- Recommendation 3: DHA should establish measurable performance goals for the inTransition program that have quantitative targets and time frames.
- Recommendation 4: DHA should implement a process for the inTransition program to use performance information to assess its effectiveness and make any needed improvements, as appropriate.
- Recommendation 5: The DoD-VA JEC should assess the effectiveness of DoD and VA programs and processes overall in facilitating access to mental health services across the transition continuum, and recommend any needed changes to DoD and VA, including changes to address any identified gaps or unnecessary duplication or overlap.

The DoD reviewed the GAO report and recommendations and a formal comment from the Department is in progress. We are committed to continuing to enhance the inTransition program and to assessing the effectiveness of transition-related programs in order to improve continuity of care for transitioning Service members.

Thank you for your continued support of the health and well-being of our Service members and for inviting me to be here with you today to discuss the important issue of continuity of mental health support services for Service members transitioning to civilian life. We recognize that we have more work to do, and much more progress to make, in support of our Service

[37] Militaryonesource.mil; "Military Transition to Civilian Life Comes with a Full Year of Support from Military OneSource."

members when they are most vulnerable as they transition into civilian life. We remain committed to enabling Service members to receive the necessary mental health support they need during this life-changing and important transition. I look forward to your questions.

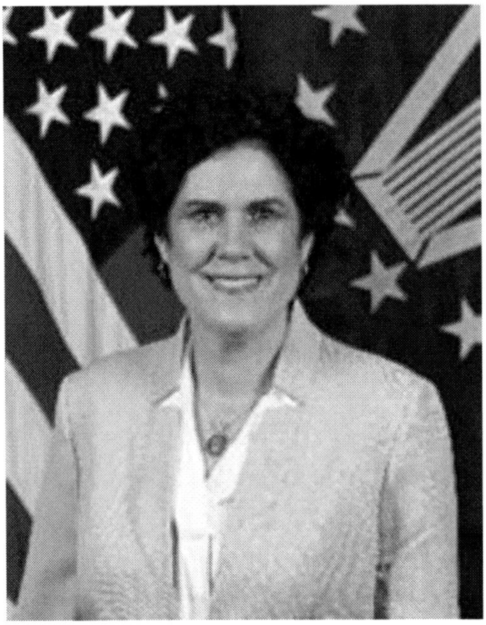

Susan Orsega
Deputy Assistant Secretary of Defense, Health Services Policy and Oversight Office
of Assistant Secretary of Defense for Health Affairs
Office of the Under Secretary of Defense for Personnel & Readiness

Susan Orsega serves as the Deputy Assistant Secretary of Defense (DASD) for Health Services Policy and Oversight (HSP&O) within the Office of the Assistant Secretary of Defense for Health Affairs in the Office of the Under Secretary of Defense for Personnel & Readiness. In this role, Orsega leads a team of subject matter experts in establishing and overseeing Military Health System (MHS) policies concerning military personnel, retirees, and their families.

DASD Orsega's HSP&O team provides medical advice and consultation to senior Defense officials, Congress, and other Department of Defense (DOD) stakeholders. HSP&O examines the MHS workforce environment and adjusts human resource policies for more than 150,000 military and civilian health professionals. Orsega and the HSP&O team serve as lead coordinators with several DOD committees, and in partnership with representatives from the Department of Veterans Affairs. Areas of policy and oversight responsibility include, as follows: Medical Quality Assurance and Clinical Quality Management, Health Information Technology, Preventive Medicine, Population Health, Warrior Care, Chronic Disease Management, Child & Women's Health, and Behavioral Health.

Prior to senior executive service appointment, DASD Orsega retired at the rank of Rear Admiral Upper Half, United States Public Health Service (USPHS) after 34 years of service as Senior Advisor to the Assistant Secretary for Health in December 2023. While serving in the USPHS, she held various assignments leading teams to build programs and improve complex global health care problems. From January 20 to March 23, 2021, she served as Acting Surgeon General. DASD Orsega is the first nurse practitioner to hold this position, chosen for her leadership and executive presence within the government, as well as her strategic operational expertise during health crises. In 2019, she was selected as the Director of USPHS and managed activation of the largest historical deployment of the U.S. Public Health Service Commissioned Corps in support of international and national COVID-19 efforts. Earlier in her career, Dr. Orsega held various positions with progressive responsibility at the National Institutes of Health (NIH).

Notably, she was selected to lead research operations partnerships in multiple African countries during periods of emerging infectious disease outbreaks.

Orsega has deployed to 15 public health crises around the world such as:

- New York City after September 11, 2001 terrorist attacks
- The US Capitol following an Anthrax terrorist event
- New Orleans following devastation from Hurricane Katrina
- Pacific region in support of Department of Defense Pacific Peleliu humanitarian mission

DASD Orsega's focus is addressing pressing issues of public health and health policy. She works to collaborate and influence people to implement necessary changes while navigating complex government regulations, legislation, policies, and organizational structures.

Orsega graduated with a Bachelor of Science from Towson University, Baltimore, Maryland in 1990. In 2001, she graduated with a Master of Science from the Nurse Practitioner Program, Uniformed Services University (USUHS), Bethesda, Maryland. Orsega later received honorary doctorates from USUHS and Georgetown University. She is a fellow in the American Academy of Nursing and in the American Association of Nurse Practitioners.

Statement of James D. Rodriguez, Assistant Secretary Veterans' Employment and Training Service, U.S. Department of Labor Before the Subcommittee on Economic Opportunity Committee on Veterans' Affairs U.S. House of Representatives September 10, 2024

Introduction

Chairman Van Orden, Ranking Member Levin, and distinguished Members of the subcommittee, thank you for inviting me to testify today. I appreciate the opportunity to discuss veteran mental health, and the "warm handover" processes that occur between agencies and programs, that help ensure that veterans receive timely and effective mental health support as they reintegrate into civilian life.

DOL is the lead federal department for employment and training programs. Successful employment is one key to economic success, and can strongly impact physical and mental health, life expectancy, and the quality of life.[38] Veterans with service-connected disabilities, including mental health conditions, often experience relatively low labor participation rates and high unemployment compared to their non-disabled counterparts.[39] Furthermore, veterans with mental health challenges, such as depression, posttraumatic stress disorder (PTSD), substance use, and anxiety, may find it difficult to maintain regular work attendance.[40] Research indicates that unemployment can adversely affect mental health and is associated with a higher risk of suicide among veterans.[41] Additionally, veterans with mental health conditions, particularly those at risk of or experiencing homelessness, may face increased risk of suicide following job loss.[42]

VETS' mission is to prepare America's veterans, Service members, and military spouses for meaningful careers, provide them with employment resources and expertise, protect their employment rights, and promote their employment opportunities. VETS administers programs designed to address the employment, training, and job security needs of over 196,000 military Service members who transition to civilian life each year, 8.6 million military veterans in the U.S. civilian labor force,[43] over 760,901 National Guard and Reserve members,[44] and 923,668 military spouses (578,952 active duty and 344,716 Guard and Reserve spouses).[45]

VETS administers the employment component of the Transition Assistance Program (TAP), which includes warm handovers (person-to-person connections) of transitioning Service members to American Job Centers and other partners when needed. DOL's American Job Centers are one-stop locations that offer a broad range of career and supportive services to the public. Veterans receive priority of service for all DOL-funded training programs in American Job Centers. Along with our partners, we are committed to ensuring the best transition for our Service members and their families and connecting them to the mental health and other services that they need.

TAP Employment Services and Warm Handovers

TAP provides training, resources, and assistance to separating and retiring Service members on active duty, Guard, Reserve, and their spouses, as authorized under 10 U.S.C. § 1144. TAP is a cooperative effort between VETS, the Department of Defense (DoD), Department of Veterans Affairs (VA), Department of Education, Department of Homeland Security (U.S. Coast Guard), Small Business Administration, and Office of Personnel Management.

There are three core VETS TAP employment workshops. First, VETS is responsible for the delivery of the Employment Fundamentals of Career Transition (EFCT) Workshop, which is a mandatory, one-day course for employment preparation. In addition, based on Service members' individual needs, VETS offers two elective tracks to acquire additional skills through

---

[38] See for examples: https://health.gov/healthypeople/priority-areas/social-determinants-health/literature-sum maries/employment.

[39] https://www.bls.gov/news.release/vet.nr0.htm.

[40] https://www.dol.gov/sites/dolgov/files/OASP/evaluation/pdf/HVRPEval-VeteranPerspectives.pdf.

[41] https://www.mentalhealth.va.gov/suicide_prevention/docs/FSTP-Employment-Status-and-Suicide-Risk.pdf.

[42] https://www.dol.gov/agencies/oasp/evaluation/completedstudies/Homeless-Veterans-Reintegration-Program-Im pact-Evaluation.

[43] https://www.bls.gov/cps/cpsaat48.htm.

[44] https://dwp.dmdc.osd.mil/dwp/app/dod-data-reports/workforce-reports.

[45] https://demographics.militaryonesource.mil/.

a two-day workshop: (1) the DOL Employment Workshop, and (2) the Career and Credential Exploration Workshop. Transitioning Service members must elect one two-day track during their individual counseling. However, they are encouraged to attend any additional track(s) and attend the courses more than once (as their unit missions allow) to prepare them for their transition.

As defined in the DoD Instruction[46] 1332.35, a warm handover is a Capstone process between the respective military department and appropriate interagency parties, resulting in the person-to-person connection of transitioning Service members to services and follow-up resources, as needed. The warm handover provides a confirmed introduction and assurance that the appropriate interagency party acknowledges that an eligible Service member needs post-military assistance, and the interagency partner follows through on providing assistance to meet the needs of transitioning Service members, mitigate risks, and assist them in attaining their post- transition goals and a successful transition.

Capstone is a two-stage process consisting of a review and verification of a transitioning Service member meeting Career Readiness Standards that takes place no later than 90 days prior to separation. Stage one is an in-depth review of the transitioning Service member's Individual Transition Plan (ITP) and Career Readiness Standards, which is conducted by the military Service's TAP staff. Stage two consists of the commander or commander's designee verifying that the transitioning Service member has a viable ITP. If the commander or their designee determines that the transitioning Service member does not have a viable ITP, he or she must confirm that a warm handover takes place with the appropriate interagency partners, as needed. For DOL, the Career Readiness Standards for those completing the employment track are either a completed resume or confirmation of employment, while a completed comparison of technical training institutions is required for those pursuing the vocational track. If a Service member fails to meet the Career Readiness Standards at Capstone, they are provided a warm handover toDOL.

DOL currently has two different warm handover procedures: (1) Employment Navigator and Partnership Program[47] (ENPP) site warm handover procedures, and (2) non-ENPP site warm handover procedures.

ENPP began as a pilot under the TAP program at 13 military installations worldwide on April 1, 2021. The pilot was designed in response to feedback from veterans who stated that, while their TAP classroom experience was educational, they desired a more personalized approach. Leveraging the Secretary's authority (10 U.S.C. § 1144), ENPP provides one-on-one, tailored services for transitioning Service members and their spouses, helping them identify and connect with meaningful employment and training opportunities. In FY 2023, 5,747 transitioning Service members and 383 military spouses received services through ENPP with more than 18,100 being served by this program to date.

Currently at 36 locations, our Employment Navigator staff and our partner organizations work with ENPP clients to assist them with their resumes, provide career direction, and provide additional employment-related personalized support. At ENPP sites, the lead Employment Navigator serves as the initial point-of-contact for those transitioning Service members who are receiving a warm handover for either an employment or vocation track. During a warm handover at ENPP sites, Employment Navigators connect transitioning Service members to a

[46] https://www.esd.whs.mil/Portals/54/Documents/DD/issuances/dodi/133235p.pdf.
[47] https://www.dol.gov/agencies/vets/programs/tap/employment-navigator-partnership.

designated American Job Center point-of-contact who verifies with DOL that they have received the contact information and reached out to the client to offer assistance. In addition to being connected with the American Job Center in the community where they plan to reside after transition, many Service members receiving a warm handover continue to receive services from our Employment Navigators and partner organizations.

ENPP partners are required to select a primary service from nine possible categories of services, which include: digital employment opportunity matching, training services, employment mentorship, hiring events, employment networking, Registered Apprenticeship opportunities, referrals to employment opportunities, placement services, and wrap-around services. Many of our ENPP partners who provide wrap-around services assist Service members in getting connected to critical healthcare-related services. ENPP partner organization services are provided at no cost to transitioning Service members or their spouses through no-cost agreements between DOL and partner organizations. A list of our current partners can be found on the VETS ENPP Partner Page,[48] and organizations that are interested in partnering with us can submit an application.[49] In coordination with our partners, VETS will continue to extend ENPP to serve as many transitioning Service members and their spouses as funding allows.

Notably, preliminary descriptive findings[50]13 show that transitioning Service members who received ENPP services have had better employment outcomes than those who did not receive ENPP services. For example, median quarterly wages were 11% higher ($11,370) for enlisted transitioning Service members who participated in ENPP compared to their counterparts ($10,248) who did not participate. And transitioning Service members who received ENPP services were employed about two months faster than those who did not. VETS will continue to gather and analyze data and will be able to provide more nuanced information as this program continues.

At non-ENPP sites, the military Service's TAP staff will connect transitioning Service members receiving a warm handover for employment or vocation with a staff member at an American Job Center near where the transitioning Service member will move to after separating. As of March 31, 2024, 3,493 transitioning Service members in FY 2024 have engaged with an American Job Center through Jobs for Veterans State Grants (JVSG) or Employment Service (Wagner-Peyser) staff, approximately 564 of whom (16.1%) indicated that they were engaging with the American Job Center as part of a warm handover.

Separate from ENPP, VETS TAP offers the Wounded Warrior and Caregiver Employment Workshop (WWCEW) to accommodate the individual needs of transitioning Service members, including individuals with mental health conditions. Each year[51] there are approximately 20,000 transitioning Service members who are considered wounded, ill, and/or injured, transitioning either through their Service branch's warrior care or military recovery units or through the Integrated Disability Evaluation System (IDES). In April 2022, VETS launched the WWCEW for those being evaluated for a disability rating through IDES as an alternative to the required one-day EFCT. Disabled Service members face barriers to completing the traditional EFCT, such as coordinating class schedules with medical appointments, long class

[48] https://www.dol.gov/agencies/vets/programs/tap/employment-navigator-partnership/enpp-partnerships.
[49] https://www.dol.gov/sites/dolgov/files/VETS/files/tap/DOLVETSENPPPotentialPartnerApplicationForm.pdf.
[50] https://www.dol.gov/sites/dolgov/files/VETS/files/ENPP-Factsheet-2024-08-05.pdf.
[51] As of 2022: https://www.militaryonesource.mil/data-research-and-statistics/military-community-demographics/2022-demographics-profile/.

duration, working with medical and health restrictions, and requiring caregiver attendance. The curriculum includes six self-paced online modules that participants can complete at their own pace, and the course interface enables users to register for a virtual meeting with a VETS facilitator to ask questions and to discuss activities and course content. As of July 31, over 9,600 participants have attended WWCEW in FY 2024.

It is also important to provide multiple pathways to assistance, so that there is no wrong door for veterans to knock on when they're seeking help. On January 11, 2022, VETS announced the launch of a five-year Off-Base Transition Training (OBTT) pilot program, in accordance with section 4303 of the Johnny Isakson and David P. Roe, M.D. Veterans Health Care and Benefits Improvement Act of 2020 (P.L. 116-315). The intent of this law was to improve health outcomes, and the OBTT pilot helps support mental health by improving economic stability for veterans and their families. Not all employment journeys are linear, and as noted above, unemployment can adversely affect mental health and is associated with a higher risk of suicide among veterans. Which is why OBTT meets veterans where they are in their post-service life to provide support whenever it's needed. OBTT provides TAP to veterans and the spouses of veterans at locations other than active military installations, in order to improve employment-related outcomes in areas with high veteran unemployment. OBTT features ten two-hour and three one-hour, instructor-led employment skills and workforce development workshops, provided in classrooms and virtually. OBTT also offers another important opportunity for veterans and their spouses to be connected to other services they may need, including mental health services in their local community. In FY 2023, 6,293 veterans or spouses of veterans were provided employment-related training through OBTT.

American Job Center Resources

DOL's Employment and Training Administration (ETA) administers the public workforce system, which includes nearly 2,250 American Job Centers across the country. These one-stop locations offer a broad range of career and wrap-around supportive services to the public, such as job training programs, employment services, adult basic education and literacy, vocational rehabilitation for individuals with disabilities, childcare, transportation assistance, housing assistance, legal aid services, unemployment compensation (including the Unemployment Compensation for ex-Service members (UCX) program), as well as referrals and linkages to physical and mental health care, suicide prevention services, addiction counseling, and other services and programs in their local communities. In most states, American Job Centers coordinate with or co-locate eligibility determination services for programs like the Supplemental Nutrition Assistance Program (SNAP), Temporary Assistance for Needy Families (TANF), and other partner programs, ensuring streamlined access for veterans and eligible persons seeking support. Veterans receive priority of service for all workforce training programs funded in whole or in part by DOL, as established by the Jobs for Veterans Act of 2002 (38 U.S.C. § 4215).

VETS administers the Jobs for Veterans State Grant (JVSG) program, which provides funding for dedicated staff who work in the American Job Centers to provide individualized career and training-related services to eligible veterans and eligible persons with significant barriers to employment, and other eligible populations[52], and to assist employers to fill their workforce needs with job-seeking veterans. This includes veterans who self-identify as having a physical and/or mental health disability, as well as veterans experiencing homelessness, or economically disadvantaged. JVSG supports Disabled Veterans' Outreach Program (DVOP) specialists, Local Veterans' Employment Representatives (LVER), and dual-role Consolidated DVOP/LVER staff, located in 50 states, the District of Columbia, Guam, Puerto Rico, and the U.S. Virgin Islands. DVOP specialists provide individualized career services and facilitate employment placements to meet the employment needs of veterans and eligible populations, ensuring that they receive the customized services that they need. Individualized career services may include comprehensive and specialized job readiness assessments, resume development, interview preparation, development of individual employment plans, career guidance, employment assistance, referrals to other programs, and other related services. LVER staff conduct outreach and advocacy efforts with local businesses to increase employment opportunities for veterans. LVER staff facilitate and support veterans in gaining and retaining employment and maintain cooperative working relationships with community organizations that provide complementary services and reciprocal referrals. Consolidated positions perform both DVOP and LVER staff functions. These services are critical to veterans, especially those struggling with unemployment, which can negatively impact mental health and create difficult experiences.

Homeless Veterans' Reintegration Program (HVRP)

Veterans experiencing homelessness and those at risk of experiencing homelessness face specific challenges, including higher prevalence rates of PTSD, a condition that can emerge from experiencing traumatic events, as well as physical disabilities and challenges in transitioning to civilian life.[53] VETS administers the HVRP program, which is designed to address these barriers and empower veterans to secure good jobs in stable and high-demand occupations paying livable wages. HVRP is the only federal grant to focus exclusively on competitive employment for veterans experiencing or at risk of homelessness. HVRP programs partner closely with their local American Job Centers, helping veterans experiencing homelessness and those at risk of experiencing homelessness reintegrate into the workforce by providing employment and wrap- around services, including mental health care, suicide prevention services, and addiction counseling. In FY 2023, HVRP awarded more than $58 million to 159 grantees and served over 17,300 veterans. Over half (55%) of participants were employed upon completion, with an average hourly wage of $18.34 at placement.

HVRP grantees work one-on-one with veterans and their families to help them obtain sustainable employment and stable housing, which in turn improves their mental, physical, and emotional well-being. One such story comes to us from a 55-year-old Navy veteran in Maryland

[52] As defined in 38 U.S.C. § 4101. In addition, beginning with the Consolidated Appropriations Act of 2014, annual appropriations for JVSG have made three additional groups eligible for JVSG services: Transition members of the Armed Forces who have been identified as in need of intensive service; members of the Armed Forces who are wounded ill, or injured and receiving treatment in military treatment facilities or warrior transition units; and the spouses or other family caregivers of such a wounded, ill, or injured member.

[53] https://www.dol.gov/agencies/oasp/evaluation/completedstudies/Homeless-Veterans-Reintegration-Program-Impact-Evaluation.

who found herself homeless after losing her job with a sub-contractor shortly after transitioning out of the military. Her recent job loss, lack of savings and support network, and inability to pay her rent caused her to experience severe bouts of anxiety and depression. After enrolling in the HVRP program, her case manager helped her enroll into mental health counseling and helped her address her immediate mental health needs, while providing her with the emotional support necessary to continue her job search with renewed energy. After participating in numerous interviews and refining her resume and job scope with the HVRP case manager, she was offered a position as a Program Analyst with an IT firm. This opportunity marked a significant turning point in her mental health journey, as the new job provided her with the stability and security she had been seeking. Her story is a testament to the power of the comprehensive support systems our agency offers to veterans facing a myriad of difficult challenges.

National Veterans' Training Institute (NVTI)

VETS established NVTI[54] in 1986 to provide specialized training and professional skills enhancement of American Job Center and other veteran service providers' staff. NVTI provides high-quality and relevant training, ensuring that veterans receive the best possible assistance in their transition to civilian careers. NVTI trains nearly 4,000 participants annually, including JVSG-funded state staff and other federal agency staff. NVTI fosters a community of practice among veteran service providers, enabling them to share best practices, resources, and innovations. This includes supporting the development and hosting of interagency resources and reports on mental health, suicide prevention, and burnout prevention.[55]

For example, NVTI offers the course, *Preventing and Healing Burnout in Veteran Service Provider,*[56] a one-day virtual course for veteran service organizations and providers to define and provide strategies for addressing burnout in veteran service providers. Course participants engage in several self-reflective activities and discussions to enable them to identify signs of burnout, understand their stress level, and understand where they are on the burnout spectrum. Participants also discuss resources and strategies for preventing and overcoming burnout.

Interagency Collaboration

President Obama's Executive Order 13625, "Improving Access to Mental Health Services for Veterans, Service Members, and Military Families," established the Interagency Task Force (ITF) on Military and Veterans Mental Health. The ITF has a primary goal of coordinating and supporting interagency programs and activities related to mental health, suicide prevention, substance use, and expanding access to mental health care. DOL is an active participant, and I serve as co-chair of the ITF's Evidence-Based Treatment Access and Engagement workgroup, which is tasked with evaluating access and engagement barriers to evidence-based mental

---

[54] https://www.nvti.org/.

[55] https://www.nvti.org/Resources/Useful-Resources/Suicide-Prevention-Mental-Health-and-Burnout/.

[56] https://www.nvti.org/training/class-descriptions/#:~:text=9612%3A%20Preventing%20and%20Healing%20Burnout% 20 in%20Veteran%20Service%20Providers.

health care for Service members, veterans, and their families. As a result of this work, NVTI has expanded its resources related to suicide and burnout prevention.

The National Defense Authorization Act (NDAA) for FY 2024 (P.L. 118-31, §1805) codified DOL as a member with DoD and VA on the TAP Joint Executive Committee. This enhanced DOL's preexisting collaboration with DoD and VA, with VETS co-chairing the Transition Executive Committee, Senior Transition Steering Group, Transition Working Group, and six functional working groups. Interagency members and the military Services meet and coordinate on a regular basis to ensure that the partners are supporting and advancing TAP, as well as to reduce redundancy, better serve unique populations, and improve coordination of services across program areas.

Conclusion

The mental health of our veterans, Service members, and military spouses is a critical concern, especially during their transition to civilian life and a post-military career.

Understandably, financial struggles, employment barriers, and the stress of reintegration can take a toll on a person's mental health and make finding meaningful employment that much more difficult. As the lead agency on veteran employment, VETS recognizes the importance of addressing these challenges and works to address them in close coordination with our interagency partners. We look forward to working with this Subcommittee and our many partners and stakeholders to create opportunities to ensure that all veterans, Service members, and their spouses can have a good job and opportunity for advancement. Chairman Van Orden, Ranking Member Levin, and distinguished Members of the Subcommittee, this concludes my statement. Thank you for the opportunity to be a part of this hearing, and I welcome your questions.

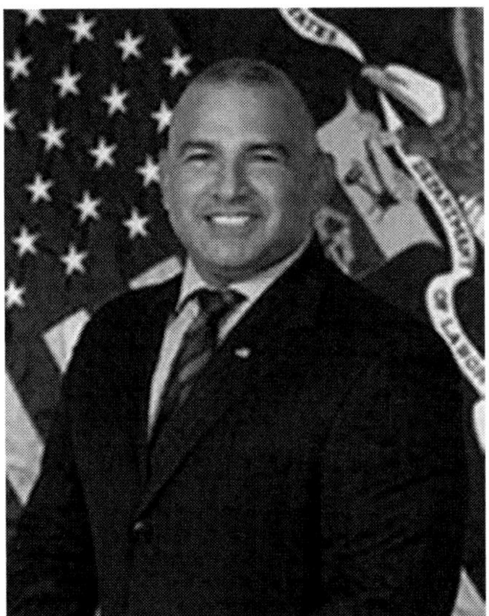

Assistant Secretary - James D. Rodriguez

The Honorable James D. Rodriguez, MA is the U.S. Department of Labor's Assistant Secretary for Veterans' Employment and Training Service (VETS). He is responsible for preparing America's veterans, service members and their spouses for meaningful careers. In this capacity and in Fiscal Year 2022, over 2,800 DOL Veterans' Employment and Training Service staff, contractors, and grantees served more than 440,000 veterans and military spouses across all Agency programs.

Mr. Rodriguez is an executive leader and proud veteran with more than 30 years of experience in the U.S. government, corporate sector, and 21 years in the United States Marine Corps. He possesses a comprehensive background in program management, interagency collaboration, and policy development. He also has extensive senior-level experience building and managing multi-million-dollar budgets and large diverse teams while meeting the expectations of the President of the United States and large corporate enterprises. Additionally, he has demonstrated experience with developing and leading large scale international and national programs with a commitment to operational excellence, risk management and quality assurance.

Mr. Rodriguez's recent executive experience includes leadership roles within Deloitte LLP's Government and Public Sector practice and BAE Systems, Inc. Government Relations department. He also previously served as the Deputy Assistant Secretary of Defense, Office of Warrior Care Policy, Office of the Secretary of Defense from 2014 through 2017.

Mr. Rodriguez earned a Bachelor of Arts in Political Science from the University of Maryland, University College and a Master of Arts in International Commerce and Policy from the George Mason University, School of Public Policy. He also serves as an adjunct faculty member in the Department of Government and Political Science in the University of Maryland, Global Campus.

September 10, 2024

The Honorable Derrick Van Orden
Chairman
Subcommittee on Economic Opportunity
Committee on Veterans' Affairs
House of Representatives
364 Cannon House Office Building
Washington, DC 20515

The Honorable Mike Levin
Ranking Member
Subcommittee on Economic Opportunity
Committee on Veterans' Affairs
House of Representatives
550 Cannon House Office Building
Washington, DC 20515

Dear Chairman Van Orden and Ranking Member Levin:

In light of the Subcommittee's September 10, 2024, hearing, Mission Transition: Evaluating Mental Health Support Programs for Separating Servicemembers, please find attached the Western Governors' Association Policy Resolution 2023-08, Veterans. The resolution emphasizes the importance of veterans' mental health care and urges the Department of Veterans Affairs (VA) to integrate peer support for traumatic brain injury and enhance staffing and training for neurological disorders. It also urges that Congress provide oversight over VA and the Department of Defense to ensure that transitioning service members receive detailed information on VA benefits and services available to them at least 12 months before they leave the military.

I request that you include this document in the permanent record of the hearing, as it articulates Western Governors' collective and bipartisan policy positions and recommendations on this important issue.

Thank you for your consideration of this request. Please contact me if you have any questions or require further information.

Sincerely,

Jack Waldorf Executive
Director

Attachment

WESTERN GOVERNORS' ASSOCIATION

Policy Resolution 2023-08 Veterans

A. Background

American military personnel often return home to a hero's welcome after completing their service, but they face a series of complex challenges. Veterans, whether they volunteered or were drafted, commonly confront a range of issues such as food insecurity, homelessness, unemployment, physical and psychological wounds, and bureaucratic barriers when seeking support services. Western Governors recognize the need to support veterans and address the challenges they face. With one-third of the known veteran population residing in western states, Governors recommend federal regulatory and statutory changes to foster an environment that facilitates access to support services for veterans and encourages further investment in initiatives tailored to assist them.

B. Governors' Policy Statement

1. Western Governors urge the Department of Veterans Affairs (VA) to prioritize the integration of peer support services and behavioral health services for Traumatic Brain Injury (TBI) into mental health care models. Additionally, Western Governors urge the VA to address staffing models to support the increasing health concerns for memory care (Dementia, Alzheimer's) and other neurological disorders. VA should also provide continuous training and support for peer specialists and focus on developing and retaining the behavioral health care workforce. Western Governors have highlighted substantive health care workforce recommendations in our health care policy resolution. Ongoing evaluations should be conducted to ensure effective implementation of these practices, which should be disseminated across all VA health care settings to ensure broad access to peer support services for all veterans.
2. Western Governors acknowledge the importance of the VA Governor's Challenge and urge VA to continue its provision of support for programs aimed at effectively addressing the issue of veterans' suicide.
3. Recognizing the need to improve health program services for women veterans, Western Governors urge VA to take urgent action to address gaps in the VA health care system. Improving the promotion of, access to, and the quality of health care for women veterans is essential and requires timely and effective measures to be implemented across VA. Western Governors recommend that VA initiate research programs to study health issues specific to women veterans.
4. Western Governors recognize the significance of expanding access to health care services for veterans, especially those residing in remote areas. VA should take action to increase the accessibility of:
   a) VA Community Care for veterans residing in areas that do not have access to VA health care facilities. It is imperative that VA consult with Governors to ensure that veterans living in rural areas are not disadvantaged in accessing health care;
   b) Vet Centers for veterans living in rural areas, to ensure that they have access to necessary health services and support;
   c) Health care professionals in rural areas, to provide flexibility for veterans and allow them to access the health care provider of their choosing; and
   d) Telemedicine services, which are a vital tool that can help bridge the gap in accessing health care services.
5. Western Governors recommend that VA seek consultation and input from tribal leaders and communities to inform the development and administration of its programs and services for American Indian, Alaska Native, and Native Hawaiian veterans.
6. To ensure that veterans have timely access to high-quality health care, Western Governors recommend that Congress prioritize providing VA with the necessary resources, authority, and ability to recruit, hire, train, and retain health care

professionals. This includes physicians, nurses, mental and behavioral health providers, long-term care professionals, and administrative staff. In addition, Western Governors believe VA should streamline the hiring process, offer competitive salaries and benefits, and provide ongoing training and professional development opportunities for health care professionals.

7. Western Governors believe VA should collaborate with states and territories to improve and expand the Highly Rural Transportation Grants program. This includes identifying counties that require assistance, simplifying the application and implementation process, and consulting early with Governors for valuable input on their state's needs. Additionally, VA should reevaluate and expand the current eligibility criteria to ensure that more veterans can benefit from the program.
8. Western Governors urge VA to conduct a comprehensive evaluation of the Veteran Transportation Services (VTS) exam and implement necessary revisions to reduce its complexity, facilitating the process for individuals to obtain a license to transport veterans to VA health care facilities and authorized non-VA health care appointments.
9. Western Governors call on VA to improve community care for veterans by enforcing timely referrals and appointments, particularly for programs like VA Community Care. VA should also streamline reimbursement processes to third-party health care providers in line with industry standards and ensure prompt access to services and increased provider participation.
10. To ensure that our nation's veterans receive the benefits and services they are entitled to in a timely and efficient manner, Western Governors urge VA to continue to improve and streamline the claims process, especially with the new Sergeant First Class (SFC) Heath Robinson Honoring our Promise to Address Comprehensive Toxics (PACT) Act (Pub. L. 117- 168) claims.
11. Western Governors recommend that VA implement a policy allowing veterans to select their own care providers, including those who are not affiliated with VA health care facilities. By doing so, veterans would have greater flexibility and choice when seeking health care services.
12. Western Governors recognize the necessity of conducting a comprehensive review of VA regulations regarding payments for State Veterans Homes and urge VA to consult with states to identify the unique needs of each state. Additionally, Western Governors recommend expanding coverage to include all specialty care services, and prioritize funding for specialized cognitive care.
13. Western Governors recommend that VA authorize and prioritize the expansion of VA programs to provide comprehensive financial support for third-party assisted living and nursing facilities, which offer varying levels of care for long-term care services to our nation's veterans.
14. Western Governors urge Congress to pass legislation that requires VA and the Department of Defense (DOD) to modernize their electronic health record-keeping systems and mandate VA to upgrade its overall technology infrastructure. These upgrades are necessary to streamline access to critical health information, enhance coordination between the two departments, and improve the claims process for veterans, which is a priority for the Governors.
15. Western Governors recommend that the federal government provide funding for state and congressionally chartered Veterans Service Organizations (VSOs) to offset the

costs of training and to enhance the workforce capacity of VSOs. This would help to improve the level of support and care provided to veterans and their families by such VSOs, ensuring that they have access to the resources and services they need to thrive.

16. Western Governors emphasize the need for VA to provide Veteran Services Officers with access to vital information, enabling them to better assist veterans in navigating VA's programs and services. This will ensure that veterans receive the support and resources necessary to thrive.
17. Western Governors recommend that VA expand its dental services to all veterans enrolled in the VA health care system, regardless of their service-connected dental issues or other narrow criteria.
18. Western Governors urge Congress to authorize and appropriate funds for VA to provide grants to state, territorial, and tribal governments. The purpose of these grants is to increase outreach and assistance to veterans and their families by raising awareness of benefits and aiding them in applying for VA benefits. Priority should be given to areas with high rates of veteran suicide and a shortage of Veteran Services Officers.
19. Western Governors support the idea that service members should be given the opportunity to receive credit or professional credentials for the training they undergo in the military, which can then be transferred to the private sector or educational institutions. This initiative will help veterans transition into civilian careers by providing them with the necessary credentials and recognition for the skills developed through their military service.
20. Western Governors urge Congress to provide diligent oversight over VA and DOD to ensure that transitioning service members receive comprehensive information on VA benefits at least twelve months prior to their transition to civilian life. This includes ensuring that service members are aware of the full range of programs and support services available to them.
21. Western Governors recommend that VA conduct a comprehensive study on their efforts to reduce homelessness and identify those programs that have provided the highest return on investment.

C. Governors' Management Directive

1. The Governors direct WGA staff to work with congressional committees of jurisdiction, the Executive Branch, and other entities, where appropriate, to achieve the objectives of this resolution.
2. Furthermore, the Governors direct WGA staff to consult with the Staff Advisory Council regarding its efforts to realize the objectives of this resolution and to keep the Governors apprised of its progress in this regard.

This resolution will expire in June 2026. Western Governors enact new policy resolutions and amend existing resolutions on a semiannual basis. Please consult http://www.westgov.org/resolutions for the most current copy of a resolution and a list of all current WGA policy resolutions.

Chapter 5

DOD and VA Health Care: Actions Needed to Better Facilitate Access to Mental Health Services During Military to Civilian Transitions*

United States Government Accountability Office

Abbreviations

DOD	Department of Defense
TAP	Transition Assistance Program
VA	Department of Veterans Affairs

Why GAO Did This Study

Thousands of service members transitioned from military service to civilian life in 2022. During this transition period, research has shown that service members are especially vulnerable. Some may face challenges, such as the loss of a sense of purpose, post-traumatic stress disorder, or other mental health symptoms.

GAO was asked to review access to mental health services for transitioning members. Among other objectives, this report examines inTransition's enrollment process and efforts to assess performance. It also examines the extent to which the DOD-VA Joint Executive Committee has assessed the effectiveness of efforts to facilitate access to mental health services.

GAO analyzed inTransition program data for calendar year 2022, the most recent available. GAO also reviewed DOD and VA information on efforts that may facilitate access to mental health services and interviewed DOD and VA officials.

* This is an edited, reformatted and augmented version of the United States Government Accountability Office Report to Congressional Requesters, Publication No. GAO-24-106189, dated July 2024.

In: Supporting Our Veterans
Editor: Gina P. Sharpe
ISBN: 979-8-89530-504-1

What GAO Recommends

GAO is making five total recommendations, including that DOD revise inTransition's enrollment criteria and outreach policy and establish performance goals, and that the DOD-VA Joint Executive Committee assess the departments' efforts to facilitate access to mental health services.VA concurred with the DOD-VA Joint Executive Committee recommendation; DOD did not provide formal comments.

What GAO Found

The Department of Defense's (DOD) inTransition program assists service members who may need support with mental health services during transitions. It automatically enrolls members transitioning from the military who received mental health or traumatic brain injury care in the year prior to separation. In 2022, inTransition identified 85 percent of its enrollees through its automatic enrollment process. (See figure.) However, GAO found that inTransition does not conduct outreach to these enrollees until 2 to 3 months after their separation.

This delayed timing may leave a gap in assistance to mental health services during a vulnerable period.

inTransition Enrollees, Calendar Year 2022

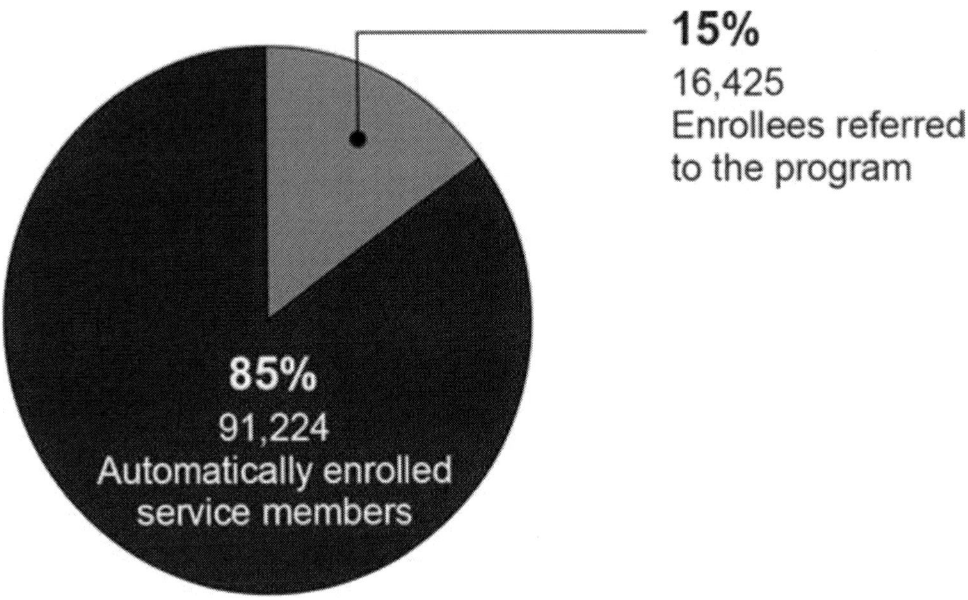

Source: GAO analysis of DOD data. | GAO-24-106189.

GAO found that the inTransition program was unable to successfully connect with over 70 percent of its automatically enrolled service members in 2022. This was due, in part, to its outreach strategy, which relies on telephone calls.

Expanding its outreach methods—such as through email, text, or the use of location services—could improve the program's ability to successfully connect with its enrollees and potentially increase participation in the program. GAO also found that the inTransition program tracks some performance data but has not defined the level of performance it aims to achieve. By establishing performance goals with measurable targets, the program could better assess its performance and use the information to make changes, as appropriate, such as to its outreach strategy.

The DOD and Department of Veterans Affairs (VA) Joint Executive Committee oversees military transition activities. GAO found that it identified an inventory of departmental efforts that may facilitate access to mental health services for transitioning members in 2022. However, it has not assessed the effectiveness of these efforts overall in facilitating access to mental health services during the transition period. As a result, the Committee does not know the extent to which there may be gaps, overlap, or other issues across these efforts. By conducting such an assessment and recommending appropriate changes, the Committee could help to better ensure that transitioning service members and veterans have access to the mental health services they may need.

July 15, 2024

The Honorable Glenn Grothman
Chairman

The Honorable Robert Garcia
Ranking Member
Subcommittee on National Security, the Border, and Foreign Affairs
Committee on Oversight and Accountability
House of Representatives

The Honorable Stephen F. Lynch
House of Representatives

Nearly 175,000 service members separated from military service and transitioned to civilian life in calendar year 2022, according to Department of Defense (DOD) data. During this transition period, research has shown that service members are especially vulnerable; for example, the suicide rate was about 2.5 times higher for veterans in the first year of separation than for the active duty population.[1] This increased risk can be attributed to the many challenges that service members face during this time, such as loss of a sense of purpose, familial and financial strain, and difficulty readjusting to social and civilian life. DOD has also seen a growing demand for mental health services among all military service members.[2]

DOD has requirements that service members are supposed to follow when they separate from active duty to help ensure a successful transition to civilian life. Service members must participate in the Transition Assistance Program (TAP), which offers counseling, employment assistance, and information on federal veterans' benefits, among other types of support. DOD also requires service members to complete its Separation History and Physical Exam to

---

[1] Chandru Ravindran, et al., "Association of Suicide Risk with Transition to Civilian Life among US Military Service Members," JAMA Network Open, vol. 3, no. 9 (2020).

[2] For more information, see GAO, Defense Health Care: DOD Should Monitor Urgent Referrals to Civilian Behavioral Health Providers to Ensure Timely Care, GAO-24-106267 (Washington, D.C.: Feb. 6, 2024).

document their medical histories—including any issues related to mental health. Once service members separate, they have the choice of seeking health care through the Department of Veterans Affairs (VA) or through DOD'sTRICARE program, if eligible.[3] Service members may also obtain coverage for care through employer-sponsored plans or through the health insurance exchanges.

DOD has a voluntary program, called inTransition, that helps facilitate connections to mental health services for service members and veterans during their transitions. For example, the program may help them find or obtain mental health resources, such as a community support group. The inTransition program can provide this assistance at various points, including when service members separate from the military.[4] Starting in 2015, the program implemented a process to identify and automatically enroll eligible service members who are transitioning from the military.[5] The program is to conduct outreach to these enrollees to determine whether they want to remain enrolled in the program and use its services, or whether they want to opt out.

The DOD-VA Joint Executive Committee, an interagency committee established in 2003, oversees the departments' coordination for health care and benefits, including programs and efforts that may assist service members and veterans during what is known as the transition continuum. The Committee defines the transition continuum period as 1-year pre- separation through 1-year post-separation from military service.

The departments' efforts to ensure that transitioning service members have continuous access to mental health care and suicide prevention services have received increased attention in recent years. For example, a 2018 Executive Order directed VA and DOD to develop a joint action plan to ensure access to mental health care and suicide prevention services for transitioning service members with an emphasis on the year following their separation.[6] However, in 2021 we and the DOD Office of the Inspector General identified concerns with DOD's and VA's efforts related to mental health and suicide prevention for this population.[7] For instance, a 2021 DOD Inspector General report found that DOD did not adequately screen for suicide risk or provide uninterrupted mental health care to transitioning service members.[8]

You asked us to review DOD's and VA's efforts to ensure continuous access to mental health services for transitioning service members. In this report, we

1. examine inTransition's processes for identifying and enrolling eligible transitioning service members and efforts to assess program performance;

---

[3] Veterans' eligibility for VA health care is based primarily on veteran status resulting from military service and meeting minimum service requirements. Military retirees may also be eligible for specific TRICARE plans depending upon a number of factors, including their age and geographic location.

[4] The inTransition program is designed to help individuals at different transition points in their military career, including a geographic relocation for a new assignment or a return from deployment.

[5] The program automatically enrolls service members who received mental health or moderate-to-severe traumatic brain injury care in the year prior to their separation.

[6] Exec. Order No. 13822, 83 Fed. Reg. 1,513 (Jan. 12, 2018). The Executive Order also identifies the Department of Homeland Security as a partner in the joint action plan.

7 GAO, DOD and VA Health Care: Suicide Prevention Efforts and Recommendations for Improvement, GAO-22-105522 (Washington, D.C.: Nov. 17, 2021). See also, Department of Defense Office of the Inspector General, Evaluation of the Department of Defense's Implementation of Suicide Prevention Resources for Transitioning Uniformed Service Members, Report No.

[8] As of January 2024, each of the report's five recommendations remained open, according to DOD Office of the Inspector General officials.

2. describe how DOD identifies transitioning service members with mental health needs prior to their separation;
3. describe how DOD and VA facilitate access to mental health services for service members across the transition continuum; and
4. examine the extent to which the DOD-VA Joint Executive Committee has assessed the effectiveness of the departments' efforts to facilitate access to mental health services across the transition continuum.

To examine inTransition's processes for identifying and enrolling eligible transitioning service members and efforts to assess program performance, we assessed relevant program documentation, including its policy, fact sheets, and marketing material. We also reviewed information related to the department's inTransition contract, including the performance work statement and reports submitted by the contractor.

In addition, we analyzed inTransition enrollment data for calendar year 2022, the most current full-year data available at the time of our review. We also analyzed 2022 data on the program's outreach phone calls to eligible service members it identified who were leaving the military. Our analysis included an evaluation of the program's unresponsive call rates and types of contacts made. We also evaluated the program's acceptance rates, that is, the number of eligible service members withwhom inTransition spoke (a successful contact) and who agreed to remain enrolled in the program. To determine the reliability of these data, we spoke with knowledgeable officials, reviewed related documentation, and tested for missing data and inconsistencies. We found the data sufficiently reliable for the purposes of our review.

In addition, we interviewed DOD officials responsible for managing the inTransition program and contract as well as officials representing the contractor, who implement the program, to determine how the program identifies and assists enrollees, how it is managed, and how they track and use any data they collect to assess program performance. We evaluated the inTransition program's processes and efforts against DOD policy, internal control standards for the federal government, and performance management leading practices identified in our prior work.[9]

To describe how DOD identifies transitioning service members with mental health needs prior to their separation, we reviewed DOD policies and information on separation protocols, processes, and programs. This included an examination of how the military services' Wounded Warrior programs and the DOD-VA Integrated Disability Evaluation System could potentially identify service members' mental health needs prior to separation. Additionally, we reviewed DOD's separation requirements— TAP and the Separation History and Physical Exam—to determine whether and how they might identify service members' mental health needs.

We also obtained and reviewed information on planned changes to these requirements, such as a new screening initiative for TAP and the implementation of a joint DOD-VA Separation Health Assessment. Lastly, we interviewed agency officials from these programs and initiatives to determine whether and how they may identify service members' mental health issues prior to their separation from military service.

---

[9] GAO, *Evidence-Based Policymaking: Practices to Help Manage and Assess the Results of Federal Efforts*, GAO-23-105460 (Washington, D.C.: July 12, 2023). Internal control is a process effected by an entity's oversight body, management, and other personnel that provides reasonable assurance that the objectives of an entity will be achieved. GAO, *Standards for Internal Control in the Federal Government*, GAO-14-704G (Washington, D.C.: Sept. 10, 2014).

To describe how other DOD and VA programs facilitate access to mental health services for service members across the transition continuum, we reviewed DOD policies on the continuity of mental health care during the transition. This included DOD Instruction 6490.10, "Continuity of Behavioral Health Care for Transferring and Transitioning Service Members."[10] Additionally, we reviewed information and available data on DOD and VA programs, processes, and services that may facilitate access to mental health services for transitioning service members. We included those that have a prominent role during the transition continuum, although there may be others that could provide assistance to this population. For DOD, we reviewed the inTransition program, the TAP warm handover process, the military services' Wounded Warrior programs, the Integrated Disability Evaluation System, the Defense Health Agency Recovery Coordination Program, and Military OneSource.[11] For VA, we reviewed the Solid Start program, Concierge for Care, the VA Liaison Program, the Post-9/11 Military2VA Case Management Program, and their Federal Recovery Consultants. Lastly, we received information from and interviewed agency officials that manage these programs, processes, and services to determine whether and how they facilitate continuous access to mental health services.

To examine the extent to which the DOD-VA Joint Executive Committee has assessed the effectiveness of the departments' efforts to facilitate access to mental health services across the transition continuum, we reviewed documentation for the Committee's activities related to mental health services for transitioning service members. This documentation included the Committee's current strategic plan, presentations, and its fiscal year 2024 joint operating plan, among other materials.[12] We also interviewed officials from the Joint Executive Committee and one of its subcommittees—the Transition Executive Committee—to better understand their roles and responsibilities related to monitoring service members' access to mental health services across the transition continuum.[13] We assessed DOD's and VA's efforts using the Joint Executive Committee's enabling statute, the Committee's strategic plan for fiscal years 2022 through 2027, as well as internal control standards for the federal government.[14]

We conducted this performance audit from August 2022 to July 2024 in accordance with generally accepted government auditing standards.

Those standards require that we plan and perform the audit to obtain sufficient, appropriate evidence to provide a reasonable basis for our findings and conclusions based on our audit objectives. We believe that the evidence obtained provides a reasonable basis for our findings and conclusions based on our audit objectives.

---

[10] Department of Defense Instruction 6490.10, Continuity of Behavioral Health Care for Transferring and Transitioning Service Members (Oct. 28, 2015).

[11] For more information see GAO, Service Members Transitioning to Civilian Life: Agencies Can Improve Warm Handovers for Additional Assistance, GAO-24-106248 (Washington, D.C.: Mar. 21, 2024).

[12] The DOD-VA Joint Executive Committee is an interagency committee established by law to oversee the two departments' coordination with health care and benefits and to provide annual reports to Congress on its efforts. National Defense Authorization Act for Fiscal Year 2004, Pub. L. No. 108-136, div A, tit. V, § 583(a)(1), 117 Stat. 1392, 1490 (2003) (codified, as amended, at 38 U.S.C. § 320).

[13] The National Defense Authorization Act for Fiscal Year 2024 added the Transition Executive Committee as a statutory committee of the Joint Executive Committee. According to DOD officials, prior to this legislation the Transition Executive Committee operated as a directed committee of the Joint Executive Committee's co-chairs. Pub. L No. 118-31, div. A, tit. XVIII, § 1805, 137 Stat. 136, 687 (2023).

[14] GAO-14-704G.

Background

Military to Civilian Transition Challenges

The transition from military to civilian life can be challenging for some veterans. Upon entering civilian life, veterans may have difficulty translating their military skills to a civilian job, and they may struggle to find employment, housing, and the other benefits that were provided as part of their military service. Additionally, veterans may struggle to reconnect with their family or relate to people who have not served in the military.

VA's research has identified many transition-related challenges—such as homelessness, family reintegration, employment, post-traumatic stress disorder, and substance misuse—that can increase the risk for suicide during the first year after separation. Recent academic research also found that certain demographic characteristics, such as length of time in service and level of education, can exacerbate these challenges.[15]

DOD's Transition Requirements

When service members prepare to separate from the military, they are required to participate in DOD's TAP, which provides assistance, training, counseling, and services to facilitate their transition to civilian life. The program provides individualized counseling sessions, tailored classes, and a final review of compliance with program requirements, also known as a capstone. TAP is separately administered by each military service branch. According to DOD's policy, service members are expected to begin TAP at least 1 year before they anticipate leaving military service, but not later than 90 days before separation.[16]

Additionally, in accordance with DOD Instruction 6040.46, all transitioning service members must undergo a Separation History and Physical Exam prior to separation.[17] The exam includes a health assessment questionnaire that is completed by the service member as well as a physical exam with a medical provider. The exam is supposed to be completed within 12 months of separation and no later than 30 days prior to separation.

DOD's inTransition Program

Established in 2010, DOD's inTransition program is intended to help facilitate connections to mental health services for individuals at various transition points, including transitioning

[15] For example, see Chandru Ravindran, et al., "Association of Suicide Risk with Transition to Civilian Life."

[16] Service members with anticipated retirement dates are expected to begin TAP as soon as possible during the 24 months preceding their retirement date, but not later than 90 days before retirement. Also, service members with short-notice separations—those who will leave the military in 90 days or fewer—are expected to begin TAP as soon as possible. However, we have previously found that 70 percent of service members did not start TAP more than 1 year in advance, as generally required. For more information, see GAO, *Servicemembers Transitioning to Civilian Life: DOD Can Better Leverage Performance Information to Improve Participation in Counseling Pathways*, GAO-23-104538 (Washington, D.C.: Dec. 12, 2022).

[17] Department of Defense Instruction 6040.46, *The Separation and Physical Examination for the DOD Separation Health Assessment Program* (April 14, 2016).

between duty stations or out of the military, to ensure continuity of needed care.[18] It is available to active- duty service members, U.S. Coast Guard personnel, National Guard members, reservists, veterans, and retirees regardless of time in service, time from service, or characterization of discharge. It is a voluntary and confidential program with coaches—licensed psychological health clinicians—who provide support services by telephone to the program's enrollees.[19] The coaches may refer service members to mental health providers, as well as provide information on community resources and support groups, among other services. Coaches do not provide telephonic mental health care or other health care services.

DOD created the inTransition program in response to a 2007 report by the DOD Task Force on Mental Health.[20] This report found that a concerning number of service members were disengaging from mental health care treatment as they transitioned between DOD's and VA's health systems, which contributed to their worsening mental health.

DOD's goal in establishing inTransition was to help service members maintain continuity of mental health care across transitions.

Individuals may enroll in the program one of two ways—through a referral or through the program's automatic enrollment process for transitioning service members.

- Referral. Providers may refer their active-duty patients to the inTransition program for enrollment. Providers may also refer service members for enrollment based on their responses to the mental health questions contained in the Separation Health and Physical Exam. Additionally, service members and other eligible individuals have the option to self-refer to the program for enrollment.
- Automatic enrollment. The program identifies eligible service members who are leaving the military for automatic enrollment using data on military separations and medical histories. Specifically, the program automatically enrolls service members who had received mental health or moderate-to-severe traumatic brain injury care in theyear prior to their separation.[21] The program conducts outreach to determine whether these individuals want to "accept" their enrollment and participate in the program or if they wish to opt out. Those who remain enrolled are assigned to a coach, who will contact them to provide support.

---

[18] Transitioning service members include those relocating to another assignment, returning from deployment, transitioning from active duty to reserve, transitioning from reserve to active duty, preparing to leave military service or recently separated from service.

[19] According to inTransition documentation, coaches are trained in motivational interviewing, understand military culture, and are knowledgeable in mental health, substance abuse, and community and military resources. Coaches are to employ interventions that are appropriate for the individual, including assistance with developing an action plan or setting goals; encouragement with the use of adapting strategies; responses to mental health questions related to diagnosis or life issues; self-management materials; decision support for treatment options; and encouragement to make healthy choices to support well-being.

[20] Department of Defense Task Force on Mental Health, *An Achievable Vision: Report of the Department of Defense Task Force on Mental Health* (June 2007).

[21] More specifically, the program automatically enrolls service members who have had a mental health or moderate-to-severe traumatic brain injury encounter in the 30 days before separation, at least two outpatient mental health or moderate-to-severe traumatic brain injury encounters in the year before separation, or at least one inpatient mental health or moderate-to-severe traumatic brain injury encounter in the year before separation.

The inTransition Program Office, within the Defense Health Agency, has a Program Manager who manages the program.[22] A contractor implements the program, and its responsibilities include hiring program coaches and managing services to enrollees, among other duties. As of February 2024, program officials stated that the contractor had a range of 25 to 27 coaches that can be adjusted as needed, based on demand.[23] Officials from the current inTransition contractor told us they started work in October 2021. The contract has an initial base year plus 4 option years, with a total value of approximately $29 million over the 5-year period, according to Defense Health Agency officials. The U.S. Army Medical Research Acquisition Activity awards and manages the inTransition contract.[24]

Enrollment in VA Health Care

Veterans must meet basic eligibility requirements to enroll in VA health care. Eligibility for VA health care is based primarily on veteran status resulting from military service (meeting minimum service requirements), which must be authenticated through the provision of discharge paperwork, specifically the DOD Form 214.[25] This form represents the complete, verified record of service members' time in the military and is generally required for enrollment in VA benefits, including health care.

Veterans enroll in VA health care by completing and submitting VA's application for health benefits. The application requests information about the veteran's military service, demographics, and (as applicable) financial status.[26]

Executive Order for Transition Support and Joint Action Plan

In January 2018, the President signed Executive Order 13822 entitled "Supporting Our Veterans During Their Transition from Uniformed Service to Civilian Life."[27] This order required DOD, VA, and the Department of Homeland Security to ensure the provision of seamless access to mental health care and suicide prevention resources for veterans, with an emphasis on the 1-year period following their separation from the military.[28] It also required

---

[22] The inTransition Program Office was previously aligned within the Defense Health Agency's Psychological Health Center of Excellence but was organizationally realigned to the Defense Health Agency's Medical Affairs under the Behavior Health Clinical Management Team in 2023.

[23] According to inTransition and its contracting officials, each coach has an average caseload of about 200 enrollees.

[24] The U.S. Army Medical Research Acquisition Activity was an Army acquisition office that became part of the Defense Health Agency in fiscal year 2023, under its Head of the Contracting Activity.

[25] Exceptions are made for veterans discharged due to service-connected disabilities, members of the Reserve and National Guard (under certain circumstances), and those eligible under special treatment authorities, such as Camp Lejeune veterans.

[26] Veterans may also separately apply for disability benefits. If needed, VA may request a medical examination—known as a Compensation and Pension Exam—to substantiate disability claims documented in the application. Veterans with service-connected disabilities may receive monthly VA disability compensation payments based on the severity of their disability. A service-connected disability has three elements, according to VA guidance: 1) a current disability; 2) an in-service event, injury, or disease; and 3) an indication that the disability had its onset in service. Department of Veterans Affairs, *M21- 1 Adjudication Procedures Manual,* V.ii.2.A.1.a (Sept. 15, 2021).

[27] Exec. Order No. 13822, 83 Fed. Reg. 1,513 (Jan. 12, 2018).

[28] The Department of Homeland Security is responsible for overseeing the US Coast Guard.

the departments to develop a Joint Action Plan to describe their actions to provide these resources. The departments submitted their Joint Action Plan to Congress in May 2018. The plan outlined three broad goals with specific actions linked to each goal. See figure 1.

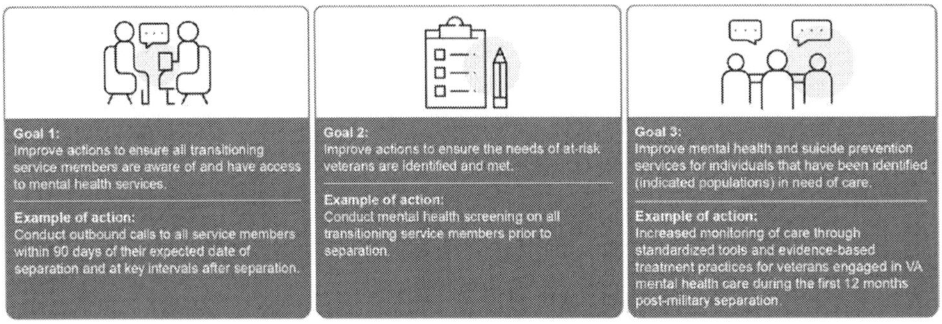

Source: GAO presentation of Department of Defense, Homeland Security, and Veterans Affairs information (information); yasnaten/stock.adobe.com (icon). | GAO-24-106189.

Figure 1. Goals from the 2018 Joint Action Plan for Supporting Veterans During Their Transition from Uniformed Service to Civilian Life and Examples of Related Actions.

In November 2021, the DOD Office of the Inspector General issued a report that assessed whether DOD had implemented the provisions required by Executive Order 13822.[29] The review also focused on the department's implementation of its related policy, DOD Instruction 6490.10, "Continuity of Behavioral Health Care for Transferring and Transitioning Service Members."

The Inspector General's report found that DOD did not adequately screen for suicide risk or provide uninterrupted mental health care to transitioning service members. The report further stated that DOD Instruction 6490.10 lacked a clear definition of a warm handoff, provider training protocols, standardized documentation, and oversight procedures to ensure compliance. The Inspector General recommended that DOD establish consistent policies and procedures to manage suicide risk screening and referrals for transitioning service members. It also recommended that DOD identify the causes for breaks in continuous mental health care and to implement solutions for those breaks. As of February 2024, DOD officials told us that they are in the process of updating DOD Instruction 6490.10. DOD Office of the Inspector General officials said that all of the report's recommendations remained open as of January 2024.

The DOD-VA Joint Executive Committee and Its Subcommittees

The DOD-VA Joint Executive Committee was established to oversee DOD and VA's coordination with providing health care and benefits and to provide annual reports to Congress on its efforts.[30] In this capacity, the Committee serves as the primary federal interagency body for overseeing military transition assistance activities. The Deputy Secretary of VA and the

[29] Department of Defense Office of the Inspector General, Evaluation of the Department of Defense's Implementation of Suicide Prevention Resources for Transitioning Uniformed Service Members, Report No. DODIG-2022-030 (Nov. 9, 2021).

[30] See 38 U.S.C. § 320(c).

DOD Under Secretary of Defense for Personnel and Readiness serve as co-chairs. The Joint Executive Committee has several subcommittees, including the Health Executive Committee and the Benefits Executive Committee. In 2020, the Transition Executive Council joined the Joint Executive Committee to focus on transition activities.

In September 2019, the Joint Executive Committee approved the "Military to Civilian Readiness" framework. This framework is a timeline that lays out the various independent processes and programs that may assist service members and veterans across the transition continuum. See figure 2.

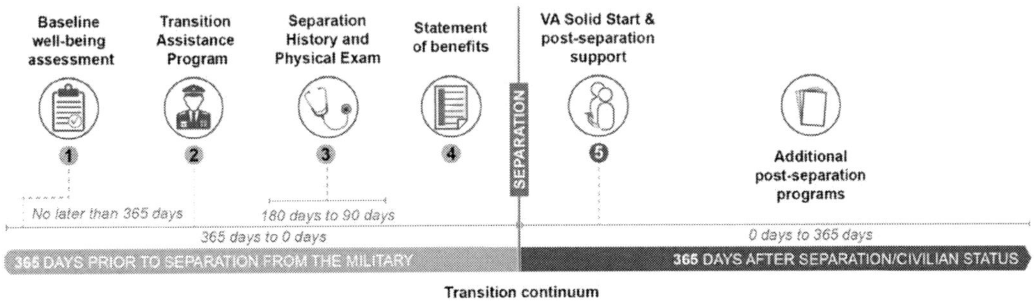

Source: GAO analysis of DOD-VA Joint Executive Committee information (information); GAO (icons); barks/stock.adobe.com (soldier icon). | GAO-24-106189.

Figure 2. Department of Defense (DOD)-Department of Veterans Affairs (VA) Joint Executive Committee's Military to Civilian Readiness Framework.

The Joint Executive Committee develops a strategic plan every 6 years. The most recent strategic plan covers fiscal years 2022 through 2027 and includes 5 goals: 1) health care collaboration; 2) integrate services and benefits; 3) enhance the transition and post-separation experience; 4) modernize shared business operations; and 5) strengthen interoperability and partnership.[31]

Each year the Joint Executive Committee develops an annual Joint Operating Plan that establishes actionable steps the departments will take to achieve these goals. In its Fiscal Year 2024 Joint Operating Plan, the Committee identified continuity of care for transitioning service members with special circumstances—including mental health needs—as a priority under its strategic goal to enhance the transition and post- separation experience. The Joint Executive Committee also provides an annual report to Congress detailing their progress against these goals.

[31] DOD-VA Joint Executive Committee, *Joint Strategic Plan Fiscal Years 2022-2027* (Washington, D.C.).

inTransition Enrolls Eligible Transitioning Service Members Several Months After They Separate and Lacks Goals to Assess Program Performance

InTransition Identifies and Automatically Enrolls Eligible Transitioning Service Members but Not Until 2 to 3 Months After They Separate

Based on our review of inTransition enrollment data and discussions with program officials, we found that the program's automatic enrollment process results in the identification of most of its enrollees 2 to 3 months after their separation from the military through its automatic enrollment process. Such timing coincides with the last 9 months of the 24-month transition continuum. This timing for enrollment may result in a gap in assistance for some service members, affecting the program's ability to ensure continuity of mental health services during times of transition.[32]

InTransition identified about 85 percent of its enrollees through its automatic enrollment process in 2022, according to our analysis of the program's enrollment data. The program identified the remaining 15 percent of its enrollees through referrals, which may include—but is not limited to—service members referred to the program prior to their separation.[33]

Automatic Enrollment Requirement for the inTransition Program

In August 2014, Presidential Executive Action "Improving Service Members' Transition from DoD to VA and Civilian Health Care Providers," directed inTransition to automatically enroll all transitioning service members receiving mental health treatment. Prior to this requirement, inTransition obtained its enrollees solely through referrals from mental health care providers as well as through self-referrals.

In October 2015, DOD updated its policy to require that all service members who had seen a mental health provider within the year prior to their date of separation be automatically enrolled in its inTransition program. These enrollees may decline enrollment at any time.

GAO review of DOD documentation and a 2014 White House Press Announcement. | GAO-24-106189.

Per InTransition's policy, the program automatically enrolls any service member who received care for mental health or moderate-to-severe traumatic brain injury within one year prior to their separation. The Defense Health Agency uses a separate contractor to generate inTransition's monthly lists of automatically enrolled service members by analyzing the department's separations data along with medical record data for these individuals. Agency officials said that accurate execution of the policy's automatic enrollment criteria requires them to conduct this process after service members have separated. According to officials, this timing allows the contractor to generate the monthly lists of automatically enrolled service members using their exact dates of separation as a reference point for the 12-month medical record review.

[32] Defense Health Agency-Procedural Instruction 6490.01, *inTransition Program* (July 12, 2019).

[33] According to inTransition officials, they do not track data on whether referred enrollees joined the program before or after their separation from the military.

Short-term Gap with the Army's Separations Data
Officials told us that the Army did not submit its separations data to the Defense Manpower Data Center from December 2022 to August 2023 due to its implementation of a new human resources IT system. According to officials, Army service members generally represent approximately one-third to one-half of all separating service members automatically enrolled in the program, resulting in a significant enrollment void during this time frame. Officials told us that in June 2023, the Army submitted a more than 7- month backlog of its separations data directly to inTransition (which included data from November 2022 through early June 2023). Then, in September 2023, the Army resumed submitting their separations data to the Defense Manpower Data Center, which included data from the rest of June and July 2023.
Source: GAO analysis of interviews with DOD and contractor officials. | GAO-24-106189.

According to the Defense Health Agency's contractor, there is a time lag with the separations data used to create the monthly lists of automatically enrolled service members. This is primarily due to when the military departments report their separations data. Based on the timing of this process, the contractor explained that a couple of months could pass before a service member's separation data is reported to DOD's Defense Manpower Data Center.[34] The Data Center subsequently provides this information to the Defense Health Agency contractor who conducts the analysis, according to officials. Consequently, the inTransition program generally identifies and automatically enrolls eligible service members about 2 to 3 months after they become veterans.

The delayed timing for automatically enrolling eligible members may leave a gap in assistance to obtain mental health services at a time that coincides with the vulnerable post-separation period. Modifying the program's criteria for identifying eligible service members for automatic enrollment prior to their separation could help address this gap and would help inTransition better ensure the continuity of any needed mental health services during the critical transition period. For example, under revised criteria, program officials could use other resources to identify transitioning service members prior to their separation, such as by tracking participation in mandatory transition processes like TAP or the Separation Health and Physical Exams.

inTransition Was Unable to Successfully Connect with Over 70 Percent of its Eligible Transitioning Service Members in 2022

We found that the inTransition program was unable to successfully connect with over 70 percent of the service members it identified through its automatic enrollment process (65,545 of 91,224), based on our analysis of inTransition data for calendar year 2022.[35] As a result,

[34] The Defense Manpower Data Center is DOD's central source for identifying, authenticating, authorizing, and providing information on personnel during and after their affiliation with DOD.

[35] This is generally consistent with the rate reported by the DOD's Office of the Inspector General in November 2021. Specifically, that report found an approximately 28 percent successful contact rate for the inTransition program's automatically enrolled service members from fiscal years 2017 through 2020. See Department of Defense Office

these service members may not have known that they were identified through inTransition's automatic enrollment process and may not have known the type of assistance it could provide. See figure 3.

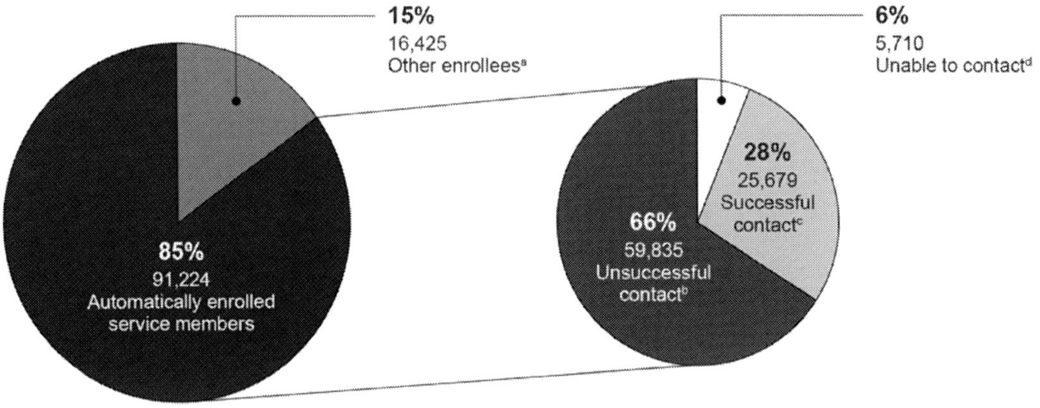

Source: GAO analysis of DOD data. | GAO-24-106189.

[a]Enrollees who were referred or who self-referred to the program.

[b]Enrollees who did not answer or return inTransition's phone calls offering assistance. [c]Enrollees who answered or returned inTransition's phone calls offering assistance. [d]Enrollees who could not be contacted due to missing or incorrect phone numbers.

Note: During this period, the inTransition program was unable to make the up to three calls provided for in the contract from April through December, according to officials. inTransition program officials said that was due to larger-than-expected enrollment lists and a shortage of contract funds. Nonetheless, the contact rate we calculated for 2022 was generally consistent with the contact rate reported by the DOD Office of Inspector General in November 2021. Specifically, that report found an approximately 28 percent successful contact rate for the inTransition program's automatically enrolled service members from fiscal years 2017 through 2020.

Figure 3. Department of Defense's inTransition Enrollees and Telephone Call Response Rates to Automatically Enrolled Service Members, 2022.

inTransition Outreach to Automatically Enrolled Service Members

The inTransition contractor is to conduct up to 3 outreach phone calls to each automatically enrolled service member to see if they would like to stay enrolled and utilize the program's services. According to officials from the contractor, inTransition will attempt a phone call within seven days of receiving the list for about 50 percent of the automatically enrolled service members. inTransition contractor officials said that they generally call all of the automatically enrolled service members within 30 days. When outreach calls to an enrollee do not result in a successful connection with them, officials said they close the enrollee's case as "unresponsive" and disenroll them from the program. Officials may attempt to provide information about inTransition by voicemail or by email, if an email address is available.

Officials said that these unenrolled service members can call back and enroll at any time.

Source: GAO analysis of inTransition documents and interviews with program and contractor officials. | GAO-24-106189.

---

of the Inspector General, *Evaluation of the Department of Defense's Implementation of Suicide Prevention Resources for Transitioning Uniformed Service Members*, Report No. DODIG- 2022-030 (Nov. 9, 2021).

The inTransition program was unable to call some automatically enrolled service members because DOD did not have up-to-date or accurate contact information to provide to the program. Our analysis of 2022 data showed that the program could not contact about 6 percent (5,710) of automatically enrolled service members because of incorrect or missing contact information. For another 66 percent (59,835), the program was unsuccessful in connecting with the enrolled service members, and therefore, they were disenrolled from the program.[36]

We also found that out of all the automatically enrolled service members inTransition attempted to contact in 2022, about 7 percent (6,390 out of91,224) opted to remain enrolled in the program and utilize its coaching services. According to program officials, some enrollees who are successfully contacted may decline enrollment because they respond that they are already connected to a mental health care provider or that they do not wish to use inTransition's coaching services.

Program officials explained that the program's method of outreach— telephone calls— may help explain the program's difficulty in successfully connecting with its automatically enrolled service members, because cold calls are an outdated form of communication. When asked about using alternative methods of outreach, program officials said that the program's policy requires telephone calls as the primary contact method.[37] Officials told us that initiating outreach via email or text would necessitate a policy revision. However, program staff said they may follow-up with email if the phone call attempts are unsuccessful, and if email contact information is available. Officials told us they may explore the feasibility of incorporating text messages and email into their initial outreach efforts in the future, but as of January 2024, specific plans to do so had not been developed. In addition to alternative methods of contact, there are services that can help locate individuals whose contact information may be outdated or incorrect.

Federal internal controls standards state that management should externally communicate the necessary quality information to achieve the entity's objective and that, as part of this, management should select appropriate methods to communicate externally.[38] Additionally, management should periodically evaluate the entity's methods of communication so that the organization has the appropriate tools to communicate quality information throughout and outside of the entity on a timely basis. Revising inTransition's policy to expand its methods for contacting automatically enrolled service members would better align its outreach strategy with these federal internal control standards. Such expansion could improve the program's ability to successfully connect with its automatically enrolled service members, potentially increasing participation among service members who may need assistance seeking mental health services. Additionally, by expanding its methods of contact, coupled with identifying and automatically enrolling service members before they separate as discussed above, the program would have more accurate contact information, as the service member's military phone number and email would likely be available as options for outreach.

---

[36] If inTransition cannot reach a service member after 3 telephone calls are made, the program closes the case as unresponsive, according to program documentation.

[37] Defense Health Agency-Procedural Instruction 6490.01, *inTransition Program* (July 12, 2019).

[38] GAO-14-704G, 63.

Additional Funding Obtained for inTransition Outreach Calls

In March 2023, inTransition program officials requested that the U.S. Army Medical Research Acquisition Authority obligate additional funds to restore the number of outreach contacts to automatically enrolled service members back to up to 3 phone calls in response to elevated demand. In April 2023, the program received $1.1 million in response to this request. However, program officials told us they ended up returning the majority of this funding—$847,224—as they could not expend the funds before the end of the contract option year for which it was provided.

Source: GAO analysis of inTransition documents and interviews with program and contractor officials. | GAO-24-106189.

In addition, we found that short-term decreases in the number of attempted outreach phone calls to automatically enrolled service members in 2022 may have also affected the program's overall rate of successful connections. Specifically, inTransition program officials told us that they did not require the contractor to make the up to three outreach calls to each automatically enrolled service member, as provided for in the contract, from April 2022 through December 2022. This was due to larger-than-expected enrollment lists and a shortage of contract funds.

InTransition officials explained that their baseline estimate of automatically enrolled service members for the existing contract was about 6,300 per month, and they considered any number over that to be elevated demand. After the new contract period began in October 2021, the program experienced elevated numbers of automatically enrolled service members that continued into calendar year 2023.[39] For those months, to try and meet this demand while staying within the contracted funding amount, program officials told us that they directed the contractor to make fewer outreach calls—one or two calls per enrollee.[40] However, inTransition program officials received additional funding for the contract in April 2023, which they said allowed the contractor to return to making up to three outreach calls for each automatically enrolled service member.[41]

We found that the months when inTransition officials directed the contractor to make 1 or 2 outreach calls for each automatically enrolled service member generally had higher unresponsive rates (fewer service members answering the calls) than months in which the contractor could make up to three calls per enrollee. These months also tended to have lower acceptance rates (fewer contacted service members choosing to stay enrolled). See table 1.

[39] his included the period that the Army was not providing its separations data, from December 2022 to September 2023, due to its implementation of a new human resources IT system. Program officials told us that they do not track reasons why the lists of automatically enrolled service members would be larger or smaller than anticipated. However, officials noted that the increased numbers likely reflect an overall increase in the use of mental health services.

[40] Additionally, at the end of February 2023, inTransition program officials advised the contractor to pause the next month's outreach calls. This caused an approximate 3-week delay in outreach, but officials told us it did not ultimately impact the number of outreach call attempts.

[41] According to these officials, this included the June 2023 list of automatically enrolled service members that included the Army's more than 7-month backlog of data. Officials said that they granted the contractor an extended time frame—approximately 2 months instead of 30 days—for completing the calls on the June 2023 list. Program officials stated that up to 3 calls were generally made to all service members on this list.

Table 1. Number of Calls DOD's intransition program made to automatically enrolled service members and the unresponsive and acceptance rates by month, 2022

Month	Number of calls made to each enrollee	Unresponsive rate (percentage of enrollees not successfully contacted)	Acceptance rate (percentage of enrollees who stayed enrolled)
January	3	63	12
February	3	51	18
March	3	58	16
April	1	71	10
May	2	68	7
June	2	60	12
July	1	70	8
August	1	73	6
September	1	83	3
October	1	88	2
November	1	85	3
December	1	90	2

Source: GAO analysis of Department of Defense (DOD) data. | GAO-24-106189.

Note: From April through December the inTransition program was unable to make the up to three calls provided for in the contract. Program officials told us that they instructed the contractor to lower the number of required phone calls to either two or one due to unanticipated elevated demand.

inTransition Program Officials Monitor Performance Information, but the Program Has Not Defined the Level of Performance It Aims to Achieve

Based on reviews of documentation and interviews with DHA and inTransition program officials, we found that the inTransition program regularly monitors a number of measures on program performance, but it has not defined the level of performance it aims to achieve. InTransition program officials said that they review the contractor's reported data.

However, despite the difficulties the contractor has faced in successfully connecting with automatically enrolled service members, program officials said they have no changes planned to improve the program, and that the program is working as intended.

The inTransition contractor submits its required reports to program officials on a monthly, quarterly, and annual basis.[42] The contract outlines 31 measures that the contractor must report to officials within the inTransition program. Some of these 31 measures track data about enrollees, such as enrollees' military service branch and the type of mental health needs enrollees have when joining the program (e.g., traumatic brain injury). Other measures track program performance, such as data on telephone contacts with enrollees, enrollees' decisions

[42] In February 2023, the Defense Health Agency modified the contract to include revised measures, which updated the data submission requirements for the monthly, quarterly, and annual reports.

about whether to stay enrolled or opt out, and the number of enrollees who schedule an appointment with a new mental health provider.

However, we found that the program does not have performance goals or associated quantitative targets and time frames against which performance can be assessed. Performance goals help assess progress towards the broader outcomes a program seeks to achieve. In our prior work, we identified three key performance management steps to help agencies measure and assess progress towards meeting their missions.[43] These steps include the following:

1. setting long-term and near-term goals, including performance goals, to identify the results they seek to achieve,
2. collecting performance information to measure progress, and
3. using the information to assess results and inform decisions to ensure further progress towards achieving those goals.

Establishing measurable performance goals that have quantitative targets and time frames would help inTransition program officials assess program performance by comparing planned and actual results. For instance, the inTransition contractor tracks and reports how many automatically enrolled service members it contacts, but the program does not have related goals for how many automatically enrolled services members it aims to successfully connect with each month (e.g., such as a targeted percentage of the monthly automatically enrolled service members).

When we analyzed acceptance rates for automatically enrolled service members who were successfully contacted and who were not already engaged with mental health services, we found that about 30 percent (6,390 of 21,647) opted to remain enrolled in 2022. This is more than four times higher than the 7 percent acceptance rate for all automatically enrolled service members during that year. This suggests that when more enrollees are successfully contacted, the program will likely see higher acceptance rates. Setting performance goals and tracking the program's progress against them could give decision-makers baseline information and longitudinal data to determine whether changes to the program's outreach approach are needed. This, in turn, could result in more enrollees participating in the program and more transitioning service members obtaining needed assistance.

DOD Has Several Programs That May Help Identify Some Service Members with Mental Health Needs Prior to Separation, with Additional Efforts Underway

Several DOD programs outside of its inTransition program may help identify service members with mental health needs prior to their separation. We found that these programs are targeted for specific populations, such as severely wounded or injured service members. Some transitioning service members with mental health needs may also be identified through the Transition Assistance Program (TAP) and the Separation History and Physical Exam, but these processes do not include a full mental health screening. DOD plans to change both of these

[43] GAO-23-105460, 9.

separation requirements—anticipated in 2025—that may better position it to more comprehensively identify transitioning service members with mental health needs prior to their separation.

DOD Programs That May Identify Some Transitioning Service Members' Mental Health Needs

Military Services' Wounded Warrior Programs

Each military service has a Wounded Warrior program to address the needs of wounded, ill, and injured service members, as well as their families and caregivers. The programs provide nonmedical care and help service members and their medical teams develop a comprehensive recovery plan that addresses rehabilitation and recovery goals. Each service has its own criteria and enrollment processes. The names of the individual programs are as follows:

- U.S. Army Recovery Care Program
- U.S. Navy Wounded Warrior
- U.S. Air Force Wounded Warrior Program
- U.S. Marine Corps Wounded Warrior Regiment
- U.S. Special Operations Command Warrior Care Program

Source: GAO analysis of Wounded Warrior program information. | GAO-24-106189.

Through our analyses of DOD program information and interviews with program officials, we found that two DOD programs—outside of inTransition—may identify some transitioning service members with mental health needs. These programs have been set up for service members with specific health care needs and include:

- Military Service Wounded Warrior programs. Each of the military services has its own wounded warrior program for severely ill or injured (e.g., cancer diagnosis, traumatic brain injury) service members. Program participants are generally assigned case managers that assist them in obtaining the care that they need, which could involve helping them obtain mental health services during the transition process. Case managers may also help connect participants with VA assistance, according to officials. In calendar year 2022 these programs collectively assisted about 16,000 service members, with more than 4,500 having a documented mental health condition or receiving mental health services.
- Integrated Disability Evaluation System. The Integrated Disability Evaluation System is jointly executed by DOD and VA to evaluate and determine appropriate disposition and compensation for service members with conditions that impact their ability to continue their military service. A service member that enters the system may have a mental health assessment conducted by a medical provider, even if a mental health condition is not the primary cause of their referral, according to officials. Officials told

us that service members who identify a mental health condition will receive a mental health exam in accordance with VA policies and procedures.

DOD Is Planning Changes to Improve Its Mental Health Screenings

DOD's Implementation of the Brandon Act

The National Defense Authorization Act for Fiscal Year 2022 required DOD to create a self-initiated referral process for active-duty service members seeking a mental health evaluation. DOD refers to this requirement as the Brandon Act. In May 2023, DOD issued guidance to establish policy, assign responsibilities, and provide procedures for service members to initiate a referral for a mental health evaluation. Specifically, service members can request a referral for a mental health evaluation through a commanding officer or supervisor for any reason or on any basis, and they do not need to provide a reason or basis to request and receive a referral.

Source: Department of Defense. | GAO-24-106189.

According to DOD officials, the department plans to make changes to TAP and the Separation History and Physical Exam, and it anticipates implementing these changes in 2025. According to DOD officials, these changes may better position the department to more comprehensively identify service members with mental health needs prior to their separation. The planned changes include the following:

TAP and the Enterprise Individualized Self-Assessment. While the current TAP's early phase includes individualized counseling to service members, DOD plans to implement a new screening tool called the Enterprise Individualized Self-Assessment in 2025. TAP currently offers individualized counseling to service members to assist them in determining the level of transition assistance they may require. According to DOD policy, multiple factors should be considered during initial counseling to identify the needed level of assistance.[44] However, TAP counselors are non-clinical administrative staff and are not allowed to conduct a mental health assessment. Instead, it is up to the service member to disclose to their counselor whether they have a mental health need. If this occurs, the counselor is supposed to refer the member to the appropriate resource, such as inTransition.

As of January 2024, DOD officials told us they are piloting a new assessment for TAP called the Enterprise Individualized Self- Assessment. The new assessment will measure transition-related readiness across nine domains, including employment, housing, and awareness of physical health and mental health resources.[45] The purpose of the pilot is to standardize how military service branches assess service members' transition-related needs at the start of TAP (more than 1 year prior to separation from the military) and again at 90 days prior to separation from the military. According to officials from the Joint Executive Committee, this new assessment will provide an opportunity for service members to self-

[44] Department of Defense Instruction 1332.35, *Transition Assistance Program for Military Personnel* (Sept. 26, 2019).

[45] The nine domains include social and relational, sense of belonging, employment, housing, hope, financial, resilience, physical health, and mental health. DOD officials said this is not a clinical tool to be used for health assessments.

identify any mental health needs prior to separation. As of February 2024, officials told us that they anticipate a department-wide rollout of the new assessment sometime in fiscal year 2025.

Separation History and Physical Exam and the Separation Health Assessment. DOD officials told us that the department plans to replace its Separation History and Physical Exam with its new Separation Health Assessment in the summer of 2025. At the time of our review, the Separation History and Physical Exam was the department's required medical exam for transitioning service members, which includes a self- assessment questionnaire for service members to document their medical histories, including any mental health conditions.[46] A credentialed health care provider is to subsequently review the completed self-assessment and then complete a separate set of questions and a physical exam for the service member. During the exam, providers will screen separating service members with any mental health or moderate to severe traumatic brain injury needs and then refer them to inTransition if the service member indicates interest in the program. In 2022, providers referred about 400 service members to inTransition through the Separation History and Physical Exam process, which was about 2 percent of the total number of referrals for that year, according to inTransition data we reviewed.

In November 2021, the DOD Office of Inspector General reported that the content of the Separation History and Physical Examination did not include mental health or suicide risk screening sections. There are nine questions (out of 92) in the self-assessment related to mental health, but the Inspector General found these questions do not constitute a mental health screening. Furthermore, the provider's set of 26 questions for the medical evaluation portion of the exam included just one question related to mental health. See figure 4 for the mental health questions from the self-assessment form.

		YES	NO
17.a.	Nervous trouble of any sort (anxiety or panic attacks)		
b.	Habitual stammering or stuttering		
c.	Loss of memory or amnesia, or neurological symptoms		
d.	Frequent trouble sleeping		
e.	Received counseling of any type		
f.	Depression or excessive worry		
g.	Been evaluated or treated for a mental condition		
h.	Attempted suicide		
i.	Used illegal drugs or abused prescription drugs		

Source: Department of Defense (DOD). | GAO-24-106189.

Figure 4. Mental Health-Related Questions from the Self-Assessment Section of DOD's Separation History and Physical Examination, as of April 2024.

DOD told us it plans to replace the Separation History and Physical Exam with the Separation Health Assessment, which it jointly developed with VA through the DOD-VA Joint Executive Committee. According to DOD and VA officials, the Separation Health Assessment

[46] Department of Defense Instruction 6040.46, *The Separation History and Physical Examination for the DOD Separation Health Assessment Program* (Apr. 14, 2016).

has multiple mental health screening sections and will serve as the department's mental health screening for all transitioning service members.

10. MENTAL HEALTH SCREENING QUESTIONNAIRES

NOTE TO THE SERVICE MEMBER: Please respond to the following screening questionnaires. Your responses will be reviewed by the Examining Clinician, and additional questions may be asked.

10.1. POST-TRAUMATIC STRESS DISORDER (PTSD) SCREEN

#	Question	Response
	Sometimes things happen to people that are unusually or especially frightening, horrible, or traumatic. In the past month, have you...	
1	Had nightmares about the event(s) or thought about the event(s) when you did not want to?	☐ Yes ☐ No
2	Tried hard not to think about the event(s) or went out of your way to avoid situations that reminded you of the event(s)?	☐ Yes ☐ No
3	Been constantly on guard, watchful, or easily startled?	☐ Yes ☐ No
4	Felt numb or detached from people, activities, or your surroundings?	☐ Yes ☐ No
5	Felt guilty or unable to stop blaming yourself or others for the event(s) or any problems the event(s) may have caused?	☐ Yes ☐ No

10.2 DEPRESSION SCREEN

#	Question	Response
	Over the last 2 weeks, how often have you been bothered by any of the following problems?	
1	Little interest or pleasure in doing things?	☐ Not at all ☐ Several days ☐ More than half the days ☐ Nearly every day
2	Feeling down, depressed, or hopeless?	☐ Not at all ☐ Several days ☐ More than half the days ☐ Nearly every day

10.3 ALCOHOL USE SCREEN

#	Question	Response
1	How often did you have a drink containing alcohol in the past year?	☐ Never ☐ Monthly or less ☐ 2-4 times a month ☐ 2-3 times per week ☐ 4 or more times a week
2	How many drinks containing alcohol did you have on a typical day when you were drinking in the past year?	☐ 1 or 2 ☐ 3 or 4 ☐ 5 or 6 ☐ 7 to 9 ☐ 10 or more
3	For men: How often did you have six or more drinks on one occasion in the past year?	☐ Never ☐ Less than monthly ☐ Monthly ☐ Weekly ☐ Daily, or almost daily
4	For women: How often did you have four or more drinks on one occasion in the past year?	☐ Never ☐ Less than monthly ☐ Monthly ☐ Weekly ☐ Daily, or almost daily

Source: department of Defence (DOD) and Veternas Affairs. | GAO-24-106789.

Figure 5. Mental Health Screening Questions from the Self-Assessment Section of the Separation Health Assessment, Estimated DOD Implementation Summer 2025.

Similar to the Separation History and Physical Exam, the Separation Health Assessment has two sections—a self-assessment questionnaire and a provider's exam that also includes a set of questions. The service member's self-assessment has an 11-question section for mental health, including specific screening sections on post-traumatic stress disorder, depression, and alcohol use. The provider's exam includes mental health screening sections to assess service members' risks for suicide and violence. The providers' questionnaire has language stating that they may refer service members to inTransition based upon their assessment of the service members' mental health needs. See figure 5 for mental health questions from the self-assessment section of the Separation Health Assessment.

DOD officials told us the department plans to pilot the new assessment starting in September 2024, with full implementation anticipated by summer 2025. Joint Executive Committee officials told us that VA has been using the new assessment since spring 2023 for transitioning service members seeking VA benefits through the Integrated Disability

Evaluation System or its Benefits Delivery at Discharge program.[47] As a result, VA may be able to identify transitioning service members with mental health needs for those seeking VA benefits prior to their separation.

DOD and VA Have Several Efforts That May Facilitate Access to Mental Health Services across the Transition Continuum

Multiple DOD and VA Efforts Can Help Facilitate Transitioning Service Members' Access to Mental Health Services Prior to Separation and across the Transition Continuum

Based on our review of DOD and VA programs, processes, and services, we found that there are a number of these efforts that can help facilitate access to mental health services before a service member separates or at any point during the transition continuum (1 year pre-separation and 1 year post-separation from military service).[48] See table 2.

Table 2. DOD and VA programs, processes, or services that may facilitate access to mental health services prior to separation and across the transition continuum

Program, process, or service name	DOD	VA
inTransition	X	-
Transition Assistance Program warm handovers	X	-
Defense Health Agency Recovery Coordination Program	X	-
Military OneSource	X	-
VA Liaison Program	-	X
Veterans Health Administration Post-9/11 Military2VA Case Management Program	-	X
VA Federal Recovery Consultants	-	X

Source: GAO review of Departments of Defense (DOD) and Veterans Affairs (VA) information. | GAO-24-106189.

Note: The DOD-VA Joint Executive Committee defines the transition continuum as 1-year pre-separation and 1-year post-separation from military service.

The characteristics of each program, process, or service are described below.

- InTransition. As discussed earlier in this report, in 2022, inTransition data show that about 15 percent of inTransition's enrollees were directly referred to the program.

[47] VA's Benefits Delivery at Discharge program allows separating service members who plan to apply for VA disability compensation to be able to file their claims between 180 to 90 days prior to separation.

[48] There may be additional programs that have a role in facilitating service members' access to mental health care across the transition continuum that we did not identify in our review. For example, the Department of Defense Office of the Inspector General's November 2021 report found that the Army created approaches within the embedded behavioral health system to arrange for uninterrupted continuity of mental health care for soldiers. See Department of Defense Office of the Inspector General, *Evaluation of the Department of Defense's Implementation of Suicide Prevention Resources for Transitioning Uniformed Service Members*, Report No. DODIG-2022-030 (Nov. 9, 2021).

These referrals may have occurred at any point in a service member's career, including during the transition continuum. Referred service members who enroll in the program prior to their separation likely benefit from program's assistance with facilitating connection to any needed mental health services during their transition out of the military.

- TAP warm handovers. According to DOD policy, a commander or commander's designee is supposed to confirm a warm handover to other agencies for transitioning service members who are anticipated to face various challenges, including services members who do not have awareness of mental health resources or self-identify a mental health concern.[49] The policy defines a warm handover as "a process between respective military services and appropriate interagency partner(s) resulting in the person-to-person connection of service members to services and follow-up resources as needed."[50] Other agencies include VA, and the warm handover process could assist service members in connecting to mental health care available through the VA.
- Defense Health Agency Recovery Coordination Program. This program, embedded in the military services' Wounded Warrior programs, supports wounded, ill, and injured service members in their recovery and reintegration back into the military or their transition to civilian life. It generally engages with service members before they separate and can assist service members with transitioning their care to the VA should that be needed. Specifically, the program provides Recovery Care Coordinators, located at military treatment facilities and installations across the country, to ensure these service members receive medical and non-medical support, which according to officials could include mental health services. As part of their responsibilities, coordinators are to work closely with each service member and their families to develop a comprehensive plan that identifies goals and resources needed to achieve them.
- Military OneSource. This program assists service members, their families, and recently separated service members by offering a wide range of individualized consultations, coaching, and non-medical counseling for many aspects of military life, including the transition to civilian life. For example, Military OneSource may offer assistance to service members as they navigate becoming a parent, filing taxes, finding a job, or if they need non-medical counseling to help deal with stress or loss.
- These services are available at any time, and service members may reach out to Military OneSource via telephone or online at any point throughout the transition continuum. Officials told us such services could include providing assistance in facilitating access to mental health care for transitioning service members, as discussed in more detail below.
- VA Liaison Program. VA Liaisons for Health Care are nurses and social workers who coordinate the transfer of health care from DOD to VA for service members separating from the military. This may include service members who need mental health services, but the program broadly assists service members navigating any type of health

---

[49] Department of Defense Instruction 1332.35, Transition Assistance Program (TAP) For Military Personnel (Sept. 26, 2019).

[50] In March 2024, we reported on DOD's implementation of the warm handover process. For more information see GAO-24-106248.

condition. As of February 2024, VA officials reported there were 43 VA Liaisons for Health Care located at DOD medical facilities and 5 liaisons support all other military installations virtually. Their responsibilities include responding to DOD referrals to coordinate inpatient care and outpatient appointments at VA medical centers near the patient's intended residence or most appropriate to the care required, including any needed mental health services. VA officials said that service members typically connect with a VA Liaison for Health Care when a DOD provider, case manager, or the Integrated Disability Evaluation System refers them to the program prior to separation. However, service members can also voluntarily reach out to the program to work with a VA Liaison for Health Care at any point prior to their separation if they think that they would benefit from the program. In fiscal year 2023, VA reported that 14,241 service members and veterans were transitioned from DOD into VA health care through the VA Liaison Program.

- Veterans Health Administration Post-9/11 Military2VA Case Management Program. Each VA medical center has a post-9/11 Military2VA Case Management team on-site to facilitate service members' transition to civilian life. Officials told us that service members are typically referred to the case management program based upon identified needs. Post-9/11 Military2VA Case Management Program Managers receive referrals from VA Liaisons for Health Care and then work with local VA staff to facilitate service members' VA registration and appointment scheduling prior to separation—including for any needed mental health care—so that the service member has appointments scheduled upon separation and enrollment in VA health care. Service members typically connect with a Post-9/11 Military2VA Case Management Program member through a VA Liaison for Health Care, and this connection is to occur prior to service members' transfer to the VA.
- VA Federal Recovery Consultants. This office provides consultation services and assistance to DOD and VA staff who are responsible for care coordination but does not provide direct case management to service members or veterans. However, the consultants may interact directly with service members and veterans who have high intensity needs. There are 9 consultants located at select VA and DOD sites, and they provide services that assist with coordinating benefits and care that align with the service member or veteran's needs; officials told us that this could include assisting service members in connecting to mental health services. They provide these services virtually regardless of the service member or veteran's location, medical treatment, geographic location of injury, place of medical diagnosis, or military or veteran status.

Several DOD and VA Programs Have Specific Components That Provide Post-Separation Assistance to Veterans Who May Need Mental Health Services

Based on our review of program documentation, our prior work, and interviews with program officials, we found that several DOD and VA programs have specific components that provide post-separation assistance to veterans. These programs also conduct outreach to certain veterans 2 months or more after their separation to offer various types of assistance, including access to mental health services.

Emergency Access to Mental Health Care for Veterans
Federal law authorizes the Department of Veterans Affairs (VA) to furnish hospital care or medical services in certain emergency situations to any individual regardless of veteran status or eligibility for VA care. These authorities are generally referred to as humanitarian care authorities and require VA emergency departments to, at a minimum, screen an individual for a medical emergency. If a facility determines that a medical emergency exists, the facility will provide care to stabilize the individual's emergency condition. A former service member with a bad conduct or dishonorable discharge who is in distress and in need of emergency mental health services may be provided services under humanitarian care provisions. Former service members can access the VA system by calling the Veterans Crisis Line or by visiting a VA emergency room, urgent care center, or VA medical center.
Source: GAO review of relevant laws. | GAO-24-106189.

- *DOD Military OneSource.* In addition to other support services, officials told us that Military OneSource provides post-separation outreach to transitioning service members who opt-in to receive information from the program during the Transition Assistance Program. This includes information about its mental health resources. Outreach for these service members occurs after separation and includes a 3-month and 6-month follow-up, according to Military OneSource officials.
- *InTransition.* As previously described, inTransition conducts post-separation outreach to automatically enrolled service members to offer the program's coaching services, which include assistance with connecting to mental health services. InTransition is to make up to 3 phone calls within 30 days to each automatically enrolled service members. Outreach for automatically enrolled service members generally occurs 2 to 3 months after their separation.
- *VA Solid Start.* Solid Start conducts outreach to recently separated veterans to share information on specific benefits and to offer personalized guidance, which could include providing assistance in obtaining mental health resources.[51] As part of this program, VA identifies "priority" veterans who have had an appointment with a mental health care professional in the year prior to separation, among other eligibility criteria, to ensure the program focuses on those veterans who may be most at risk of self-harm.[52] Solid Start representatives email eligible veterans to notify them that Solid

[51] An additional VA outreach initiative—Concierge for Care—was another effort until it ceased to function as a standalone effort as of August 2023. Under this initiative, VA contacted recently separated service members and answered questions about VA health care, explained eligibility, helped with enrollment, and helped schedule appointments. According to VA officials, to improve the efficiency of post-separation outreach efforts, in August 2023, VA Solid Start assumed sole responsibility for offering Solid Start-eligible veterans the option to enroll in VA health care.

[52] VA Solid Start designates service members for "priority" outreach if they had any two of the following six risk factors in the 12 months prior to separation: 1) suicide attempts or self-harm; 2) admission to an inpatient psychiatric facility; 3) diagnosis of a mood disorder; 4) diagnosis of an anxiety disorder; 5) diagnosis of an adjustment disorder; or 6) diagnosis of a substance abuse or substance use disorder.

Start representatives will call them soon and to provide a link to the VA Welcome Kit, which is a guide to VA benefits and services. Solid Start personnel are then to make seven telephone outreach attempts at three different points in time, at 90-, 180-, and 360-days post- separation.[53] According to VA officials, Solid Start representatives must discuss VA mental health benefits for these priority veterans during every answered call.

DOD-VA Joint Executive Committee Has Not Assessed the Effectiveness of the Departments' Efforts to Facilitate Access to Mental Health Services

We found that the DOD-VA Joint Executive Committee has not assessed the effectiveness of the departments' efforts overall in facilitating access to mental health services for transitioning service members. Officials told us the Committee directed the Transition Executive Committee (its subcommittee focused on transitioning from the military) to identify DOD and VA mental health-related programs and processes across the transition continuum.[54] The Transition Executive Committee identified mental health "touchpoints"—programs or processes that could support the mental health of transitioning service members and veterans—across the transition continuum and presented the results to the Joint Executive Committee co-chairs in June 2022. The Transition Executive Committee identified multiple DOD and VA programs and processes that may provide mental health touchpoints for service members prior to separation. Such programs include TAP pre-separation counseling, the Enterprise Individualized Self-Assessment, inTransition, pre- and post- separation VA health care registration, and the Separation Health Assessment. The Transition Executive Committee also identified Military OneSource and VA Solid Start as programs that may provide mental health touchpoints once service members have separated from the military.

Officials told us that the Transition Executive Committee limited its review to an inventory of available mental health resources and did not assess the effectiveness of those efforts overall in facilitating access to mental health services during the transition period. Specifically, the officials involved in the review said that they did not evaluate whether or how these programs and processes collectively facilitate continuous access to mental health services across the transition continuum. However, officials described two issues they identified that could result in a gap in accessing mental health services for some transitioning service members.

- Transition Executive Committee officials identified a potential gap in mental health care coverage prior to separation for some service members. Officials explained that a service member who is scheduled to separate in 60 days may take "separation leave" and relocate from their installation to another location. In this scenario, the service

[53] According to VA officials, this calling strategy was informed by private industry consultants with expertise on the number of calls needed to successfully connect with people. For more information about VA's Solid Start program, see GAO, *Veterans Benefits: VA Could Enhance Outreach for Its Solid Start Program by Increasing Collaboration with Veterans Organizations*, GAO-23-105699 (Washington, D.C.: Jan. 5, 2023).

[54] The Transition Executive Committee provides oversight and direction related to transition assistance to service members and veterans. The National Defense Authorization Act for Fiscal Year 2024 added the Transition Executive Committee as a statutory committee of the DOD-VA Joint Executive Committee. Prior to this legislation, the Transition Executive Committee operated as a directed committee of the DOD-VA Joint Executive Committee's co-chairs. Pub. L No. 118-31, div. A, tit. XVIII, § 1805, 137 Stat. 136, 687 (2023).

member can no longer access the military medical treatment facilities on their base at their former location, and they are not yet eligible for VA health care because they have not separated from the military.[55]

- Joint Executive Committee officials also identified a potential post- separation delay in obtaining VA health care benefits, which could affect veterans' access to mental health care.[56] Officials noted that a delay in the receipt of DOD Form 214 would affect a veteran's ability to apply for VA benefits because VA uses this form to authenticate an individual's military service. For example, DOD officials told us that the Army experienced problems with its new personnel processing IT system that prevented the production of many DOD Form 214s from late December 2022 to late January 2023. These officials told us that nearly 5,000 service members who separated or retired during that period may have experienced delays in their post-separation benefits. As of January 2024, DOD officials reported that issues related to the delayed receipt of DOD Form 214 have been resolved.

Mental Health Resources Available to Veterans Encountering Health Care Enrollment Delays

According to Joint Executive Committee officials, transitioning service members could potentially encounter delays with accessing mental health care during the process for enrolling in health care benefits with the Department of Veterans Affairs (VA). Should veterans encounter such delays, they could obtain immediate attention to urgent mental health needs through VA's emergency access provisions and the Veterans/Military Crisis Line. They could also obtain care through Vet Centers, if eligible. Vet Centers are community-based counseling centers that provide a wide range of social and psychological services, including professional counseling, to veterans and their families.

Lastly, DOD's Military OneSource provides counseling resources to service members up to 1-year post-separation.

Source: GAO review of DOD and VA documentation and interviews with department officials. | GAO-24-106189.

In its fiscal year 2024 Joint Operating Plan, the DOD-VA Joint Executive Committee identified continuity of care for transitioning service members with special circumstances—which includes those with mental health needs—as a priority for its strategic goal of enhancing the transition experience. However, Joint Executive Committee and Transition Executive Committee officials said that they do not plan to assess the effectiveness of the programs and processes they identified through the 2022 review, and that work is complete. Joint Executive

---

[55] According to VA officials, transitioning service members can obtain VA care while on "separation leave" in an emergent situation or if they have received an authorization from their DOD provider. Furthermore, while not eligible for enrollment in the VA health care system, transitioning service members on active duty can be registered in the VA health care system. A future appointment to occur once in veteran status can be scheduled while the transitioning service member is in this registered, "not enrolled," status.

[56] According to VA officials, if the transitioning service member connects to a program such as the VA Liaison Program, the service member can register for VA health care prior to separation from the military and be referred to the Post-9/11 Military2VA Case Management Program for coordination of care, to include scheduling future VA appointments to occur once in veteran status.

Committee officials explained that they do not have authority over the individual DOD and VA programs and lack expertise to evaluate the programs.

Nevertheless, the responsibilities outlined in the Committee's enabling statute include identifying changes in policies, procedures, and practices that promote mutually beneficial coordination or sharing of resources between the two departments.[57] Given the Joint Executive Committee's statutory authority and responsibilities, it is the entity best positioned to assess the departments' overall efforts and assess how well—taken together—they provide coverage of mental health services across the transition continuum. The Committee could then use the results of this assessment to make recommendations to the DOD and VA programs that have authority to make changes, as appropriate.

Such an assessment would align with the Joint Executive Committee's strategic goal of enhancing the transition experience. It would also align with federal internal controls standards, which state that management should periodically review policies, procedures, and related control activities for continued relevance and effectiveness in achieving an agency's objectives or addressing related risks.[58]

Specifically, this assessment would provide the Committee with a more comprehensive understanding of how and when service members can access mental health services through the departments' programs across the transition continuum. For example, in 2022 the Transition Executive Committee identified the inTransition program as a pre-separation resource. However, we found that most service members are not enrolled in the program until several months after their separation, which could result in a gap in services. Such an assessment could also be used to help address gaps already identified by the Joint Executive Committee and the Transition Executive Committee, including those related to service members taking separation leave or the potential post-separation delay in obtaining VA health care benefits. A more comprehensive assessment of the timing and availability of the programs, processes, and services that can assist the transitioning population would better position the Joint Executive Committee to identify and address service gaps. This would help to ensure that service members and veterans can receive the assistance they may need in accessing mental health services when they need it.

Additionally, such as assessment would help the Joint Executive Committee identify and address any unnecessary duplication or overlap across the various efforts. For example, we found that two programs with mental health touchpoints—DOD's inTransition program and VA's Solid Start program—have overlap with the population they assist and the timing of their outreach. Both programs' outreach lists include individuals who had an appointment with a mental health provider in the year prior to their separation. During our review, we found that approximately 95 percent of the veterans on VA's Solid Start lists of "priority" veterans also appear on DOD's inTransition lists of automatically enrolled service members for calendar year 2022.[59] As a result, almost all of these veterans may have received multiple outreach calls from both programs during the same post-separation time period—starting approximately 2 to 3 months after they have left the military. This could be confusing for veterans who may have

---

[57] See 38 U.S.C. § 320(d)(1).

[58] GAO-14-704G, 56.

[59] Officials told us the same Defense Health Agency contractor prepares both DOD's monthly list of service members automatically enrolled to inTransition and VA's monthly list of Solid Start "priority" veterans. According to the contractor, the lists are provided to the programs at approximately the same time, 2 to 3 months after the veterans have separated from the military.

difficulty determining which program is best suited for their needs. The Transition Executive Committee's 2022 identification of mental health touchpoints also found that service members and veterans may be unaware of the various programs offering touchpoints, unable to distinguish the difference between them, and could be confused by multiple programs.

Conclusion

Ensuring service members have access to mental health care is essential during their transition out of the military, especially in light of the many challenges they may face in readjusting to civilian life. DOD's inTransition program is designed to offer specialized coaching and assistance to those who may need access to mental health services, including transitioning service members. However, the delayed timing for automatically enrolling eligible members into the program—late in the transition continuum—may leave a gap in assistance to mental health services during the vulnerable post-separation period. Modifying the program's criteria for identifying eligible service members for automatic enrollment prior to their separation could help address this gap and would help inTransition better ensure the continuity of any needed mental health services during the critical transition period.

The inTransition program aims to contact all automatically enrolled service members to determine whether they would like to participate in the program, but the program has faced difficulties in successfully connecting with a significant portion of eligible service members due, in part, to its reliance on telephone calls. Revising the program's policy to expand its outreach methods, such as by adding requirements for outreach through email, text, or exploring the use of services to help locate enrollees, could improve the program's ability to successfully connect with eligible service members and increase participation in the program.

Additionally, inTransition program officials track some performance information, such as data on contacts with enrollees, but the program has not defined the level of performance it aims to achieve. Setting measurable goals that have quantitative targets and time frames will better allow the program to assess its performance. Importantly, implementing a process to use such information to make any needed improvements will help the program accomplish its primary objective of ensuring continuity of mental health services during times of transition.

Furthermore, the DOD-VA Joint Executive Committee is uniquely positioned to assess overall how well DOD and VA's many programs, processes, and services facilitate access to mental health services across the transition continuum. The 2022 identification of an inventory of mental health programs and processes by the Transition Executive Committee— one of its subcommittees—was a critical first step. By also assessing the effectiveness of these efforts overall in facilitating access to mental health services, the Joint Executive Committee would be better positioned to identify and recommend appropriate changes to the departments to address any identified gaps or unnecessary duplication or overlap across the transition continuum. Such an assessment would help the departments better ensure that transitioning service members and veterans have access to the mental health support they may need when they need it.

Recommendations for Executive Action

We are making a total of five recommendations, including four to DOD's Defense Health Agency and one to the DOD-VA Joint Executive Committee. Specifically:

The Defense Health Agency should revise the inTransition program's criteria for auto-enrollment as outlined in its policy to identify and enroll eligible service members prior to their separation from the military. (Recommendation 1)

The Defense Health Agency should revise the inTransition program's policy to expand the outreach methods used by the program to contact automatically enrolled service members, such as by adding requirements for outreach through email, text, or the use of location services. (Recommendation 2)

The Defense Health Agency should establish measurable performance goals for the inTransition program that have quantitative targets and time frames. (Recommendation 3)

The Defense Health Agency should implement a process for the inTransition program to use performance information to assess its effectiveness and make any needed improvements, as appropriate. (Recommendation 4)

The DOD-VA Joint Executive Committee should assess the effectiveness of DOD and VA programs and processes overall in facilitating access to mental health services across the transition continuum, and recommend any needed changes to DOD and VA, including changes to address any identified gaps or unnecessary duplication or overlap. (Recommendation 5)

Agency Comments

We provided a draft of this report to DOD and VA for review and comment. VA's comments are reproduced in appendix I; DOD did not provide formal comments. VA concurred with our recommendation directed to the DOD-VA Joint Executive Committee. In its response, VA agreed that the Joint Executive Committee is the appropriate body to assess the effectiveness of mental health services across the transition continuum. To address our recommendation, VA said the Joint Executive Committee will ensure the proper executive subcommittees are coordinated and establish plans of action, milestones, and metrics to identify gaps or duplicative efforts. DOD and VA also provided technical comments, which we incorporated, as appropriate.

We are sending copies of this report to the appropriate congressional committees, the Secretary of Defense, the Secretary of Veterans Affairs, and other interested parties. In addition, the report will be available at no charge on the GAO website at https://www.gao.gov.

If you or your staff have any questions about this report, please contact me at (202) 512-7114 or hundrupa@gao.gov. Contact points for our Offices of Congressional Relations and Public Affairs may be found on the last page of this report. GAO staff who made key contributions to this report are listed in appendix II.

Alyssa M. Hundrup
Director, Health Care

Appendix I: Comments from the Department of Veterans Affairs

DEPARTMENT OF VETERANS AFFAIRS
WASHINGTON

June 7, 2024

Ms. Alyssa M. Hundrup
Director
Health Care
U.S. Government Accountability Office
441 G Street, NW
Washington, DC 20548

Dear Ms. Hundrup:

The Department of Veterans Affairs (VA) has reviewed the Government Accountability Office (GAO) draft report: **DOD AND VA HEALTH CARE: Actions Needed to Better Facilitate Access to Mental Health Services During Military to Civilian Transitions** (GAO-24-106189).

The enclosure contains technical comments and the action plan to implement the draft report recommendation. VA appreciates the opportunity to comment on your draft report.

Sincerely,

Kimberly Jackson
Chief of Staff

Enclosure

Enclosure

The Department of Veterans Affairs (VA) Response to the
Government Accountability Office (GAO) Draft Report:
DOD and VA HEALTH CARE: Actions Needed to Better Facilitate Access to Mental Health Services During Military to Civilian Transitions
(GAO-24-106189)

Recommendation 5: The DOD-VA Joint Executive Committee should assess the effectiveness of DOD and VA programs and processes overall in facilitating access to mental health services across the transition continuum, and recommend any needed changes to DOD and VA, including changes to address any identified gaps or unnecessary duplication or overlap.

VA Response: Concur. The Department of Defense (DOD)-Department of Veterans Affairs (VA) Joint Executive Committee (JEC) is the appropriate governing body to assess the effectiveness of mental health services across the transition continuum. The JEC will ensure the proper executive subcommittees are coordinated and establish plans of action, milestones, and metrics to identify gaps or duplicative efforts. Mental health services during this difficult transition from military to civilian life are critical and will be highlighted in the upcoming JEC Co-Chair Annual Priority Guidance Memorandum and the JEC Joint Operating Plan.

Appendix II: GAO Contact and Staff Acknowledgments

GAO Contact

Alyssa M. Hundrup at (202) 512-7114 or HundrupA@gao.gov.

Staff Acknowledgments

In addition to the contact named above, Bonnie Anderson (Assistant Director), Nick Bartine (Analyst in Charge), Amy Andresen, and Ester Weir made key contributions to this report. Also contributing to this report were Deborah Healy, Roxanna Sun, Cathy Hamann Whitmore, Jennifer Whitworth, and Bobby Younce.

GAO's Mission

The Government Accountability Office, the audit, evaluation, and investigative arm of Congress, exists to support Congress in meeting its constitutional responsibilities and to help improve the performance and accountability of the federal government for the American people. GAO examines the use of public funds; evaluates federal programs and policies; and provides analyses, recommendations, and other assistance to help Congress make informed oversight, policy, and funding decisions. GAO's commitment to good government is reflected in its core values of accountability, integrity, and reliability.

Connect with GAO

Connect with GAO on Facebook, Flickr, Twitter, and YouTube. Subscribe to our RSS Feeds or Email Updates. Listen to our Podcasts. Visit GAO on the web at https://www.gao.gov.

To Report Fraud, Waste, and Abuse in Federal Programs

Contact FraudNet:

Website: https://www.gao.gov/about/what-gao-does/fraudnet Automated answering system: (800) 424-5454 or (202) 512-7700

Congressional Relations

A. Nicole Clowers, Managing Director, ClowersA@gao.gov, (202) 512-4400, U.S. Government Accountability Office, 441 G Street NW, Room 7125, Washington, DC 20548.

Public Affairs

Sarah Kaczmarek, Acting Managing Director, KaczmarekS@gao.gov, (202) 512- 4800, U.S. Government Accountability Office, 441 G Street NW, Room 7149 Washington, DC 20548

Strategic Planning and External Liaison

Stephen J. Sanford, Managing Director, spel@gao.gov, (202) 512-4707
U.S. Government Accountability Office, 441 G Street NW, Room 7814, Washington, DC 20548

Index

Q

R

S

T

U